THE A TO Z OF

SPORTS MEDICINE

Elizabeth H. Oakes

Foreword by
Connie Lebrun, M.D., MDCM, MPE, CCFP, Dip. Sport Med.,
Director of Primary Care Sport Medicine,
Fowler Kennedy Sport Medicine Clinic,
London, Ontario, Canada

Checkmark Books®
An imprint of Facts On File, Inc.

The A to Z of Sports Medicine

Checkmark Books
An imprint of Facts On File, Inc.
132 West 31st Street
New York NY 10001

Library of Congress Cataloging-in-Publication Data

Oakes, Elizabeth H., 1964–
[Encyclopedia of sports medicine]
The A to Z of sports medicine / Elizabeth H. Oakes; foreword by Connie Lebrun.
p. ; cm.
Originally published: The encyclopedia of sports medicine.
New York : Facts On File,© 2005, in series: Facts On File library of health and living.
Includes bibliographical references and index.
ISBN 0-8160-6692-2 (pb : alk. paper)
1. Sports medicine—Encyclopedias. I. Title.
[DNLM: 1. Sports Medicine—Encyclopedias—English. QT 13 O11e 2005a]
RC1206.O355 2006
617.1'02703—dc22
2005025988

Text design by Cathy Rincon

Printed in the United States of America

VB Hermitage 10 9 8 7 6 5 4 3 2 1

This book is printed on acid-free paper.

CONTENTS

Acknowledgments   vii

Introduction   ix

Entries A–Z   1

Appendixes   227

Bibliography   289

Index   293

ACKNOWLEDGMENTS

I am particularly grateful to Connie Lebrun for her expert and thorough guidance in the writing of this book. I would also like to thank my editor, James Chambers, and his assistant, Vanessa Nittoli, for their unfailing and always good-natured support. For patience and perseverance on the home front, my heartfelt thanks as always to my littlest readers, Colter and Ella. Finally, for giving me horses and ballet lessons and inspiring in me a love of what the body can do, I thank my parents, Bob Oakes and Jeraldine Kellison.

INTRODUCTION

With the exponential increase in participation in sports and recreational activity over the past few decades has come the concomitant need for specialized knowledge in sports medicine, not only for diagnosis and treatment of common injuries and conditions, but, more important, for prevention. Stores selling running shoes and other athletic equipment are rife with do-it-yourself books, magazines, etc., and almost any topic can easily be "researched" on the Internet. The difficulty arises in sifting through the mass of information available through all these sources. How to verify the accuracy of information, how and when to access which type of sports medicine practitioner, when to just "push through the pain," and when to back off from the offending activity to allow an injury time to heal—these are just some of the challenges facing the would-be athlete, as well as scores of active men and women of all ages already enjoying the health benefits of exercise.

Many of the medical and orthopedic considerations in the field of sports medicine have gender and/or age-specific epidemiological features. Female athletes have unique anatomy and, with their changing physiology throughout the reproductive lifespan, may face special challenges not encountered by their male counterparts. Similarly, children and adolescents who partake in sporting activities are not "little adults" and frequently have different patterns of injuries. In order to achieve competitive excellence, intensive training practices often begin at an early age, thereby increasing the risks of over-training and overuse injuries. In addition, the external pressures from coaches and parents, particularly on the younger athletes, are quite significant and can have profound and long-lasting psychological effects. At the other end of the spectrum, older adults are looking more toward recreation and exercise to fill their increased leisure time—to help manage chronic medical conditions and to help stave off the untoward effects of aging. They are usually also contending with a host of underlying disease processes that may impact their ability to exercise successfully and to gain cardiovascular, respiratory, and muscular fitness. Then again, it is not uncommon to encounter older "master's" athletes, who vehemently wish to continue with vigorous training and competition, despite multiple injuries, and even following hip- or knee-replacement surgery!

Sport specificity is another important characteristic of this emerging body of medical knowledge related to sports. Some sports are inherently more risky for the participants, irrespective of age or physical fitness. The wave of new "endurance" sports and extreme or combination sports, for example, has done nothing to decrease the occurrence of injuries. In the workplace, "repetitive strain"–type injuries are commonplace, but fortunately many of these problems of the "industrial athlete" can be managed using good sports medicine principles, such as accurate diagnosis and adequate rehabilitation. Similarly, musicians and performing artists have a variety of musculoskeletal concerns that are frequently analogous in etiology and pathophysiology to those found in more traditional athletes. For all of these special populations, an understanding of the exact demands of their profession is critical in helping them back to their chosen or requisite activities.

Equipment is an additional variable that has allowed athletes to go "higher, stronger, faster." Technological improvements in footwear, playing surfaces, protective padding, and sports clothing have modified the patterns of injuries. For example, the "boot-top" fractures of the tibia (lower leg) that were previously seen with the older style of ski boots, have given way to an increased incidence of ligamentous tears, specifically of the anterior cruciate ligament. Shoe design is becoming more focused toward anatomical configuration, as well as the specific needs of certain sports. The addition of over-the-counter or custom-made orthotics can alter the weight-bearing surface of the foot, improve gait patterns, and possibly help with prevention and rehabilitation of certain common injuries. There are specialized knee braces for ligamentous problems and osteoarthritis, wrist and elbow braces, and other protective equipment, such as helmets and mouthguards. Some of these have strict regulatory criteria for safety purposes and have played a major role in reducing certain types of head, facial, and dental injuries. Sport nutrition, or the "fuel" that athletes place into their body, is another huge topic. Supplements are "big business," but can be confusing to the average consumer, particularly as the science and research lag somewhat behind the commercial aspects.

Advances in technology include improvement in current imaging techniques for the visualization of more detailed anatomy. The traditional X ray can now be supplemented with diagnostic ultrasound, nuclear medicine bone scans, computed tomography (CT scans), and magnetic resonance imaging (MRI) studies to confirm suspected diagnoses or exclude other pathology. Each imaging modality has its own inherent advantages and indications. As there are varying costs to these procedures, it is essential that they are ordered by a physician knowledgeable about specific sports injuries in order to get "the most bang for the buck."

Although the health benefits of physical activity generally outweigh the risks, there are nevertheless many injuries and illnesses that can befall the unwary person, from the precontemplative "couch potato" to the "weekend warrior," through to the seasoned competitor or elite professional athlete. This *A to Z of Sports Medicine* is written for the layperson in search of a comprehensive yet simple to use source of information. More than 200 topics, from "head to toe," are covered in a concise and readable format. These are organized in alphabetical order, for ease of reference. Each section consists of a general overview, followed by causes, diagnosis, treatment, and prevention. Many nonorthopedic or medical concerns for active people are covered as well. Several sports are dealt with in more detail in terms of typical injuries and problems. An appendix at the back of the book lists many of the different sports medicine organizations as additional resources.

Optimal management of medical conditions related to sports, however, requires the skills and expertise of a trained professional. The information in this book should not be utilized in isolation. Definitive diagnosis of the problem, as well as potential treatment options, should be deferred to a suitably qualified practitioner. As the field of sports medicine continues to evolve, there are many professions that lay claim to the name. It is essential to understand the differences, the advantages, and disadvantages of the various branches of sports medicine. In the early years, most care to athletes was provided by orthopedic surgeons, but more recently primary-care sports physicians (including osteopathic physicians), physiotherapists, athletic therapists, chiropractors, sport nutritionists, and sport psychologists have all entered the field.

In many instances, the primary-care physician is the initial access point, as more than 90 percent of sports injuries can be managed non-operatively. These providers can initiate treatment, order appropriate imaging studies, and expedite referral to the most appropriate specialist (including orthopedic surgeons). In the United States, sports medicine specialists are physicians with a primary certification in family medicine, internal medicine, emergency medicine, pediatrics, or physical medicine and rehabilitation who obtain one to two years of additional training in sports medicine through recognized fellowship (subspecialty) programs. Eligible physicians then take a subspecialty certification examination in sports medicine. To maintain their expertise, they must also participate in continuing medical education and must be recertified every 10 years.

Other countries, as well, have special criteria, training programs, and examinations that distinguish certified sports medicine specialists from other doctors without specialized training in this area. Importantly, in addition to being able to deal with common sports injuries, these physicians have all received extra training in nonmusculoskeletal aspects of sports medicine, such as mild traumatic brain injury and other head injuries, chronic or acute illnesses (such as infectious mononucleosis, asthma, and diabetes) in the athlete, exercise prescription, and promotion of a healthy lifestyle, just to name a few. The latter two skills, in particular, are critical in this era of increasing obesity and sedentary behavior. A wealth of supplemental resources for the active individual can also be found through the American College of Sports Medicine, a large multidisciplinary organization dedicated to the advancement and integration of scientific research to provide education and practical applications of exercise science and sports medicine.

The widespread use of arthroscopic surgery for treatment of injuries to the knee, elbow, wrist, and ankle has greatly widened the scope of orthopedic practice and enhanced the management of sports injuries. The specialty of orthopedic surgery has also recently acknowledged that additional expertise in sports medicine beyond traditional orthopedic training is both beneficial and desirable. In March 2003, the American Board of Medical Specialties (ABSM) approved the application of the American Orthopedic Society for Sports Medicine (AOSSM) for orthopedic sports medicine subspecialty status. A task force of experts has been estab-lished to develop a suitable examination or certificate of added qualification (CAQ), with the first tests projected to take place in 2006. This process is hoped to boost standards for orthopedic sports medicine fellowship programs and, as the field evolves, to drive the educational process.

Of course, diagnostic and surgical specialists in sports medicine do not and cannot function in isolation. The importance of rehabilitation and ancillary services such as pedorthics, bracing, massage therapy, and others should not be underestimated. Many of these other professional groups, such as physical therapists, have standard curricula and examinations to document proficiency in sports medicine. There is an ever-increasing trend toward evidence-based practice, with the use of standardized and validated outcomes to evaluate new devices and treatment programs, as well as the old tried and true remedies. The complexity of expertise within the field of sports medicine also offers the interested student a multiplicity of educational choices and career options.

In summary, sports medicine is a fascinating area, which flourishes best in a multidisciplinary setting, where practitioners can work together to provide care for active people of all ages. The goal of sports medicine is ultimately to treat the athlete in each person. This *A to Z of Sports Medicine* will provide a window into this exciting and expanding area, with an entry-level roadmap and directions for further exploration. Read it and enjoy!

—Dr. Connie Lebrun
MDCM, MPE, CCFP, Dip. Sport Med.,
Director of Primary Care Sport Medicine,
Fowler Kennedy Sport Medicine Clinic,
London, Ontario, Canada

ENTRIES A–Z

abrasions (road rash) Abrasions are common sports injuries that often result from the friction of an athlete falling and or sliding against a hard surface, such as pavement, which rubs off layers of skin, creating an abrasion. Cyclists call this "road rash," since it commonly occurs from wrecking a bike on pavement. While bike wrecks can potentially cause very serious and painful abrasions, most abrasions are fairly shallow scrapes that do not take off many skin layers or cause much bleeding. Abrasions can still be extremely painful, since many nerve endings are exposed when the skin is torn off.

Causes

Anything that forces the skin to slide against a hard surface can create an abrasion. Bike wrecks may be the most common causes of these injuries, but they occur in rollerblading, skateboarding, and other sports as well.

Diagnosis

A minor abrasion may be treated without consulting a doctor, but a doctor should see any severe abrasion. An abrasion is typically defined as an injury in which layers of skin are rubbed off, including the epidermis, which is the outer layer of skin that provides protection, and the dermis, the deep inner layer that provides the firmness and flexibility of the skin.

Treatment

Conventional treatment involves cleaning the wound and dressing it with an antibiotic ointment followed by a dry dressing. Historically, people cleaned such wounds with mild soap and water or a mild antiseptic wash, but recent studies suggest that using antiseptics may actually increase the tissue damage and necessary healing time. The best approach is to clean the wound, using a syringe for increased pressure in applying a nontoxic surfactant (detergent) so that it does not become infected. Remove any dirt and debris that may be stuck in the skin. The area should be completely clean before a dressing is applied. If necessary, it is acceptable to use a clean gauze to gently scrub the area, as long as care is taken not to scrub hard. It is best to use a semipermeable dressing, such as Tegaderm or Second Skin, to cover the wound and attach the dressing to dry, healthy skin with adhesive tape. The dressing should be changed every few days, and the wound should be kept moist, which will promote healing.

The skin will heal from the deeper layers to the surface layers, and from the outer edges of the wound toward the center. As it begins to heal, the wound will look pink and raw, but over time new skin will form that is pink and smooth.

Tetanus is a concern with abrasions. If the last tetanus booster was more than 10 years ago, see a doctor to get a tetanus immunization. Tetanus is a serious infection that can develop in wounds in which the flesh is torn or burned.

Deep cuts that continue bleeding after 15 minutes of applying direct pressure may need to be stitched up in order to heal properly. It is best to see a doctor if there are any doubts about the need for stitches.

Prevention

Protective pads and covering skin with a layer of clothing will aid in the prevention of abrasions. It is also helpful to keep the necessary first aid supplies available when the risk of an abrasion is present. That way the wound can be cleaned and treated quickly, which will aid in the healing process.

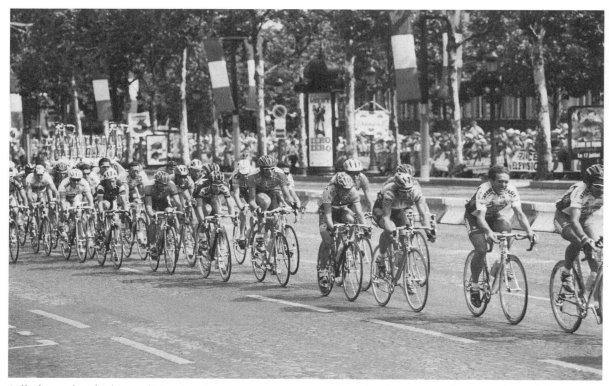

Called "road rash" by cyclists, abrasions are common sports injuries that occur when an athlete falls or slides on a hard surface. Spectacular crashes often occur during bike races, leaving numerous cyclists with abrasions that range from minor to severe. In the worst cases, abrasions are treated with stitches to encourage the wound to heal. *(Fogstock, LLC)*

Achilles tendon rupture   A loud "pop" in the back of the ankle followed by a sharp pain that makes it impossible to walk properly on the foot may signal an Achilles tendon rupture. Some describe it as feeling like being kicked, or even shot, in the back of the foot. A strong band of tissue named after the indestructible mythological Greek warrior, the Achilles tendon is the continuation of the large calf muscles, and it connects these muscles in the back of the lower leg to the heel bone, serving as the power source for pushing off with the foot. It helps point your foot downward, rise up on the toes, and push off in walking. Basketball, tennis, and football players are especially vulnerable to Achilles tendon ruptures, since their sports require so much jumping and abrupt start-and-stop footwork. But anyone, even garden-ers who may overstress the tendon while kneeling in one position too long on an ambitious spring day, can suffer this painful injury.

Causes

Achilles tendon ruptures and partial tears most often occur during sports that require quick cutting and jumping motions. In these cases, the tear or rupture results from a violent contraction of the large calf muscles. Rarely does it involve contact with another player. Achilles tendon injuries, including ruptures, also result from repeated stress on the tendon. This repeated stress may develop from the following conditions:

• simple overuse

• failure to stretch properly

- running on hills and hard surfaces
- worn-out shoes
- flat feet
- weak or tight calf muscles

Achilles tendon ruptures are more likely to occur in people who have a long history of ACHILLES TENDONITIS, or inflammation of the Achilles tendon. In addition, poor conditioning, advanced age, and overexertion put people at risk of experiencing an Achilles tendon injury. Despite these risk factors, it is not uncommon for well-conditioned athletes to experience Achilles tendon ruptures.

Diagnosis

Achilles tendon ruptures, which can be partial or complete, usually occur just above above the heel bone, although they can occur anywhere along the tendon. They are diagnosed by a history of a sudden injury followed by a "pop" felt behind the ankle. The injury is confirmed by squeezing the calf muscles. If the foot does not move, the tendon is probably torn. In addition, pain and swelling near the heel and an inability to bend the foot downward or walk on it normally indicate a torn or ruptured Achilles tendon. If the tendon is completely ruptured, the patient will be unable to rise up on the toes on the injured leg. The pain is sometimes severe.

Occasionally, a MAGNETIC RESONANCE IMAGING (MRI) scan may be ordered. The computer image created by the MRI shows the soft tissues of the body and allows the doctor to determine if the injury is a partial tear of the tendon or a complete rupture.

Treatment

Treatment for Achilles tendon rupture may involve surgery. In most cases, a complete rupture is treated with surgery, which involves making an incision at the back of the leg and stitching the torn tendon together. The recovery period lasts about six to 12 weeks, during which time the leg is placed in a walking boot, cast, brace, or splint. Sometimes the foot may initially be pointed slightly down in the boot or brace, and then gradually moved to a neutral position, in order to prevent the tendon from healing in a stretched position, which would render it useless.

The benefits of surgical versus nonsurgical treatment include a lower risk of re-rupture and a greater chance of restoring full strength to the leg, making surgery the preferred treatment for active patients. Risks of complications with this treatment are very low but do include infection, scarring, and poor healing of the wound.

The nonsurgical treatment for Achilles tendon ruptures usually involves wearing a cast or walking boot until the ends of the torn tendon have had a chance to reattach themselves. This method can be effective, but the incidence of re-rupture is higher with nonsurgical treatment and the recovery period usually lasts longer.

Prevention

As with many sports-related injuries, the keys to avoiding a tear or rupture of the Achilles tendon are proper stretching and warm-up exercises. Gently stretch the Achilles tendon before participating in physical activities. Stretching exercises should be performed slowly, and the stretch should be held until you feel a pull, but not pain.

An excellent stretch for the Achilles tendon is the following:

- Stand at arm's length from a wall and place the palms of the hands flat against it.
- Step one leg back, keeping the knee straight and the heel flat on the floor.
- Lean toward the wall, slowly bending the elbows and the front knee.
- Hold the stretch for 30 to 60 seconds.
- Switch legs and repeat.

Achilles tendonitis   The largest and strongest tendon in the body, the Achilles tendon gets much use and abuse, but it is not, like its Greek mythological namesake, indestructible. It is susceptible to a number of injuries, ranging from inflammation to ACHILLES TENDON RUPTURE, many of which are generally referred to as Achilles tendonitis. In general, Achilles tendonitis refers to inflammation of the tendon behind the ankle that connects the leg and ankle to the heel bone. Specifically, the range of Achilles tendon inflammation and degeneration is classified as follows:

- *Peritenonitis.* Characterized by a burning pain during or following activity, this occurs when the paratenon is inflamed and thickened. As the disease gets worse, the pain may occur during periods of little activity and even at rest. Prolonged peritenosis may result in a ruptured Achilles tendon.

- *Tendinosis.* People with tendinosis often describe feeling a "nodule" or sensation of fullness at the back of the leg. There is no swelling and no pain, but the condition is degenerative of the tendon fibers.

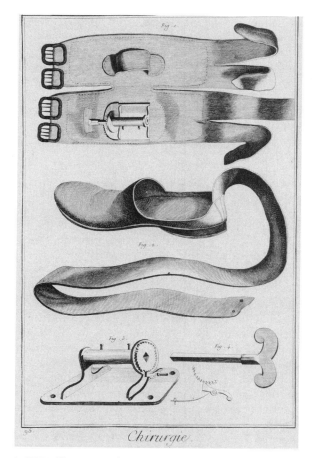

A 1772 illustration by Frenchman Louis-Jacques Goussier proves that Achilles tendonitis has been a source of pain for centuries. Treatment approaches, however, have evolved a bit during this time.
(Courtesy History of Medicine Collection, United States National Library of Medicine)

- *Peritenonitis with tendinosis.* A combination of the two diseases above, this condition usually causes activity-related pain and diffuse swelling, as well as the "nodule" sensation.

Achilles tendonitis usually sets in following sudden changes in activity or training level, use of inappropriate footwear, or training on inappropriate running surfaces. It is commonly seen in runners; some estimates in the United States report an incidence of Achilles tendonitis in 6.5–18 percent of all runners.

Causes

Achilles tendonitis is most often caused by excessive running or jumping without proper stretching and strengthening. Uphill running in particular can cause inflammation of the Achilles tendon. Injuries to the tendon often occur in older, recreational athletes, though they may occur in younger, well-conditioned athletes, too. The following are common causes of injury:

- overuse
- increased intensity of activity
- increased duration of training
- stairs
- hill climbing
- poor conditioning
- improper shoes
- improper training surfaces
- improper or lack of stretching exercises

Intrinsic causes may include the following:

- age
- tight Achilles tendon
- varus heel
- varus forefoot
- cavus foot
- tibia vara
- medical diseases that may affect tendon tissue, which include diabetes mellitus, and diseases

that require corticosteroid treatment, which include lupus, asthma, and transplants

Diagnosis

Doctors diagnose Achilles tendonitis based on the patient's experience of pain behind the ankle when running or jumping. Tenderness in the area over the Achilles tendon and weakness in the calf muscles further indicate Achilles tendonitis. To ensure that the Achilles is not ruptured, doctors will often ask the patient to try to rise up on the toes of the injured leg, which is impossible if the tendon is not at least partially intact.

Treatment

Achilles tendonitis can usually be treated without surgery, using rest, anti-inflammatory medications, and stretching exercises. Physical therapy and orthotics for the shoes may also be needed.

Some patients, however, will require surgery. Those with severe tendonosis may need to have the degenerated portions of the tendon removed. The surgery is then followed by a strenuous rehabilitation program.

Prevention

Warming up before exercising and proper stretching are essential to the prevention of Achilles tendonitis. Avid runners should take precautions against developing problems with the Achilles tendon by not only stretching properly but also by running on soft surfaces, wearing shoes with adequate cushion, and making gradual changes in mileage, speed, and terrain, as opposed to abrupt and severe changes.

acromioclavicular (AC) joint injury Acromioclavicular (AC) joint injuries are extremely common, accounting for 40 to 50 percent of all athletic shoulder injuries. An AC joint injury is one that disrupts the group of ligaments that holds the clavicle to the portion of the scapula known as the acromion. They occur in many different kinds of sports, but especially in collision sports such as hockey, rugby, football, and cycling, and are precipitated by a blow to the tip of the shoulder. The severity of the disruption can vary, resulting in different degrees of AC separation, from Type I to Type V, each requiring its own specific treatment.

They are most common in males, due to their greater participation in collision sports.

Cause

Falls on, or hard blows to, the tip of the shoulder are the most common causes of AC joint injury, which is classified according to the severity of the damage to the ligaments, with Type I being a strain and Type V describing the most severe form of separation and disturbance of the ligaments.

Diagnosis

A patient who complains of acute or chronic shoulder pain, either in the front or back of the shoulder, will normally be considered a candidate for AC joint injury. Often there is acute pain, tenderness, and swelling around the shoulder right after the injury occurs. Once the generalized pain dissolves, the point over the AC joint remains tender. An ABRASION or prominence may be visible at the clavicle. If the patient is involved in WEIGHT TRAINING, he or she will usually experience pain with certain exercises, especially bench presses and dips. In addition, patients often report pain during the night, when they roll onto the shoulder while sleeping. Although not common, there is sometimes a popping noise or catching sensation associated with the AC joint injury.

The doctor will question the patient concerning his or her experience of pain. When there is pain and swelling over the joint, it may be difficult for a doctor to determine the stability of the AC joint. If the patient stretches the injured arm across his or her chest it will normally produce pain. If the ligaments are actually torn, as opposed to strained, it may be difficult to rule out a ROTATOR CUFF TEAR due to limitations in the movement of the shoulder.

Imaging studies, primarily radiographs, are used to evaluate the severity of the AC joint injury. A minimum of two views is necessary. In some cases, it may also be helpful to take a stress radiograph of the AC joint, in which the patient holds a certain amount of weight while moving the injured shoulder. Since this is usually painful, the test is not recommended unless it is the only way to determine if the ligaments have been completely torn.

Bone scans are not recommended as initial screening tools, but they have been proven extremely effective in demonstrating AC joint injury in patients whose plain radiographs returned negative results.

MAGNETIC RESONANCE IMAGING (MRI) scans are rarely used in diagnosing AC joint injuries, but in some cases they may be required. In middle-aged and older patients who have disabling shoulder pain after the acute pain of an AC injury subsides, an MRI may be useful to rule out a rotator cuff tear. In athletes with persistent pain over the AC joint, an MRI may help determine if there is irreversible damage to the cartilaginous disk or if osteoarthritis has set in.

Treatment

During the acute phase of the injury, a conservative treatment may involve PHYSICAL THERAPY to help restore normal FLEXIBILITY and range of motion. Exercises may also be prescribed to help strengthen the rotator cuff, which has been reported to improve the symptoms associated with AC joint injury. Type I and type II injuries are always treated conservatively, and there is little controversy about these treatments. In type III injuries, there are conflicting opinions concerning the use of surgery. The complications involved in the surgery and the realization that the recovery time for surgery was as long as the recovery time of the conservative treatment have led many orthopedic surgeons to reconsider surgical approaches that were once common, especially in athletes such as baseball players, who use overhead movements. Type IV and V injuries require some type of reconstruction in order to prevent further complications. Surgeries for AC joint reconstruction may be done arthroscopically, which has the potential advantage of offering a shorter period of post-surgery symptoms and a quicker recovery of strength. One major risk involved in the surgical approach is failure to complete an adequate resection of the ligaments. This is the most common cause of post-surgery pain.

Patients are ready to return to their normal activities when there is an absence of significant symptoms. For those who have undergone surgery, healing of the wound and muscles, as well as a return of strength to the shoulder, dictate when normal activity may be resumed.

Prevention

Prevention is managed simply by avoiding the maneuvers that may cause the injury. In addition, proper diagnosis of the AC joint pathology from the start helps in the prevention of greater injury to the area. Those with osteoarthritis in the AC joint must refrain from engaging in the movements that cause pain in order to gain relief from symptoms.

acute mountain sickness (altitude sickness) A common and usually minor illness that typically affects mountain climbers, skiers, hikers, and others who ascend too rapidly to high elevations, acute mountain sickness is the result of problems associated with lack of oxygen. Most people will experience some symptoms of this illness if they travel rapidly by car, train, or plane from sea level to 11,500 feet, but practicing proper acclimatization techniques will allow most healthy people who are accustomed to living around sea level to climb to high altitudes with only minimal symptoms of altitude sickness. The illness does occasionally become a medical emergency when serious symptoms develop. These include pulmonary edema and cerebral edema which can, if untreated, lead to death.

Causes

Acute mountain sickness is caused by reduced atmospheric pressure and a lower concentration of oxygen at high altitudes. These conditions affect the nervous system, lungs, muscles, and heart, producing symptoms that can range from mild to life threatening.

Diagnosis

Most people experience only mild symptoms and recover from these in two to three days. These include headache, dizziness, inability to sleep, shortness of breath, rapid heart rate, fatigue, loss of appetite, and nausea. In severe cases, however, the symptoms are quite serious. Fluid can collect in the lungs, a condition called pulmonary edema, which causes extreme shortness of breath and even less oxygenation. Swelling may also occur in the brain, which is called cerebral edema and can cause confusion, coma, and even death. Coughing, chest congestion, bluish discoloration of the skin, and gray or pale complexion may also be symptomatic of severe illness. The risk of experiencing these more serious symptoms is greater at higher altitudes and with faster rates of ascent.

Often the diagnosis of acute mountain sickness must occur outside the reach of medical help. If a doctor is present or the patient can go in for treatment, listening to the chest with a stethoscope will reveal crackling in the lungs of patients with pulmonary edema. A chest X ray may also confirm the diagnosis.

Treatment

The main treatment for all forms of altitude sickness is to descend to a lower altitude as quickly and safely as possible. Those with fairly minor symptoms can be given acetazolamide (Diamox) to stimulate breathing, speed acclimatization, and diminish the discomfort. Patients should consume plenty of fluids, excluding alcoholic beverages, while taking Diamox since it increases urination.

Patients with more serious symptoms should be given supplemental oxygen if possible and taken to a hospital as soon as possible. Pulmonary edema is treated with oxygen, nifedipine (a high-blood pressure medication also effective for this disorder), and in severe cases, mechanical ventilation. If cerebral edema is present, the doctor may administer the steroid drug dexamethasone (Decadron), which is sometimes helpful. A delay in treatment for serious cases of altitude sickness may negatively affect the chances of recovery. Swelling of the brain and the respiratory distress that can evolve from pulmonary edema may lead to death.

Prevention

Education about the proper techniques for ascending to high altitudes is the key to preventing acute mountain sickness. The basic guidelines to follow include:

- ascending gradually
- stopping for a day or two of rest every 2,000 feet above 8,000 feet
- sleeping at lower altitudes whenever possible
- learning to recognize early symptoms so that you can return to lower altitudes before symptoms worsen
- carrying several days worth of oxygen when climbing above 11,500 feet
- taking acetazolamide prior to rapid ascents
- correcting anemic conditions before ascending to high altitudes
- drinking and eating sufficiently to prepare the body for the stress of the climb
- avoiding high altitudes if you have heart or lung disease

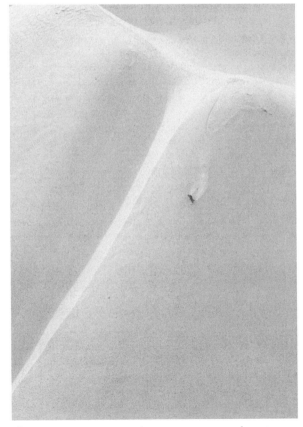

Skiers sometimes experience symptoms of acute mountain sickness when they climb to elevations above 11,000 feet too rapidly. It is important to acclimatize oneself gradually when ascending to high altitudes. *(Fogstock, LLC)*

aerobic training Aerobic exercise uses large muscle groups, such as the legs and arms, which raises the heart rate and increases breathing.

Whether a person is walking, swimming, or dancing the tango, the body will benefit from the resulting increase in oxygen intake and the conditioning effects of getting the heart pumping. Participating in some form of regular aerobic training also increases strength and endurance. Even if it is just a brisk walk around the block, aerobic exercise can improve the overall functioning of the body and make a person feel happier.

Benefits of Aerobic Exercise

- *Weight loss.* Combined with a healthy diet and appropriate strength training, aerobic exercise will help lose weight. Loss of excess weight has numerous beneficial side effects, but one of the most important is its contribution to reducing the risk of disease. Many major diseases, such as heart disease, high blood pressure, stroke, and diabetes, are associated with being overweight. As a person loses excess weight, the risk of developing these life-threatening diseases decreases.

- *A more efficient heart rate.* A stronger heart pumps more blood with each heartbeat, which means that the heart does not need to beat so fast. This slower, more efficient heart rate contributes to living a longer, healthier life.

- *Improved mental health.* Aerobic exercise releases the body's natural painkillers, called endorphins, which help reduce stress, anxiety, and depression.

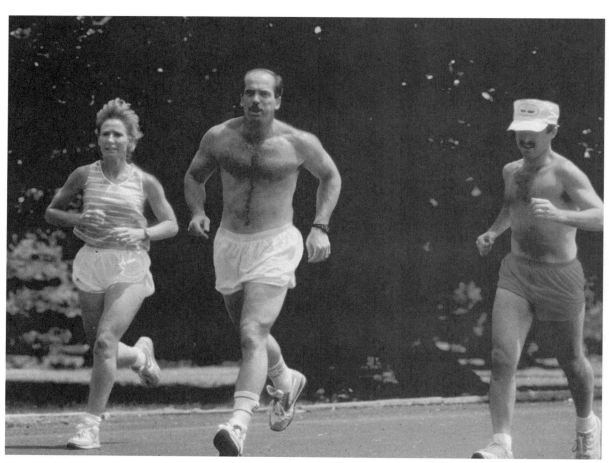

Running is the most popular form of aerobic conditioning. *(Courtesy Public Health Image Library)*

- *Improved immune system.* It is believed that aerobic exercise helps to activate the body's immune system, readying it to fight off infection. Consequently, regular exercisers are less likely to contract viruses, such as colds and the flu.
- *Increased stamina.* Although exercise sometimes makes a person feel tired during or immediately following the activity, in the long term it increases stamina and reduces the amount of fatigue experienced.
- *Increased life span.* Studies have shown that exercise is definitely linked to an increase in life span.
- *Improved muscle health.* Capillaries, the tiny blood vessels in the muscles, grow more readily in those who exercise aerobically. A greater number of capillaries translates into more oxygen for the muscles and less lactic acid and other metabolic wastes. Especially for those who experience chronic pain or fibromyalgia, aerobic exercise can help lessen pain.

Cautions about Aerobic Exercise

Since aerobic exercise is widely touted for its effects on weight loss, it is important to understand a little bit about how this works. The body loses weight by using more energy than is required to maintain its base metabolic rate. This energy is found in the form of glycogen, which is the name for stored carbohydrates, and fat. The body will burn either glycogen or fat in its attempt to find energy to fuel its additional activities. But in order to lose weight most efficiently, it is preferable to have the body burn fat.

To burn fat calories, as opposed to glycogen calories, choose moderately paced activities, such as brisk walking, swimming, or leisurely tennis, that can be sustained over longer periods of time. These lower-intensity sports are easier on the body and more effective at burning fat calories and helping to lose weight. Higher-intensity activities, such as running sprints, are called anaerobic, as opposed to aerobic, and tend to burn glycogen calories. They are also more stressful to the body in general, creating a greater risk of injury unless you are conditioned for the activity.

How to Begin an Aerobic Exercise Program

- Consult with a doctor first. This is especially important for those over 40, overweight, have a chronic health condition, or who are a smoker or drinker.
- Pick something you enjoy doing. More than 60 percent of all Americans do not get enough exercise. Choose to be among the 40 percent who do. If you pick an activity you enjoy, the chances of continuing are much greater.
- Modify your activity to fit your lifestyle. If you really don't want to miss the evening news but find that is the only time you have for exercising, try placing a treadmill or stationary bike in front of the TV, so that you can enjoy both activities. If you don't have any 30-minute time slots open, try three, 10-minute periods of exercise throughout the day. Studies show that this can be just as effective as one continuous 30-minute session.
- Start out with moderate expectations. Thirty minutes a day of aerobic exercise is an excellent goal. But when you first begin, it may take several weeks to build up to 30 minutes of continuous activity. Start slowly and give the body a chance to get conditioned to the new activity, and be flexible with goals. Many people quit because they set their goals too high in the beginning and become discouraged.
- Be sure to stretch the muscles, but not when they are cold. Warm up a bit by starting out slowly in the exercise, then stop and stretch once the muscles have had a chance to limber up a bit. Runners, for example, may want to stretch in the middle or end of the run instead of at the very beginning.
- Do not be concerned about purchasing expensive equipment and apparel. For most activities, a good pair of athletic shoes is all that is required.

anabolic steroids Anabolic steroids are manmade drugs that are similar to the male hormone testosterone. Doctors sometimes prescribe steroids to treat men whose bodies do not naturally produce enough testosterone or to increase weight gain in people with diseases such as AIDS, where loss of muscle mass and weight is a severe problem. They also have been shown to improve the symptoms of arthritis.

The use of anabolic steroids in the United States is legal only if prescribed by a doctor; however, they are often purchased illegally by athletes who consume them in the hopes of gaining weight, muscle mass, strength, power, speed, endurance, and aggressiveness. Their use is often reported in sports such as weightlifting, track and field, and American football, where muscle mass is most associated with successful performance.

Some of the most common anabolic steroids include dehydrochlormethyl-testosterone (Turnibol), metandienone (Dianabol), methyltestosterone (Android), nandrolone phenpropionate (Durabolin), oxandrolone (Oxandrin), oxymetholone (Anadrol), and stanozolol (Winstrol).

Athletes with asthma are sometimes prescribed a class of drugs called anabolic agents that includes salmeterol (Serevent) and metaproterenol (Alupent), which are usually administered with an inhaler.

How They Work

Male hormones, specifically testosterone, are partially responsible for the tremendous developmental changes that occur during puberty and adolescence. Male hormones have androgenic and anabolic effects. Androgenic effects are changes in primary and secondary sexual characteristics. These include enlargement of the penis and testes, voice changes, hair growth on the face, axilla, and genital areas, and increased aggressiveness. The anabolic effects of androgens include accelerated growth of muscle, bone, and red blood cells, and enhanced neural conduction.

Anabolic steroids are created to provide the anabolic properties of male hormones without producing the sex-linked (androgenic) effects. However, none of the steroids has been very successful in doing this. The steroids that work most effectively at building muscle are also the ones that produce the most changes in sexual characteristics. An increase in facial hair and a deepening of the voice are often side effects of taking steroids.

Steroid hormones work by stimulating receptor molecules in muscle cells, which activates specific genes to produce proteins. They also increase the rate of protein metabolism, allowing the body to synthesize more protein and inhibiting the natural rate of protein degradation in the body.

Heavy-resistance training seems to be necessary for anabolic steroids to exert any beneficial effect on physical performance. This is because the effectiveness of anabolic steroids is dependent upon unbound receptor sites in the muscles. Intense strength training may increase the number of unbound receptor sites, which in turn would increase the effectiveness of anabolic steroids, allowing the athlete to build more muscle.

Many athletes have stated that anabolic steroids help them train harder and recover faster. It is possible that anabolic steroids have an anticatabolic effect, which means that they block the effects of hormones such as cortisol, which actually break down tissue following exercise. This indeed speeds recovery following exercise. However, when the athlete goes off the steroids, he experiences a faster than normal rate of muscle loss, as well as symptoms of addiction.

Cortisol is secreted during exercise to help the body use its protein for fuel and to suppress the inflammation that occurs in response to tissue injury. The hormone actually binds to receptors sites in the muscles. When the steroids interfere with the cortisol binding, the body responds by secreting more cortisol and creating more and more receptor sites. This rebound effect means that it is very difficult for the athlete to sustain gains in muscle mass when he or she goes off the drug. This difficulty may then encourage the athlete to become addicted and to become psychologically dependent. Long-term use of anabolic steroids increases the chance of experiencing serious side effects. In addition, the increased cortisol in the body suppresses the immune system, making the athlete more susceptible to illnesses of all kinds.

Some researchers have also hypothesized that anabolic steroids work by producing a psychosomatic state that allows athletes to feel better and train harder. According to this theory, the benefits come from increased feelings of well-being, greater tolerance to stress, and increased aggressiveness, all of which make it easier for the athlete to train harder.

Side Effects

Anabolic steroids can help athletes gain size and strength, but not without a price. In addition to the drugs being illegal without a prescription, there are numerous serious side effects associated with their use.

Men may develop prominent breasts, baldness, decrease in sperm count, erectile dysfunction, and shrunken testicles. Women may experience a deeper voice, enlargement of the clitoris, increased body hair, baldness on the head, and female hormone problems. Both sexes might experience severe acne, liver abnormalities and tumors, increased low-density lipoprotein (LDL) and lower high-density lipoprotein (HDL) cholesterol, psychiatric disorders including severe mood swings and aggressive behavior, and chemical dependence on the drug. If an injected form is used, there is higher risk of infections and diseases that are transmitted in blood, including HIV and hepatitis. The use of steroids by teenagers can interfere with normal growth and development, sometimes even causing the bones to stop growing too soon, and put the teenagers at risk for future health problems.

Be Aware

In addition to all the health risks involved with steroid use, anabolic steroids are not legal in organized sports. They are probably the best-known banned substances in sports. The International Olympic Committee (IOC), National Collegiate Athletic Association (NCAA), and many professional sports organizations regularly test athletes for steroid use. Those who test positive are suspended or disqualified from competition. Famous athletes have had their careers ruined or negatively affected by steroid use. Ben Johnson, the Olympic sprinter, and Ken Caminiti, the baseball player, are two athletes whose names will forever be associated with illegal use of steroids.

Athletes must also be aware that the effects of anabolic steroids on physical performance are unclear. Although the mystique of steroid use suggests that they have tremendous power to increase muscle mass and strength, scientific studies have produced conflicting results. It is likely that steroids have the greatest effect on athletes who are already

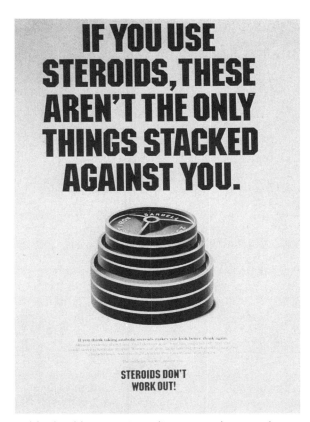

IF YOU USE STEROIDS, THESE AREN'T THE ONLY THINGS STACKED AGAINST YOU.

If you think taking anabolic steroids makes you look better, think again.

STEROIDS DON'T WORK OUT!

Public health campaigns discourage the use of steroids, but their popularity among athletes persists despite the legal and health risks associated with them. *(Courtesy History of Medicine Collection, United States National Library of Medicine)*

highly trained and who consume dosages that are considered unhealthy by scientists. Most studies have not used the same drug dosage used by athletes. Institutional safeguards prohibit administration of high dosages of possibly dangerous substances to human subjects. In addition, subjects in research experiments seldom resemble accomplished weight-trained athletes. Consequently, the subjects given a safe dosage of steroids over a limited time period showed some beneficial effects, but nothing as impressive as what many athletes claim to achieve in their uncontrolled experiments with steroids.

ankle fracture The ankle is a hinge-type joint that connects the leg to the foot. It consists of one large bone (tibia), one small bone (fibula), and one square-shaped bone (talus), all of which fit snugly together and are supported by strong ligaments. The ankle joint is the most commonly injured joint in sports, but ankle fractures, a break of one or more of the bones that make up the ankle, occur in only 15 percent of the cases where the ankle joint is injured. The Danis-Weber classification for ankle fractures is commonly used among primary care physicians and grades the fracture based on the level of the fracture in relationship to the joint mortise of the distal fibula. Fractures are classified as Type A, Type B, or Type C.

Causes

Basketball players are especially vulnerable to ankle fractures due to the jumping and cutting aspects of the game, but many activities can lead to this injury. In general, when a fracture occurs, there has been some external force acting on the ankle, forcing it inward or outward past its normal range of motion. But fractures of the ankle can also occur when a person is jumping or running and lands on an uneven surface, or when the foot is firmly planted and the body gets twisted.

Diagnosis

The first step in diagnosing an ankle fracture involves questioning the patient about the injury. A patient who describes a history of "turning" or "rolling" the ankle should be considered for a diagnosis of ankle fracture. It is helpful if the patient can recall the placement of his or her foot when the injury occurred. How much weight a patient can bear on the injured foot is important as well. If the patient cannot bear any weight, the likelihood of a clinically significant unstable fracture is greater. The patient may also recall a popping sound when the injury occurred. Any history of previous injury to the ankle is also relevant in helping the doctor assess the current injury.

The physical examination includes inspecting the ankle for swelling and fluid accumulation, as well as thoroughly palpating the ankle to determine the location of the tenderness. Normally, the more severe the injury, the greater the swelling will be. The doctor will also determine the range of motion in the ankle, as well as its strength when moving in each direction. In addition, the doctor will examine the tension in the ligaments.

Checking the joints and the soft tissue around the point of injury is also important to rule out the possibility of additional injury in other areas.

The results of this physical exam will indicate whether or not an X ray is needed. If the fracture is an unstable one, as opposed to a stable fracture, it is possible that a COMPUTERIZED AXIAL TOMOGRAPHY (CAT) or MAGNETIC RESONANCE IMAGING (MRI) scan will be necessary to assess possible damage to the cartilage or tendon around the ankle.

Treatment

Initial treatment following the injury involves immobilization of the injured foot and measures to reduce pain, such as administering analgesics. Some Type A injuries can be treated with a walking cast or stirrup brace, allowing the patient to walk as long as there is no pain. Casting is usually for four to six weeks. Patients who have not healed in eight weeks should be referred to an orthopedic physician. The cast should not be applied until the initial swelling has subsided. During this time, the patient should apply ice to the injury for 20 minutes every three to four hours during the first 24 hours following the injury and then every four to six hours thereafter until the cast is put on. The ankle should also be elevated above the level of the heart during this time to reduce swelling.

Patients with Type B and Type C unstable fractures should be referred for consultation with an orthopedic physician, where the treatment will range from various types of immobilization to possible surgical treatments, which involve the placement of screws and plates in order to stabilize the ankle.

Surgery is followed by casting or splinting for a length of time determined by the severity of the fracture. Weight bearing may not be allowed for four to eight weeks until there is evidence that healing has begun.

Rehabilitation following the immobilization period should include exercises for increasing strength and flexibility. Younger patients may not need supervised PHYSICAL THERAPY, since they tend to regain strength and range of movement easily, but older patients may require formal physical therapy. Once there is documentation to support that the fracture has healed and that strength and motion have returned to the injured ankle, the patient may resume normal activities.

Prevention

Taping or bracing of the ankles and wearing high-top shoes may help prevent some ankle fractures. Exercises to maintain excellent ankle muscle strength and balance should also help.

ankle sprain   Ankle sprains are the most common sports-related injuries in the United States, occurring in nearly all types of sporting events and accounting for significant time away from games and practices. An ankle sprain occurs when the ligaments that support the ankle joint are stretched or torn. The ligaments around the ankle are strong bands of tissue. They surround the ankle, both outside the bones, in between the bones, and on the inside of the three bones that make up the ankle. Ankle sprains are graded according to the severity of the injury, with a Grade I injury referring to stretched ligaments, a Grade II injury referring to a partial tear of the ligaments, and a Grade III injury describing a complete tear of the ligaments.

Causes

Ankle sprains occur for the same reason as ankle fractures—something has forced the ankle inward or outward past its normal range of motion. This can occur in a number of different situations, and may be the result, for example, of an external force applied to the ankle, such as another athlete landing on the ankle, or of the injured person landing on an uneven surface, which causes the ankle to twist. In any case, ankle sprains are especially common among basketball players but also occur with some frequency in football, baseball, and soccer, as well.

Diagnosis

A history of "turning" or "rolling" the ankle accompanied by sudden pain and swelling may indicate an ankle sprain. The patient may report hearing a popping sound at the time of the injury, as well. Tenderness over the injured ligaments with bruising will be noticeable. The doctor will test the ligaments to determine if the range of motion is abnormally increased due to stretching. X rays are usually needed to rule out an ankle fracture, and occasionally a MAGNETIC RESONANCE IMAGING (MRI) scan will be necessary to examine the cartilage and tendons around the ankle.

Treatment

Most ankle sprains can be treated conservatively by protecting the ankle from further injury, resting and icing the ankle, applying a compression wrap, and elevating the ankle to reduce swelling. A short program of rehabilitative exercises to increase strength and balance is necessary in order to prevent further sprains.

In rare cases, surgery is needed to stabilize the ankle. In these cases, there are a number of different procedures that have been used to repair or reconstruct the ligaments.

Prevention

To prevent sprains, athletic trainers and sports medicine professionals routinely tape and brace athletes' ankles, a practice that has been common for more than 50 years. Most ankle sprains occur when landing from a jump, with the foot in an inverted position. Several studies support the theory that ankle sprains frequently involve disruption in ankle proprioception, or the ankle's sensitivity to stimuli, preventing the ankle from being able to protect itself. Eversion ankle sprains, on the other hand, usually are not related to inadequate proprioception but are the result of outside forces, such as contact with another player.

In either case, studies examining the effectiveness of external ankle stabilization have had conflicting results. While some show no change in injury rates, most have found at least some decrease in inversion sprains although the mechanism for this protection is still somewhat unclear. It seems logical that taping and bracing the ankle should increase its structural stability and make it less susceptible to inversion. While this is true to some extent, at least one study has shown that regular taping can lose most of its supportive effect after only short periods of exercise. Although studies regarding effectiveness and technique are not all in agreement, it seems clear that bracing or taping of the ankle will continue to be a mainstay in the prepractice and precompetition routine.

Despite this, it is important to remember that ankle bracing and taping should not be used in place of aggressive rehabilitation including strengthening and other therapeutic exercises.

When taping an ankle, the lower leg, ankle, and foot should be cleaned and dried before applying a layer of prewrap (a thin foamlike material) to the area to be taped. Some athletes go as far as shaving the hair from around the area so that they can apply the tape directly to the skin. In this case, a quick-drying adherent is recommended and may be sprayed onto the skin to allow for better tape adhesion. Often, heel and lace pads are applied to areas of high friction to prevent blisters.

anorexia   Anorexia is an eating disorder that is both a physical and a mental illness. It occurs when a person is morbidly afraid of being overweight, which leads to eating as little as possible and possessing a distorted body image. There are two types of anorexia: restrictive anorexia does not involve any regular bingeing and purging; bingeing-purging anorexia involves regular use of this behavior during an anorexic episode. Although the illness is associated almost solely with girls and women, about 10 to 15 percent of all anorexics are men. A very severe illness, anorexia usually leads to a loss of regular menstruation, which results in hormone changes that can, among other things, result in permanent loss of bone mass. Other health complications associated with anorexia include heart problems, endocrine system problems, and even death.

Causes

It is not clear exactly what causes anorexia, but it is believed that external social pressure and internal pressure to conform to expectations for thinness play a significant role. Some researchers also believe that eating disorders may be related to problems with the chemicals in the brain that regulate mood and appetite. In either case, girls and women who are determined to achieve a lean appearance and who believe their athletic success is tied to this achievement may try to reach this goal through excessive exercise and dieting. Such an approach may eventually lead to development

of the FEMALE ATHLETE TRIAD. In addition, a tendency toward perfectionism, compulsive behavior, and being extremely goal-oriented make an athlete more susceptible to the illness.

Risk factors associated with anorexia include:

- a family history of anorexia nervosa or other eating disorders

- a family or personal history of mood disorders, such as major depression and bipolar disorder (manic depression), anxiety disorders, or obsessive-compulsive personality disorder

Diagnosis

Recognizing and diagnosing anorexia may be difficult, but awareness of the symptoms is the first step in recognizing the illness and getting help. Symptoms of anorexia include morbid fear of fatness, distorted body image, refusal to maintain a weight at least 85 percent of that expected for height and age, and amenorrhea, or loss of menstruation. Symptoms may also include the following:

- weight loss from strict dieting, usually severe

- binge eating (eating large amounts of food in a short period of time) and/or purging (using laxatives or making yourself throw up)

- weakness and dizziness

- feeling depressed or anxious

- insomnia

- fasting or eating very little

- seeing oneself as being overweight when one is not

- too much exercise

- fearing weight gain even when underweight

- thinking about food all the time

Diagnosing anorexia will involve both a medical history of the patient and a physical examination. The doctor will ask about eating habits, as well as about other behavior patterns that might include the following:

- extreme selectiveness in choosing food that is low in calories

- purging, taking laxatives

- ritualistic eating
- denying hunger or denying any problem at all

The physical examination may reveal erosion of tooth enamel from frequent vomiting and enlarged parotid glands. If there is any history of stress fractures, especially those that occur in unusual places such as femurs, ribs, or pelvis due to minimal trauma, this may indicate the possibility of osteoporosis. The consequences of untreated eating disorders are serious. They include the possibility of irreversible bone loss, disturbances of the cardiovascular, endocrine, and gastrointestinal systems, disruption of temperature regulation, and death.

Treatment

Anorexia can be a very difficult illness to treat. Patients are often reluctant to seek care and may deny that they have any nutritional or health problems. Quite often, it takes a team of professionals and friends to get patients the help they need. A physician, nutritionist, and psychologist may each be helpful, in addition to friends, parents, and coaches. An individual who needs help may be more open to it if the risks of her illness are explained in a nonjudgmental way and if she is convinced that treatment would probably help her athletic performance. This type of intervention is often more successful in the early stages of the illness than it is later on.

A treatment plan for anorexia may include nutritional monitoring, hormone replacement, and reduced training. The doctor will help the patient to start eating normally again and may prescribe medicine to assist in overcoming the patient's fear of becoming fat and to reduce the depression and anxiety the patient is experiencing. The patient will probably need individual psychotherapy and family therapy as well.

When discussing the patient's diet, it is helpful to emphasize increasing lean-body mass and sustaining the lean-body mass by eating a well-rounded, high-carbohydrate diet. The patient should understand that she needs sufficient calories to meet both her routine daily needs and her sport needs. It is likely that the physician or nutritionist will recommend taking supplemental calcium to provide some protective effect for the bones. Sufficient vitamin D is also important.

People with anorexia may have symptoms for many years and will probably need ongoing treatment. Any stressful situation can cause a relapse. After reaching a normal weight, the patient may need to continue having psychotherapy or taking medicine for months or years. In addition, he or she may be weighed regularly to make sure the illness is not returning.

Treatment will likely involve the following:

- eating a nutritious, well-balanced diet
- limiting exercise programs as advised by the treatment team
- getting plenty of rest and sleep
- maintaining a realistic weight for height and body frame
- taking mineral and vitamin supplements, if recommended by the health care provider
- seeing a doctor regularly to have weight, blood pressure, heart rate, and temperature checked
- keeping an optimistic outlook
- with a therapist, working out areas of conflict and learning healthy coping strategies
- balancing work with recreation and social activities
- learning to communicate feelings

Prevention

Although the social pressures on women, and athletes in particular, to be thin will not likely change soon, parents, coaches, teachers, and friends can have a mitigating effect by refraining from focusing on the athlete's weight or from suggesting that he or she lose weight for any reason. In addition, alertness to symptoms will help interested parties intervene early, which increases the chances for successful treatment.

The following are helpful guidelines for athletes and others who feel vulnerable to developing an eating disorder:

- keep appointments with your health care provider or therapist;
- avoid skipping meals;
- avoid using laxatives;

- avoid excessive exercise;
- avoid drinking alcohol;
- avoid smoking cigarettes.

anterior cruciate ligament (ACL) injury   A strong band of tissues located in the center of the knee, the ACL's function is to prevent the shinbone from extending too far beyond the thighbone. One of four primary stabilizers of the knee—the others are the posterior cruciate ligament (PCL), the medial collateral ligament (MCL), and the lateral collateral ligament (LCL)—the ACL and its partners work together with the muscles and cartilage of the knee to control the knee's motion. Injuries to the ACL are common, especially among skiers and those who play basketball and football. They may result in partial or complete rupture of the ligament.

Causes

When a violent twisting motion of the knee occurs, the risk of an ACL injury is high. This can easily happen in stop-and-start sports and in activities that involve jumping, cutting, or twisting. The ACL may also be torn if the knee is hyperextended, or bent backward.

Diagnosis

Patients who describe a twisting or hyperextension of the knee often have an ACL tear. They sometimes feel a popping sensation in the knee that is followed by immediate swelling. Significant build-up of excess fluid inside the knee usually follows the injury. Most people with an ACL tear will be unable to fully straighten the affected knee. But even if all these symptoms exist, a complete examination of the knee is warranted to rule out other injuries such as a fracture or meniscus tear. If there are other injuries in conjunction with the ACL tear, the knee may actually lock.

Treatment

Conservative treatments that avoid surgery are appropriate for some patients with partial ACL tears and those whose lifestyle involves limited activity. Initially, the treatment involves the application of ice and anti-inflammatory medication to minimize the pain and swelling. In some cases, draining fluid off the knee may also be recommended.

Once the acute phase of the injury has passed, the patient should be prescribed a rehabilitative program aimed at strengthening the quadriceps, the large muscles in the front of the thigh, and the hamstrings, the large muscles at the back of the thigh. This will help take some of the work off the ACL as it heals. For athletes, PHYSICAL THERAPY should include sports-specific drills and possibly the use of a brace when returning to the sport.

Most athletes who wish to participate in cutting and twisting sports should strongly consider ACL reconstruction so that they avoid doing further damage to the injured knee. This is also true for patients whose knee gives way during ordinary daily activities. The success and ease of ACL reconstruction have increased greatly in recent years, further increasing the attractiveness of this treatment approach.

There are many methods a surgeon can use in reconstructing a ligament, but all involve the grafting of tissue from either the patient or a cadaver. The three most common types of grafts are a bone-patellar tendon-bone autograft, a hamstring autograft, or an allograft, the use of a cadaver's tissue. In the allograft, the patellar tendon and the Achilles tendon are the most common sources of the tissue. Screws or other fastening devices are used to secure the tissue graft inside the knee.

Rehabilitation following surgery is quite similar to rehabilitation with nonsurgical treatment. It focuses on restoring full range of motion to the knee, with the patient picking up exercises to enhance strength, coordination, and endurance as the knee heals. The typical recovery time following surgery is one to three weeks before resuming normal daily activities and about six months before resuming complete sports activities.

Prevention

Strong quadriceps and hamstrings go a long way in helping to avoid some ACL tears. In addition, skiers who have studied ski injury prevention techniques have a lower rate of ACL tears than those who have not studied ski injury prevention.

arch pain   There are two arches in the foot. The longitudinal arch runs the length of the foot, and the transverse arch runs across the width of the foot. The arches are made up of ligaments, whose job is to keep the bones of the feet in place. Although arch pain can occur in one or both arches, it most commonly occurs in the longitudinal arch.

Causes

Arch pain is most often experienced by athletes who participate in activities such as running, hiking, walking, and jumping. Considered an OVERUSE INJURY, it occurs when the ligaments are strained by repeated use without enough rest and time for recovery. People who have flat feet, or people whose feet flatten and roll inward when walking, a condition called overpronation, are more prone to arch pain. Arch pain usually comes on slowly. However, it can occur suddenly if the ligaments are stretched or torn during a forceful activity such as sprinting or jumping.

Diagnosis

Arch pain is easy to diagnose. Athletes will complain of pain along the arch of the foot. Usually the pain is worse when participating in activities that involve weight-bearing on the injured foot. Rest normally alleviates some or all of the symptoms. In a physical exam, the doctor will ask questions to get an accurate history of the patient's activities and to determine how long the arch pain has been present. The physical exam will be concentrated on palpating the arch and checking for levels of pain and tenderness there.

Treatment

Treatment for arch pain is like treatment for other overuse injuries. The athlete should place ice packs on the arch for 20 to 30 minutes every three to four hours for two or three days or until the pain goes away. If there is swelling, the doctor may prescribe an anti-inflammatory medication. During the recovery period, the arch needs extra support. Taping the arch or using an extra arch support in the shoe may provide enough support to help alleviate the problem. If over-pronation is a problem, or the athlete's feet are particularly flat, the doctor may prescribe custom-made arch supports, also called orthotics, to be worn in the shoes.

The goal of rehabilitation is to return to sports activities as soon as is safely possible. With an over-use injury, however, it is very easy to worsen the injury by returning too soon, so it is important to wait until the pain is gone and full range of motion has returned to the affected foot. There should also be full strength in the injured foot, and the athlete should be able to run, sprint, and jump without any pain or limping.

Prevention

Arch pain can be prevented by wearing shoes that fit properly and have proper arch support. Stretching the feet and arches before any strenuous activity will also help prevent this injury. Some athletes will need orthotics while playing sports, and others will need to wear them all the time in order to ensure that the arches are not repeatedly injured.

arthroscopy Arthroscopy is a minimally invasive surgical technique that allows for more precise evaluation and quicker treatment and rehabilitation of many joint injuries that commonly occur in sports, such as strains or tears in the ligaments and tendons of the shoulders, knees, wrists, elbows, and ankles. These injuries that formerly required large incisions during complicated operations, long hospital stays during recovery, and extensive physical therapy during rehabilitation can now be handled effectively and quickly with fewer risks and side effects.

How Does It Work

The arthroscope is a fiber optic instrument that is narrower than a pen and can be put into a joint through small incisions less than five millimeters in length. A camera is attached to the arthroscope, and the image is viewed on a television monitor. Small instruments ranging from three to five millimeters in size may be inserted through additional portals. These instruments allow the surgeon to feel the various joint structures, diagnose the injury, and then repair, reconstruct, or remove the damaged structure.

One of the great benefits of arthroscopic surgery is that it requires such tiny incisions. In any operation, the length of the incision is directly related to the amount of pain that the patient is going to experience after surgery because a greater amount of healing needs to take place inside the joint to recover from the trauma of the operation. The arthroscope allows for much smaller incisions, which translates into a faster, less painful recovery period for the patient.

Although many sports injuries are effectively treated with arthroscopic surgery, some are still better handled in traditional surgery. Good candidates for arthroscopic surgery in the knee joint include cartilage injuries, ANTERIOR CRUCIATE LIGAMENT (ACL) tears, synovial injuries involving the inner lining of the joint, loose bodies that may be inside the joint, and even certain problems that deal with patellar instability. In the shoulder, one can address a huge number of problems with the arthroscope. Loose bodies, calcium deposits, and certain types of rotator cuff injuries can be addressed arthroscopically. If the patient has a significant ROTATOR CUFF TEAR, it is still a little controversial to use arthroscopy exclusively, so at this point the injury is probably better taken care of through open surgery. Yet if there is a partial tear or impingement where the rotator cuff is inflamed or compressed, then the arthroscope is very valuable.

For almost any operation, the arthroscope is an effective diagnostic tool, regardless of the type of surgery needed. Doctors often see things that were not seen with plain X rays or even MAGNETIC RESONANCE IMAGING (MRI) scans. Occasionally, doctors find a significant tear or injury when they use the arthroscope diagnostically on an injury they were planning to repair arthroscopically. In these cases, they may change their minds and decide to repair the injury through open surgery instead.

Risks

As with any type of surgery, there is some risk of infection and nerve damage, but the risks are generally considered to be low in arthroscopy due to the minimal invasiveness of the procedure.

History of the Procedure

Arthroscopy remained a relatively underutilized procedure until the late 1970s and early 1980s when three events occurred that brought the concept into practical use.

An explosion of interest in sports and fitness, combined with the advent of fiber optics and the invention of new surgical instrumentation led to the development of arthroscopy as a practical and mainstream surgical technique. New applications for arthroscopic surgery have continued to be developed on an almost monthly basis. In 2003 approximately 98 percent of all knee surgeries were being performed arthroscopically. Arthroscopic treatments for shoulder stabilization have also become commonplace. The procedure has evolved from a diagnostic tool into a highly specialized surgical technique.

Patients with torn knee cartilage, for example, formerly underwent open surgery, which involved making a two- to three-inch incision in the knee and removing the entire cartilage. Those patients would remain in the hospital for nearly a week, and then be immobilized in a splint and on crutches for another three weeks. If they were fortunate, they might be running again in three to six months.

Today patients with the same injury are treated on an outpatient basis with three small incisions, each about one quarter inch in length. After three or four days on crutches, they begin walking again, and in two to three weeks, they are running and playing sports.

asthma, exercise-induced Asthma is a lung condition that causes the small airways of the lungs to spasm or constrict. Exercise-induced asthma is a form of asthma that some people have during or after physical activity. It is one of the most common conditions among active children, adolescents, and young adults, occurring in almost 90 percent of people who have chronic asthma and in 40 percent of individuals who have certain types of common allergies.

Exercise-induced asthma develops when vigorous physical activity triggers airway narrowing in people whose bronchial tubes are especially sensitive. It is a reversible airway obstruction that occurs during or after exertion and can occur in otherwise healthy people who do not have chronic asthma. In these people, exercise is the only stimulus for their asthma symptoms. However, exercise-induced asthma can also occur in people who have chronic asthma and may not be aware that their symptoms during exercise are a manifestation of asthma.

Causes

There are several theories concerning the cause of exercise-induced asthma, but none have been proven.

Exercise-induced asthma most often occurs in the following conditions:

- during or after physical activity and usually when breathing is hard, heavy, or fast
- when the air is cold
- when the humidity is very low or high
- when there is a lot of air pollution
- when there are a lot of allergens in the air

Winter sports, such as cross-country skiing, and bicycling in cold air often trigger symptoms of exercise-induced asthma.

Diagnosis

The most common symptoms of exercise-induced asthma include the following:

- wheezing
- coughing
- shortness of breath
- chest tightness
- fatigue
- decreased athletic performance

Although the above symptoms are seen most often, some individuals will experience more subtle symptoms, such as chest discomfort, stomachache, fatigue, feeling out of shape, inability to keep up with peers, or poorer performance than training would predict. These symptoms may occur during or after exercise. A doctor will take a medical history that includes a history of breathing problems during or after exercise. In addition, the patient history can help the physician identify subtle exercise-induced asthma clues such as fatigue or poorer performance than training would predict. It is important that the doctor distinguish between a patient with chronic asthma who also experiences asthma symptoms after exercising and a patient who experiences asthma symptoms only after exercising because the treatments for these two types of asthma are different.

A careful physical exam can help rule out conditions that mimic exercise-induced asthma such as respiratory infections or cardiac conditions. Pulmonary function testing is often useful for assessing severity and establishing a baseline for assessing the patient's progress during treatment. The patient may be asked to run on a treadmill or to exercise outside the office so that the doctor can listen to the lungs with a stethoscope following the exercise to see if there is any wheezing. The doctor may also give the patient a peak-flow meter, a small instrument that measures how fast he or she can exhale air in one breath. When the patient experiences the exercise-induced asthma, the amount of air exhaled in one breath will decrease from the normal measurement.

Treatment

Treatment options include measures that address the exercise environment and warm-up routines, so that the patient avoids the conditions that tend to cause the asthma. Exercise-induced asthma can also be successfully treated with medication. Normally, patients are given a bronchodilator and instructed to take two puffs of the prescribed medication, such as albuterol or pirbuterol, about 15 to 30 minutes prior to exercising. The doctor may also instruct the patient to use the medication during the exercise if needed.

Prevention

One key to preventing exercise-induced asthma is knowing what kind of conditions bring it on. If strenuous activity in cold, dry air seems to be the biggest culprit, the patient may need to exercise indoors during cold weather or wear a mask when exercising outside so that the air is warmed before entering the lungs. In addition, breathing through the nose warms the air more than breathing through mouth and should be emphasized for patients who have trouble with the cold. The presence of air pollution or pollen may also play a role in determining where and how the patient exercises. Although special consideration may need to be made for those who experience exercise-induced asthma, it is possible to stay physically fit and enjoy an active lifestyle as long as the patient takes the proper precautions. Many elite athletes have exercise-induced asthma and yet have participated in their sports at the highest levels and even won Olympic medals, so there should not be any expectations that the exercise-induced asthma will limit the patient's athletic performance.

athlete's foot (tinea pedis) A common skin problem caused by fungus, athlete's foot is associated with athletes and locker rooms, since it likes to grow in warm, moist environments. It usually begins on the skin between the toes and becomes scaly and itchy. Over time the infection may cause a break in the skin and become sore.

Causes

The fungus that causes athlete's foot is everywhere in the environment, but one of the most common places to pick it up is the locker room. The floors of showers, locker rooms, and exercise facilities are a hospitable environment for the fungus, which prefers to grow on sweaty, constantly wet, or improperly dried feet, especially in shoes or socks that do not have good ventilation.

Diagnosis

A person with athlete's foot will normally complain of itching, cracked and peeling skin, often between the last two toes on the foot, soreness on the bottom of the foot, and sometimes blisters.

A doctor can normally diagnose athlete's foot quite easily after examining the skin. Sometimes he or she may swab or scrape off a skin sample to test for fungus. If the doctor suspects a bacterial infection, the skin sample may be tested for bacteria as well.

Treatment

Athlete's foot can often be treated successfully with a nonprescription antifungal medicine such as Micatin, Tinactin, or Desenex. These medicines are creams that are applied to the skin of the foot. In cases of severe athlete's foot, when the infection has spread over a wide area, the doctor may prescribe oral medication.

Some people contract mild athlete's foot infections occasionally but are able to get rid of them quickly with over-the-counter medication. Other athletes contract infections regularly and may even keep the infection continuously for months or years. People who have frequent and chronic problems with athlete's foot that are resistant to treatment should consult with their doctor to obtain medication that will help with the constant itching and discomfort and also help prevent a more serious bacterial infection from developing.

Prevention

Prevention of athlete's foot is focused on keeping the feet clean and dry, especially in hot weather. Athletes should dry their feet well after showering, paying particular attention to the space between the toes where moisture can accumulate. It is also important to wear shower shoes to avoid picking up the infection from the floor, and to ascertain that shower and locker room floors are disinfected on a regular basis.

It helps to use an antifungal powder on the feet if there are parts of the feet prone to infection. Athletes should wear either cotton or wool socks, since they breathe best, and they should change their socks daily to avoid wearing dirty or damp socks. Shoes with ventilation are particularly helpful since they help to keep the feet dry. Another good practice is to dry out shoes after they have been worn in situations in which the feet were sweating.

athletic amenorrhea Common among runners, athletic amenorrhea is defined as the cessation of menstruation for six or more months due to a combination of factors, such as inadequate nutrition and low body fat. There are two main kinds of amenorrhea, primary and secondary. Primary amenorrhea is not having menstrual periods by the age of 16. Secondary amenorrhea is the absence of three or more periods in a woman who has had regular menstrual periods. Although many of these girls and women who are participating heavily in sports enjoy the reprieve from their monthly period, the condition is actually dangerous due to the lack of circulating estrogen in the body and can pose serious long-term health risks, such as premature osteoporosis, infertility, increased risk of injury, and an increased risk of cardiovascular disease and endometrial cancer, as well as impaired athletic performance.

Causes

There are probably several primary causes of athletic amenorrhea. The most recent research suggests that a low percentage of body fat, weight loss, poor nutrition, and excessive training all contribute to the development of menstrual cycle abnormalities that come about due to hormonal imbalances in the body. Although these seem to work together to make the body cease menstruation, it is believed that poor nutrition may be the leading factor in amenorrhea. Studies have shown that exercise combined with a low-calorie diet causes abnormal menstruation more frequently than just exercise alone.

Another factor that often contributes to the development of athletic amenorrhea is participation in a sport that places significant emphasis on leanness. Runners and ballet dancers, as well as gymnasts, figure skaters, divers, and others, are vulnerable to developing an eating disorder because their sports place such emphasis on maintaining a thin physique. Eating disorders inevitably result in poor nutrition, which can easily lead to amenorrhea. The association between amenorrhea and anorexia is so strong, in fact, that the American Psychiatric Association lists amenorrhea as one of the criteria for diagnosing anorexia.

Another possible influence on menstruation may be vegetarianism. Researchers have speculated that vegetarian diets contain amounts of trace elements and plant hormones that may negatively affect the menstrual cycle. There also may be a lack of protein in the diets of women who develop amenorrhea. Although lack of protein may just indicate a poor overall diet, it is possible that eating enough protein plays an important role in sustaining menstruation.

Diagnosis

Amenorrhea is diagnosed by taking a detailed history of the patient and conducting a physical examination that includes various tests to determine why the periods have stopped. The doctor will ask questions about the patient's diet and exercise habits, as well as the history of menstruation. If the patient is 16 years old and has never begun menstruating, or if the patient has gone three months without menstruating when her history of menstruation was regular, she may have athletic amenorrhea.

Tests performed include a pregnancy test to ensure that the patient is not pregnant, since preg-

nancy is the main cause of period cessation. The doctor may also request a DEXA scan, which is a special type of X ray to measure bone density and determine if the patient is developing osteoporosis.

Patients with amenorrhea may develop osteoporosis, a condition in which the bones have become brittle and weak and may become broken. This occurs because the lack of estrogen in the body results in a lack of calcium in the bones, rendering them weak. In addition, intense exercise puts a great deal of stress on the bones, making athletes with osteoporosis vulnerable to stress fractures.

In addition to checking for osteoporosis, the doctor will also want to determine if an eating disorder exists. When women athletes have a combination of athletic amenorrhea, osteoporosis, and an eating disorder, it is called FEMALE ATHLETE TRIAD.

Treatment

A common treatment for athletic amenorrhea includes a prescription for estrogen replacement in the form of an oral contraceptive. Patients may also need to increase their overall caloric intake, gain 2 to 3 percent of their body weight, add resistance training to their workouts to strengthen their bones, and take supplemental calcium, usually 1,500 milligrams a day.

Prevention

Eating a well-balanced diet with adequate calories helps prevent athletic amenorrhea. If the patient tends to eat too little and exercise too much for the amount she is eating, she may need to be treated for an eating disorder as well.

athletic trainer Athletic trainers work more closely with athletes than anyone else on the sports medicine team. They see all the injuries and illnesses first. Their judgment determines which cases are referred to the team physicians and which are treated by first aid measures. They also carry out or supervise much of the reconditioning and rehabilitation of the athletes. The athletic trainer is the contact between the athlete, coach, and team physician.

Training

An athletic trainer has a bachelor's degree as well as hundreds of hours of approved "on-field" training before becoming certified as an athletic trainer by the National Athletic Trainers Association. In many cases, athletic trainers have degrees in physical therapy or exercise physiology. Student athletic trainers who may work in a high school or university setting are often people interested in pursuing a career in the field but lacking in any formal credentials or qualifications.

Career

Typically, athletic trainers can be found providing services for pro sports teams, colleges and universities, high schools, and sports medicine clinics. In addition to their formal training in sports medicine, they should have good communication skills because they are responsible for establishing and maintaining the network of communication among athletes, coaches, physicians, and the athlete's family.

The job of an athletic trainer often necessitates that he or she work long and irregular hours. Frequent travel is often involved.

Working with an Athletic Trainer

Athletic trainers have the skills to administer emergency care. They are usually the first ones onto the field when an injury occurs. They are specialists in the rehabilitation and prevention of injuries, which means that most of their work happens behind the scenes, in the locker rooms and in training sessions with athletes.

avascular femoral head necrosis Avascular femoral head necrosis is a common debilitating disorder affecting the hip that usually leads to osteoarthritis of the hip joint in relatively young adults. It occurs when the tip of the hipbone loses its blood supply and dies. It is frequently seen among corticosteroid users and also occurs as a complication of other diseases.

Avascular necrosis means "death from lack of blood." Although avascular necrosis can affect various joints in the body, including the knees and shoulders, it most often affects the hips. Avascular necrosis of the femoral head occurs in bone tissue in the femoral head, or the knob at the end of the thighbone that connects to the hip. When the tissue in this knob dies, the bone can gradually collapse under the weight that the hip joint bears. As weight-bearing portions of the femoral head collapse, the joint operates less smoothly and the patient experiences pain in the joint. This is most often felt as groin pain, but can also cause pain in the thigh, buttock, or knee. If left untreated, avascular necrosis can lead to severe degeneration of the hip joint. It may become necessary to replace the patient's hip joint with an artificial one, a procedure known as total hip replacement.

Causes

The exact cause of avascular necrosis of the femoral head remains unknown. Trauma to the hip joint, including femoral head fractures and hip dislocations, can impair blood circulation and lead to bone death. While other possible causes of avascular necrosis remain uncertain, there are a number of factors that are known to increase the risk of suffering from avascular necrosis.

The most common risk factor for avascular necrosis is the use of steroids, with even a single large dose of steroids increasing the risk of avascular necrosis. Systemic lupus (a chronic inflammatory disease of the connective tissue) and chronic alcohol consumption are also known to increase the risk of avascular necrosis. About 25 percent of avascular necrosis cases cannot be traced to any known risk factor.

One theory holds that the loss of circulation to the femoral head may be due to an increase in pressure within the bone. If the pressure surrounding the vessels supplying blood to the femoral head is greater than the pressure within the vessels, the vessel walls collapse and blood can no longer flow through them. It is thought that this increase in pressure can cause hip pain.

Traumatic avascular necrosis is simply a result of mechanical disruption of blood flow to the femoral head. During sports endeavors, hip dislocation or subluxation is the most frequently reported traumatic means of avascular necrosis. A tackle from behind may cause an anterior hip subluxation in a ball carrier. Likewise, extreme abduction or external rotation may result in an anterior dislocation in a fallen water-skier.

Traumatic causes include the following:

- FEMORAL NECK FRACTURES
- HIP DISLOCATION
- SLIPPED CAPITAL FEMORAL EPIPHYSIS

Most cases of avascular necrosis are not caused by traumatic circumstances. Following are some of the common atraumatic causes:

• excessive corticosteroid usage and alcohol abuse that account for as many as 90 percent of new cases
• intravascular coagulation appearing to be the central event associated with nontraumatic AVN
• coagulation that may occur from other conditions, such as marrow fat enlargement, vessel wall injury from chemotherapy or radiation, or some type of blood clot
• chronic liver disease
• decompression sickness
• Gaucher's disease
• gout
• metabolic bone disease
• pregnancy
• smoking
• systemic lupus
• vasculitis

Diagnosis

Although the condition is painless in early stages of the disease, there is eventually pain and limited motion associated with it. The pain normally includes pain in the groin area, but it may also be present in the buttock, knee, or thigh. The patient will normally describe greater pain with weight-bearing activities and lesser pain when resting. The doctor will take a complete medical history of the patient that includes a history of any pain or weakness associated with the hip.

The physical examination will include the following:

• Passive range of motion (PROM) of the hip is limited and painful, especially forced internal rotation.
• A distinct limitation of passive abduction usually is noted.
• A straight-leg raise against resistance provokes pain in most symptomatic cases.

Routine laboratory studies are of little value other than to rule out other conditions that may cause

hip pain (e.g., rheumatoid arthritis). MAGNETIC RESONANCE IMAGING (MRI) is the study of choice in patients who demonstrate signs and symptoms suggestive of avascular necrosis but have normal radiographs. Bone scans may be used but should be supplemented by (MRI). Other potentially useful procedures may include biopsy, measuring bone marrow pressure, and angiography.

Treatment

If avascular necrosis of the femoral head is detected early enough, before significant bone collapse occurs, it may be possible to avoid a total hip replacement.

Treatments may then include the following:

• *Core decompression.* A hole is surgically drilled through the femur and into the femoral head to remove dead tissue and reduce pressure within the femoral head. The goal is to restore blood flow and encourage new bone growth to replace the dead bone that was removed. This procedure is effective for 70 percent of avascular necrosis cases detected in early stages.

• *Vascularized fibula graft.* As with core decompression, a hole is drilled through the femur to remove dead bone in the femoral head. At the same time, a section of healthy bone from the fibula (the smaller of the two bones in the lower leg) is removed, along with the vessels that supply it with blood.

This bone segment is inserted in the hole drilled in the femoral head and is reconnected to the circulatory system. The bone graft provides support to compensate for the bone that was drilled away and, because it is well supplied with blood, encourages new bone growth in the femoral head.

The section of fibula removed for this procedure is not necessary to support the lower leg. Its removal puts no additional limitations on the patient's activity after recovery from surgery.

In some cases, the vascularized fibula graft will be supplemented with the use of a special protein that can promote bone formation. This protein can enhance bone formation.

• *Osteotomy.* A wedge-shaped piece of bone is removed from the femur to change the position of the femoral head in the hip joint. The bone wedge removal rotates the femoral head so that an undamaged portion of the femoral head bears the weight that had been supported by the diseased portion.

This procedure works best in patients with limited damage to the femoral head, and is often used to treat avascular necrosis that follows trauma to the hip.

If one of the above treatments fails to preserve the femoral head or is deemed unsuitable, a total hip replacement is the next option. Because of its complexity, this procedure is the last choice for treating avascular necrosis. There is also always the chance that the artificial hip will need to be replaced more than once since artificial joints wear out with use. Young, active patients may have to undergo additional replacements of the joint over time.

With nonsurgical treatment, the patient will likely be prescribed a PHYSICAL THERAPY program to help control symptoms of the disease, but the therapy does little to alter the disease's progression. If there is surgical intervention, the rehabilitation will depend upon the type of surgery done but will include physical therapy and a program that emphasizes a very gradual return to nonimpact activities. The athlete should focus on maintaining fitness through participation in sports that are easy on the joints, such as swimming, biking, and the use of elliptical training machines.

Prevention

Because early detection is the most important factor in successfully treating avascular necrosis, awareness of risk factors and symptoms is essential. In addition, it is important to abstain from excessive use of alcohol and use the lowest possible dose of corticosteroids when prescribed, since these play a major role in development of avascular necrosis.

Baker's cyst   A bursa is a fluid-filled sac that serves as a cushion between tendons, bones, and skin. If the bursa in the space just behind the knee swells and causes pain, it is called a Baker's cyst.

Causes

It is not known exactly what causes a Baker's cyst, although the cysts can occur following an injury to the knee or when the lining of the knee joint produces too much fluid, as in rheumatoid arthritis.

Diagnosis

When there is pain, swelling, or a feeling of fullness in the area behind the knee, a Baker's cyst may be the culprit. A physical examination will reveal a bulge in the back of the knee. An MRI (MAGNETIC RESONANCE IMAGING) or an arthrogram may be needed to determine if you have a Baker's cyst. In an arthrogram, dye is injected into the knee and an X ray is taken to examine the membrane surrounding the knee joint.

Treatment

Initial treatment may involve simply wearing an elastic bandage around the knee, which often relieves the discomfort. Anti-inflammatory medication may also be helpful. If the cyst does not go away on its own, a doctor may recommend draining the cyst or operating to remove the cyst. Sometimes, a Baker's cyst will form without causing any discomfort, in which case it normally goes untreated.

Prevention

There is no way to prevent the formation of a Baker's cyst.

baseball finger (mallet finger)   A painful injury to the tip of the fingertip, baseball finger, or mallet finger, occurs when the tendon that controls muscle movement in the finger is torn or detached from the bone. If the force that pushes the finger down is great enough, as in a batted ball, it may even pull tiny pieces of bone away as well, creating a fracture. If the tendon is detached, the tip of the finger will hang down abnormally.

Causes

The usual cause is some kind of injury that jams the tip of the finger, often a really hard blow to the fingertip. This is so often associated with baseball, that it has borrowed that sport for its name.

Diagnosis

The patient may lose the ability to straighten the injured finger. There is normally pain and swelling at the fingertip, and if the injury is old before it is addressed, the patient may permanently lose the ability to straighten the end of the finger. A review of the symptoms, including a history of trauma to the finger, will normally determine the diagnosis. Fractures are not uncommon with baseball finger, because when the tendon is damaged, it tends to pull off a piece of the bone to which it is attached at the fingertip. Consequently, if there is any suspicion of a fracture in the finger, the doctor may take an X ray. Other injuries may be associated with baseball finger. Cartilage damage can result from the finger joints being jammed together, and the joint can also be dislocated, so the doctor should check for these injuries as well.

Treatment

The usual treatment in either a stretched or torn tendon or a fracture is to straighten the finger and place it in a splint for about six weeks until the tendon has a chance to reattach to the finger bone or, in the case of a fracture, the bone has a chance to heal. The splint must be worn at all times in order for healing to occur. In addition to wearing the splint, the finger should be iced on a regular schedule for the first few days following the injury, until the pain subsides. Icing for 20 to 30 minutes every three to four hours should reduce the inflammation. The patient should also try to keep the injured hand elevated above the level of the heart whenever possible. When lying down, the hand should rest on a pillow, and when sitting it should be placed on the back of the chair or couch.

The patient should not resume normal activities until the splint is removed and the injured finger is completely healed. Failure to wear the splint as prescribed or a return too soon to physical activity may incur permanent damage or deformity of the finger.

Prevention

Since baseball finger is normally caused by an accidental trauma to the fingertip, it is usually not preventable.

basic sports medicine practices at home   The most common sports injuries involve the knee, shoulder, and elbow in that exact order. Many of these injuries, as well as injuries to other parts of the body, are minor enough to be treated successfully at home, using the following general treatment principles. Often following these steps will allow athletes to return to their sports safely and quickly. Sometimes, however, an injury that appears minor may not heal despite these treatments, and the athlete should see a doctor. In addition, many injuries are not considered minor and should be seen by a doctor immediately. These injuries can cause obvious deformity, inability to move a limb or joint, numbness in an extremity, or severe pain at the place of injury.

If an injury appears to be minor, try the following steps and see if symptoms improve. If they do not, see a doctor for further treatment.

- *Rest.*   The athlete should avoid the irritating activity or sport until he or she can go through a normal daily routine (not including sports or heavy physical activity) without pain or diffi-

culty. This may be only several days, although more severe injuries may require several weeks or even months.

- *Ice.*   Ice helps when applied for 10- to 20-minute periods several times a day for two to three days after the injury. Ice slows the blood flow at the place of injury and thereby decreases swelling; it also has mild analgesic effects that help diminish pain.

- *Medication.*   Nonsteroidal anti-inflammatory medications, such as Motrin or Advil, help to decrease inflammation, and thereby pain and swelling at the injury site.

- *Maintain endurance.*   While resting an injury, maintain endurance by cross training. This includes choosing another form of exercise that does not stress the injured area (i.e., stationary cycling after an elbow injury).

- *Rehabilitation.*   Once there is no pain at the injury site, begin to move the injured area. This is done by slowly increasing its movement to match that of another uninjured joint or muscle. Once full motion (compared to the other side) is achieved, the patient may begin to strengthen the area. Light weights can be used and slowly increased until the strength of the other side is matched.

basic sports performance tips   Athletes focused on improving their performance may bring plenty of desire and willpower to their efforts, but an organized and comprehensive strategy is probably more important than sheer determination. Such a strategy involves some attention to the following aspects of training.

The Basics

Every sport has a fundamental set of skills and conditioning required for success. Runners and cyclists must build base mileage if they hope to work on speed and endurance. Athletes who play team sports must practice in order to develop the core skills of the game and their working relationships with other teammates. Whatever the sport may be, the athlete must be sure to have the basics covered before trying to move to more advanced training.

Interval Training

It is easy to get into a rut when training. Athletes tend to put in time in their given sport without much attention given to the quality of the time. While steady pace training is necessary, it is important to amp up the effort and have at least 10 percent of the workouts each week be high-intensity efforts. For runners, this may mean covering half the distance at a faster speed or doing speed intervals at the track. Although this kind of training is essential, it is also easy to overdo it. Athletes must be careful not to do too much too fast since this can easily cause an injury if the body is not conditioned for the effort it is required to make.

Nutrition and Hydration

It is critical that athletes eat healthy, nutritious food that will provide adequate fuel. A solid training program requires proper nutrition, as well as refraining from alcohol and smoking. Adequate fluid intake is an extremely important aspect of optimal performance, too. Research shows that losing as little as 2 to 4 percent of body weight in water can lead to decreases in maximum speed and endurance. Adequate fluid intake means that the athlete needs to drink about a cup of fluid every 15 minutes or so during exercise. In general, the athlete needs to align his or her lifestyle with the goals he or she hopes to achieve.

Carbohydrate Replacement

For athletes whose event lasts longer than 90 minutes, it is important to replace carbohydrates. Drinks, gels, and solid food are all possible ways to do this. The particular method really depends on the sport and personal preference.

Strength Training

Building strength can provide the extra boost of power and endurance an athlete needs to set a new personal best. Strength exercises three times a week are enough to build power and mass, and they do not have to require lots of time. A well-planned routine of as little as five exercises can be enough to condition the muscles throughout the body and improve strength.

Stretching

Stretching exercises have also been linked to improved performance and reduced risk of injury.

One study demonstrated a 5 percent increase in power just from doing hamstring stretches. Increased flexibility in the hamstrings apparently leads to better utilization of the quadriceps muscles.

Rest

Never underestimate the value of rest when trying to achieve an optimal performance. Overtraining is a significant problem in athletes who have hit a training plateau. It is important to pay attention to signs of physical and psychological fatigue, lack of motivation, little aches throughout the body, and declines in skill.

Training Log

Athletes who monitor their training in a log book have a record of what works and what does not. They record the content of their workouts, their resting heart rates, and their body weight. They can then see fluctuations that take place during training. When the resting heart rate rises for two or more consecutive days, most athletes are advised to adjust their schedule to include more rest so that they avoid becoming overtrained. A decrease in body weight may indicate dehydration or loss of muscle glycogen repletion, which requires increased consumption of carbohydrates and drinking more fluids.

Relaxed Breathing

Learning to breathe deeply from the belly will help all athletes stay relaxed when competing and training. The benefits of overall relaxation in the body are immense and lead to enhanced performance.

Visualization

Visualization is a great way to get an edge on the competition and improve performance. Mental rehearsal for competition has been shown useful in improving performance in tennis, golf, and other skill sports. It creates a positive attitude and can strengthen muscle memory so that the body is more likely to make the correct movements automatically. Practicing visualization requires a quiet, calm environment. The idea is for the athlete to imagine in minute detail the competition as it unfolds from beginning to end with the athlete achieving exactly the performance that is desired.

biceps tendonitis (bicipital tendonitis) The biceps muscle, located in the front part of the upper arm, attaches at the elbow and in two places at the shoulder. When the tendons that attach this muscle to the bones becomes inflamed, there is pain in the front part of the shoulder or the upper arm, depending on which tendons are irritated. Commonly seen in throwing sports, such as football and baseball, biceps tendonitis is also known as bicipital tendonitis.

Causes

As with all tendonitis, biceps tendonitis results from overuse of the arm and shoulder or from an injury to the biceps tendon.

Diagnosis

A doctor will first take a history of the patient's symptoms, which normally include pain with movement of the arm or shoulder, especially when the arm is raised over the height of the shoulder. In addition, the area in the front of the shoulder is usually quite sensitive to the touch. Tenderness along the biceps muscle and biceps tendon indicates either tendonitis or some type of break in the tendon.

Treatment

Icing the shoulder every 20 to 30 minutes, every three to four hours for several days until the pain subsides is necessary. Anti-inflammatory medication may also be helpful in relieving the pain and reducing swelling in the tendon. Surgery may be necessary to reconstruct a torn tendon. Rehabilitation exercises involve strengthening the biceps and increasing flexibility in the shoulder.

When the patient no longer experiences pain with the aggravating activity and normal strength and range of motion have returned to the shoulder and biceps, he or she may begin a gradual return to normal activities. In throwing sports, the patient must gradually rebuild tolerance to throwing. This means starting with gentle tossing and gradually throwing harder. In contact sports, the shoulder must not be tender to the touch, and contact should progress from minimal contact to harder contact. Returning to activities too soon can result in a worse injury and an even longer recovery period.

Prevention

Proper warm-up and stretching exercises for the arm and shoulder will help prevent biceps tendonitis. Rest and icing whenever any pain occurs may also prevent mild inflammation from developing into full-blown tendonitis.

bicycle seat neuropathy (saddle numbness, erectile dysfunction) One of the most common injuries in cyclists, bicycle seat neuropathy occurs as a result of the cyclist supporting his or her weight on a narrow, hard seat, which causes either vascular or neurological damage to the pudendal nerves, the primary nerves of the genitals. Commonly implicated in impotence among male cyclists, some doctors estimate that up to 50 percent of men who ride a bike for two to three hours at a time experience pain or numbness in the perineal region. According to these doctors, those who ride a bike for longer than three or four hours at a time increase their risk of impotence. Not all doctors, however, agree that bicycle riding creates a major risk for impotence. Some suggest that erectile dysfunction in cyclists is more directly related to the cyclist's history of a fall onto the top tube of a bicycle frame. Perineal numbness has also been reported in women.

Causes

Studies, which have usually focused on long-distance, multiday rides, suggest that long-distance cycling creates indirect pressure on the pudendal nerves, as well as the entire perineal region, which includes the surrounding soft tissues, bony structures, and associated sexual organs. Over extended periods of time, this kind of pressure and compression can lead to nerve damage and sexual dysfunction.

Diagnosis

Cyclists who complain of numbness, pain, decreased orgasm sensitivity, and impotence, all of which can occur temporarily or chronically, may have bicycle seat neuropathy. It is important to note that numbness may be a warning sign for further problems, but impotence can occur without any preceding experience of numbness. In addition, doctors need to determine the severity of these symptoms. Some cyclists experience mild numbness, while others experience impotence or urinary incontinence.

Doctors will normally question a cyclist about the amount of time he or she spends cycling, although time on a bike before the onset of symptoms varies greatly between patients. Doctors will also attempt to rule out other causes of impotence, such as a history of diabetes, metabolic disorders, endocrine or vascular disease, perineal trauma, or cancer. Questions concerning changes in training or bicycle setup are also pertinent.

The physical examination will probably include observation and palpation of the penis, testicles, and perineal area, as well as testing of motor and sensory function in these areas.

Normally, there are no lab tests or X rays needed in diagnosing bicycle seat neuropathy. However, in order to rule out certain other disorders, such as hypothyroidism or diabetes, lab studies may be called for. In addition, a Doppler ultrasound of the vascular structures in the perineal region may be necessary. If there is any history of acute trauma to the pelvis, an X ray may be ordered to rule out pelvic fracture.

Treatment

Rest from biking and equipment changes are the main types of treatment available for bicycle seat neuropathy. Cyclists can switch to riding a recumbent bike, which relives pressure from the perineum. They can also switch to a wider bike seat or to one of the new bike seats designed to take pressure off the perineal nerves and arteries. Changing in riding practices may also be helpful. Rising out of the seat every 10 minutes while riding will relieve pressure in the perineal area. Some doctors go further in suggesting that children never be given bikes with top tubes and that all seats be designed without "noses."

Rehabilitation should include an evaluation of the cyclist's position in the saddle and adjustments where necessary to the seat height and position. Cyclists need to be sure to rest long enough so that they do not experience symptoms upon returning to the bike. Continuation of neuropathy can lead to permanent damage and long-term impotence.

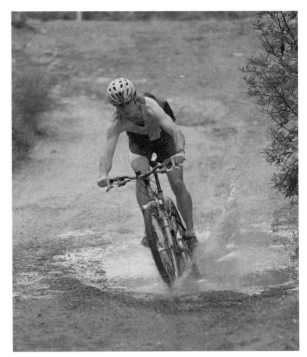

Commonly called saddle numbness, bicycle seat neuropathy occurs frequently in male cyclists, causing pain and numbness in the genitals. The condition may be implicated in erectile dysfunction and, ultimately, infertility. *(Fogstock, LLC)*

Prevention

Avoid long-distance cycling or any cycling that produces pain or numbness in the perineal region. Using an anatomically correct bicycle seat and changing positions frequently while riding will also help to prevent the development of this condition.

blisters   A blister is a bubble of fluid under the outer layer of skin. The fluid may be clear or filled with blood or pus. Blisters most commonly occur on feet or hands.

Causes

Blisters are caused when skin rubs against something (friction). First, a tear occurs within the upper layers of the skin forming a space between the layers while leaving the surface intact. Then fluid seeps into the space. Soles of the feet and palms of the hands are most commonly affected for several reasons. The hands and feet often rub against shoes, skates, rackets, or other equipment. Athletes and hikers often get foot blisters, while gymnasts and baseball players often get blisters on their hands and fingers. Blister formation usually requires thick and rather immobile epidermis, as is found in these areas. In addition, blisters form more easily on moist skin than on dry or soaked skin, and warm conditions assist blister formation. Blisters may form on feet if shoes or socks don't fit well and rub uncomfortably.

Blisters most often occur at the start of a new sports season or exercise program, after wearing new shoes, or when the weather is hot and humid.

Diagnosis

When the skin becomes irritated, fluid collects underneath the outer layer of skin. This can be quite painful. The surrounding area may be red, sore, or swollen. Blisters can be very small or quite large.

Most blisters are filled with clear fluid. If the fluid is bloody, it usually means that a lot of force caused the blister. If the blister is filled with pus, it is probably infected. The blister as well as the tissue around the blister can get infected. Infected blisters are very painful. They may be swollen and hot. Symptoms may include a fever.

Treatment

The goal of treatment is to relieve pain, keep the blister from enlarging, and avoid infection. Signs of infection include pus draining from the blister, very red or warm skin around the blister, and red streaks leading away from the blister. Small, intact blisters that don't cause discomfort usually need no treatment, so it is best to leave most small blisters alone. They should be kept clean and covered with an antibiotic ointment and a bandage. Putting a little petroleum jelly around the blister or the part of a shoe that causes the irritation may reduce friction.

Moleskin, available at the drug store, may also be used to protect a blister. The best way to do this is to cut a hole in a piece of moleskin that is bigger than the blister. Then put the moleskin on the skin with the "donut hole" over the blister. Cover the moleskin with a bandage. Blisters usually drain by

themselves. The overlying skin is a natural protective layer. It should be left in place until it is very dry and the underlying skin has become tough and painless. Then trim off the layer of dry skin.

Large blisters may need to be drained. It is important to do this in a way that does not cause an infection. Always use a sterilized needle to drain a blister. The needle should be sterilized by heating it with a flame until it is red-hot and then allowed to cool. Rubbing alcohol can also sterilize a needle. Use the needle to puncture the edge of the blister in several places. Make the punctures wide enough so they do not reseal.

If a blister becomes infected, see a health care provider. He or she may prescribe an antibiotic.

Most blisters last about three to seven days. Sometimes blisters are so large or painful that they preclude a few days of activity. Athletes can play a sport if they can tolerate the discomfort of the blisters and they are well protected. Athletes should not play if blisters are infected.

Prevention

In order to prevent getting blisters, athletes must minimize all rubbing against the skin. The following guidelines suggest ways to avoid this friction.

- Make sure that shoes fit well.
- Don't wear wet shoes.
- Wear two pairs of socks.
- Put petroleum jelly (Vaseline) on spots that tend to rub or use a foot powder.
- Put athletic tape or a bandage over sore spots.
- Wear gloves to protect hands.

blowout fracture A direct blow to the eye or cheek can result in a fracture of the bones of the eye socket, the cavity containing the eyeball and its associated muscles. This cavity is called the orbit, and it connects to one of the sinuses. If the orbit is fractured, the patient will be unable to blow hard through the nose without the eye swelling shut as air seeps into the tissues directly under the eye.

Causes

A direct blow to the eye or cheek can cause a blowout fracture. Racquetball, tennis, baseball, lacrosse, and soccer players are all at risk of a blowout fracture, since they play with hard balls that can come into contact with the face. Most blowout fractures are the result of an impact to the front of the eye from something bigger than the eye opening, such as a baseball or clenched fist.

Diagnosis

In addition to bruising and swelling around the eye socket and possible redness are areas of bleeding in the white of the eye, the patient may experience double vision if the orbit is displaced and has trapped one of the eye muscles, which happens easily in this type of injury. A trapped eye muscle will usually mean that the eyes do not move in conjunction with each other, which causes double vision. There may also be difficulty in looking up, down, right, or left, and the eye may be abnormally positioned, either bulging out or sunken in. Numbness may occur in the forehead, eyelids, cheek, upper lip, or upper teeth on the same side as the injured eye if there is nerve damage. Finally, there may be deformity in the cheek or forehead, with the area over the broken bone appearing to be dented. The cheek may be abnormally flat in appearance, and the patient may have severe pain in the cheek when attempting to open the mouth.

Checking for all these symptoms in a physical examination with a doctor will determine the diagnosis. The doctor will also look inside the eye with an ophthalmoscope to check for signs of internal damage. Diagnosis will be confirmed with an X ray or COMPUTERIZED AXIAL TOMOGRAPHY (CAT) SCAN of the area around the eye.

Treatment

The severity and exact location of the injury will determine the treatment. A small fracture that does not affect the movement of the eye may heal with ice packs, decongestants, and an antibiotic to prevent infection. In such cases, the patient will usually be advised to rest for several days and avoid blowing the nose.

In more serious fractures, the patient may be referred to a plastic and reconstructive surgeon who specializes in eye injuries. The specialist will determine if surgery is needed. Reasons for treating with surgery include removing bone fragments, freeing trapped eye muscles, restoring the normal structure of the eye socket, and repairing deformities of the eye rim that affect appearance.

Prevention

Most eye injuries can be prevented by taking proper precautionary measures. Those who risk eye injury on the job should always wear protective face shields and goggles. Baseball and basketball cause the greatest number of sports-related eye injuries. Players in these sports should also use protective eyewear. Amateur boxing is another cause of serious eye injury, and, according to the American Academy of Pediatrics, children and adolescents should not be allowed to participate in the sport of boxing. Finally, wearing a seat belt in the car will help protect the eyes, face, and upper body in the event of an accident.

boxer's fracture (fifth metacarpal fracture) The metacarpals are the long bones in the hand. The fifth metacarpal is the bone in the hand that attaches to the pinky finger. A boxer's fracture occurs when there is a break in this metacarpal.

Causes

Although a fifth metacarpal fracture usually occurs from hitting a hard object with the fist, hence its common name, boxer's fracture, it can also occur from falling onto the hand if the pinky finger bears much of the weight of the fall.

Diagnosis

An athlete with a boxer's fracture will normally complain of pain, swelling, and tenderness on the pinky finger side of the hand. There may be a bump on the side of the hand or the side of the hand or pinky finger may look crooked. As with any broken bone, the pain will usually be significant enough to cause the athlete to stop using the hand and seek treatment.

A doctor will take a medical history to review all the symptoms and determine the cause of injury. A physical examination may be enough to make the diagnosis, but the doctor will want to take an X ray as well to determine the severity of the break and check for any surrounding damage that may have occurred to the ligaments.

Treatment

If the broken bone is crooked, the doctor will straighten it before applying a cast or splint. The cast or splint will provide protection and support for the broken bone until it has time to repair itself, which normally takes four to six weeks. In addition to wearing the cast or splint, the athlete will need to keep the injured hand elevated as much as possible. This includes placing it up on a pillow while sleeping. Icing the injury over the cast or splint for 20 to 30 minutes every three to four hours for the first two to three days will help to keep the swelling down. In addition, anti-inflammatory medication or other medication may be prescribed by the doctor.

The doctor will take follow-up X rays to determine that the bone has healed properly. When the fracture has closed, the athlete may begin rehabilitation. Range of motion and strengthening exercises for the hand should be done until the injured hand has full range of motion and strength compared to the uninjured hand.

Prevention

Since most boxer's fractures happen as a result of hitting hard objects with the fist, the most simple form of prevention is to avoid hitting things. Boxers should be careful to wear protective gloves and to tape the finger and hands as much as possible.

bulimia Bulimia nervosa is an eating disorder. People with this illness engage in a pattern of disordered eating that includes eating larger amounts of food than most people would eat in a short time, then purging, fasting, or exercising excessively to compensate for the bingeing. There are two types of bulimia: purging and nonpurging. Patients with purging bulimia may purge by vomiting or using laxatives or diuretics. Those with nonpurging bulimia may fast or exercise excessively following the binge eating. Most bulimics have a normal weight, but feel a marked lack of control over their eating behavior. They often feel that their life is controlled by their conflicts over eating and the seesaw effects of the disorder on their moods. Although the disorder can affect men, most people with bulimia are young women.

Causes

The exact cause of bulimia is not known, but some researchers believe that eating disorders may be related to problems with the chemicals in the brain that regulate mood and appetite. Others stress the negative impact of the external social pressure on women to be thin and the corresponding internal pressure to conform to these expectations for thinness that many women feel. In either case, girls and women who are determined to achieve a lean appearance and who believe their athletic success is tied to this achievement may try to reach this goal through excessive exercise and dieting. Such an approach may eventually lead to the development of bulimia. A tendency toward perfectionism, compulsive behavior, and being extremely goal-oriented make a person more susceptible to the illness.

Diagnosis

A doctor will diagnose bulimia by taking a complete medical history of the patient and then conducting a physical examination. The focus will be on the patient's eating patterns and on identifying the presence of the behaviors that are associated with bulimia. These behaviors include the following:

- repeated episodes of binge eating followed by purging
- alternate bingeing and fasting
- secretive eating and bingeing
- exercising excessively to prevent weight gain

Other sign and symptoms of bulimia include

- excessive weight loss or gain
- repeated weight loss and gain of more than 10 pounds
- dehydration
- weakness
- heartburn or reflux from the stomach acid contained in vomit
- swollen cheeks from repeated vomiting
- damaged teeth from stomach acid contained in vomit
- being overly concerned with one's weight

- visiting the bathroom after meals
- depression
- excessive dieting, followed by binge eating
- always criticizing one's body
- scratches or scars on the backs of fingers or hands from self-induced vomiting
- menstrual irregularity

Patients diagnosed with bulimia average about 14 episodes per week. In general, people with bulimia have a normal to high-normal body weight, but it may fluctuate by more than 10 pounds because of the binge-purge cycle.

Treatment

Eating disorders can be very difficult to treat. Patients are often reluctant to seek care and may deny that they have any nutritional or health problems. Quite often, it takes a team of professionals and friends to get the patient the help he or she needs. A physician, nutritionist, and psychologist may each be helpful, in addition to friends, parents, and coaches. An individual who needs help may be more open to treatment if the risks of her illness are explained in a nonjudgmental way and if she is convinced that treatment would probably help her athletic performance. This type of intervention is often more successful in the early stages of the illness than it is later on.

A treatment plan for bulimia may include nutritional monitoring, hormone replacement, and reduced training. The doctor will help the patient to start eating normally again and may prescribe medicine, such as antidepressants or mood stabilizers, to assist in overcoming the patient's fear of becoming fat and to reduce the depression and anxiety the patient is experiencing. The patient will probably need individual psychotherapy and family therapy as well.

When discussing the patient's diet, it is helpful to emphasize sustaining the lean-body mass by eating a well-rounded, high-carbohydrate diet. The patient should understand the needs for sufficient calories to meet both routine daily needs and sport needs. It is likely that the physician or nutritionist will recommend taking supplemental calcium to provide some protective effect for the bones. Sufficient vitamin D is also important.

People with bulimia may have symptoms for many years and will probably need ongoing treatment. Any stressful situation can cause a relapse. After normalizing eating patterns, the patient may need to continue psychotherapy or medicine for months or years.

Treatment will likely involve the following:

- eating a nutritious, well-balanced diet
- limiting an exercise program as advised by the treatment team
- getting plenty of rest and sleep
- maintaining a realistic weight for height and body frame
- taking mineral and vitamin supplements, if recommended by the health care provider
- seeing a doctor regularly to have weight, blood pressure, heart rate, and temperature checked
- keeping an optimistic outlook
- with a therapist, working out areas of conflict and learning healthy coping strategies
- balancing work with recreation and social activities
- learning to communicate feelings

It is important that patients understand that bulimia is a serious illness, especially for athletes who routinely put greater than normal stress on their bodies through their participation in a sport. Bulimia has numerous harmful long-term side effects if left untreated. These include the following:

- laceration of the oral cavity (injury due to self-induced vomiting)
- esophageal inflammation (acid from vomiting irritates the esophagus)
- esophageal tears and ruptures (force from vomiting may cause the tears in the esophagus)
- dental erosion (acid from vomiting erodes the dental enamel)
- cardiac arrest
- dehydration
- electrolyte imbalance

- major depression
- suicide

Prevention

Many bulimics do not feel good about themselves and consequently do not take good care of their bodies. They can help prevent the development of bulimia by following the guidelines for self-care below and by seeking help from a therapist or doctor if they feel they are developing the illness:

- Try to resolve areas of conflict.
- Try to achieve a balance of work, social activities, recreation, rest, and exercise.
- Create a support group of good friends.
- Keep a positive outlook on life.
- Stop judging oneself and others.
- Eat well-balanced, nutritious meals.
- Schedule meals regularly, but not too rigidly. Avoid irregular eating habits and avoid fasting.
- Take vitamin and mineral supplements if recommended by a health care provider.
- Avoid using laxatives and diuretics. These can have serious side effects if taken inappropriately.
- Seek professional help to lose weight slowly and to a healthy level.
- Exercise regularly and in moderation.

bunion (hallux valgus) A bunion is an abnormal bony bump that forms on the joint at the base of the big toe. The big toe joint becomes enlarged and the big toe points toward the other toes. The medical term for the deformity where the big toe angles toward the other toes is hallux valgus. People with weak or flat feet and women who wear high heels a lot tend to develop bunions.

Causes

Bunions can result from wearing shoes that do not fit properly or from wearing high-heeled shoes with narrow, pointed toes. When a shoe rubs against the toe joint, it irritates the area and makes it swollen, red, and painful. A tough, callused covering grows over the site. The tendency to have bunions may be inherited. Runners and others who put a lot of stress on their feet may be more vulnerable to developing bunions.

Diagnosis

Patients with bunions have a bony bump at the base of the big toe that can vary in size from rather unnoticeable to extremely large. There is swelling, redness, and soreness of the big toe joint and a thickening of the skin at the base of the big toe. The doctor diagnoses a bunion by examining the affected foot. In some cases there may be a reason to take X rays of the affected joint.

Treatment

Conservative treatment includes trying to relieve pressure on the big toe by wearing roomy, comfortable shoes; wearing a corrective device that forces the big toe back into its proper position and holds it in that place; and placing a pad on the bunion to alleviate the aggravation to the skin when the bunion rubs against shoes.

Athletes with significant bunions may need to take anti-inflammatory medication, such as aspirin or ibuprofen, for pain relief. Custom-made arch supports called orthotics may also help reduce bunion pain.

In cases where the bunion gets worse and causes too much discomfort, the doctor may suggest a surgery called bunionectomy. This type of treatment removes the swollen tissue, straightens the toe by taking out part of the bone, and permanently joins the bones of the affected joint.

For patients who try conservative treatment, there is no complete recovery. A bunion is a permanent problem. It remains unless removed in surgery. But the treatments mentioned above may be enough to alleviate the discomfort so that the patient can live with the bunion. If the patient has surgery, recovery may take two or more months, and sometimes the surgery is not completely effective in eliminating the pain and discomfort.

Prevention

The best way to prevent bunions is to avoid wearing high heels or shoes that are uncomfortable and do not fit well. If the toes become irritated or cramp while wearing certain shoes, that is a sure sign that pressure is being applied to the big toe joint, which makes it vulnerable to developing a bunion. If the athlete has a history of bunions in his or her family, this advice is particularly important, since a predisposition to bunions may be an inherited condition.

burners/stingers   Common among football players, burners and stingers occur when the neck is forced one way and the arm the other way, stretching or pinching the bundle of nerves that run from the back of the neck into the arm. It feels like an electric shock and usually goes away in a few minutes or less.

Causes

Burners and stingers can occur in all contact sports, such as hockey, wrestling, and football, and are usually the result of a hit to the top part of the shoulder. They may also come about when carrying a backpack that is too heavy or cradling a phone under the neck while reaching for something. Any forced twisting of the head and neck that stretches this bundle of nerves, known as the brachial plexus, is capable of producing burners and stingers.

Diagnosis

The patient will feel an acute pain or shocking sensation that runs from the shoulder down into the arm and fingers. Numbness or weakness in the arm may follow the pain, which usually lasts just a few minutes before it is completely gone.

Treatment

Normally this injury resolves itself on its own, but if the patient continues to experience the pain and sensation of burners and stingers, he or she should see a doctor to rule out the possibility of a slipped disk or injury to the spinal cord. If both arms are affected by the injury, there is neck pain that continues beyond a few minutes, or a loss of consciousness, the patient should immediately see a doctor.

Return to the sport should happen when all the pain has subsided and there is normal strength in the neck and arm. If the patient returns too quickly to the sport, further injury to the neck could occur.

Prevention

Once the patient has experienced this injury, it is extremely important to avoid recurrent stingers because subsequent injuries tend to be increasingly severe and can eventually do permanent damage to the nerve. In contact sports, players should always make sure to use proper techniques, such as in tackling, and avoid awkward head and neck positions in order to prevent injuring the neck. Warm-up and strengthening exercises for the neck, back, and shoulders will also help. Football and hockey players, especially, should use protective equipment such as shoulder pads and neck rolls that are in good condition and properly fitted.

bursitis   There are bursa sacs located all over the body, anywhere that there is a major prominence in a bone. The purpose of the bursa is to provide a smooth surface that allows the skin to slide over these bony prominences. If there is trauma to a bursa sac, either through injury or through repeated contact with a hard surface, the bursa may become inflamed, causing pain to the joint where it is located. Since bursitis is an overuse injury, it can potentially affect anyone who incurs repetitive stress to a joint. The knees, elbows, and shoulders, however, are particularly vulnerable to developing bursitis, so athletes who stress the joints in these parts of the body may be at more risk of developing bursitis than are others.

Causes

Anything that causes trauma to a bursa sac, forcing the cells of the bursa to secrete a liquid that fills the sac and causing the joint pain, can bring on bursitis. Javelin throwers, baseball pitchers, and tennis players are just a few of the athletes who are at higher risk of developing bursitis as a result of the type of stress they place on their shoulders and elbows. Others prone to developing bursitis include secretaries, who get bursitis in their elbows, and plumbers who tend to get it in their knees.

Diagnosis

Patients normally experience pain and discomfort, possibly swelling, in the area where the bursa is inflamed. When the tissue of the bursa sac stretches to fill with fluid due to its inflammation, this stretching causes pain in the joint. The doctor will take a complete medical history and do a physical examination that, among other things, will focus on determining just how much fluid is built up in the fluid sac.

Treatment

The basic treatment for bursitis is rest, ice, compression, and elevation (RICE) to combat the swelling. Anti-inflammatories also help to relieve the discomfort and swelling. Once the swelling has been reduced, the patient may be prescribed exercises to strengthen muscles in the problem area, since sometimes muscle weakness is the reason the joint was overused in the first place. In some cases, usually with the elbow, the fluid will build up so much that it will not go away on its own. These are unsightly and quite uncomfortable and will require that a doctor drain the fluid from the bursa sac in order for the swelling to go down. Bursitis usually heals completely with proper treatment, although in some cases the bursa can become infected. Proper medical attention is necessary in order to treat the infection.

Prevention

Protection of the joints is the best way to prevent bursitis. Using the appropriate equipment, such as knee pads and shoulder pads, and warming up the joints and muscles adequately before participating in strenuous activity will help to avoid trauma or overuse injuries that lead to bursitis.

caffeine and athletic performance Many people, not just athletes, like caffeine because it makes them feel alert, energetic, happier, and more productive. If taken in moderation, caffeine can provide some benefits, but in order to enhance athletic performance, athletes normally have to take very high doses of caffeine, which like any other drug has numerous negative side effects. Athletes who want to use caffeine to help them perform in training or in competition must be aware that the drug can cause an array of unwanted side effects and that it is banned at certain levels in the urine. The International Olympic Committee (IOC) allows up to 12 mcg/ml of urine tested, which means that even a couple of high-powered espresso drinks could potentially put in athlete over the legal limit of caffeine allowed in competition.

How It Works

Caffeine is a stimulant, which means that it works by reviving the central nervous system. Historically, researchers thought that caffeine also has endurance-enhancing properties, encouraging the body to burn its stores of fat while preserving the glycogen stored in the muscles, but recent research has failed to find any support for this theory. It is now generally assumed that any endurance benefits of taking caffeine are a result of its effects as a stimulant.

Side Effects

At high dosages, caffeine can cause sleeplessness, anxiety, headache, a wired or jittery feeling, nausea, and muscle tremors. In addition, too much caffeine can make the body produce more urine, which has a dehydrating effect. For athletes performing in hot weather, this could have serious negative consequences.

Sources

Caffeine occurs naturally in some foods, such as coffee, tea, and chocolate, and can also be found in numerous pain medications, including Anacin and Excedrin. NO DOZ, an over-the-counter drug designed to prevent sleep, contains significant amounts of caffeine.

Be Aware

- Many soft drinks, but especially Coke, contain substantial amounts of caffeine.
- Caffeine is among a long list of stimulants that are banned at certain levels in the urine.
- Caffeine can cause urination, which can lead to dehydration.

calf injuries Calf muscle injuries can happen to runners, walkers, and all sorts of ballplayers, but they are painfully common in racket sports that require a lot of quick starts and stops. If calf muscles are too tight, they cannot take the sudden stress, so they strain, they pop, and they can end up causing real grief. Some women are especially vulnerable, because years of wearing high heels leave them with short, contracted calf muscles.

Calf muscle injuries are almost always tears of the juncture between the medial half of the calf muscle (the inner part, technically called the gastrocnemius) and the Achilles tendon.

Causes

In most cases, the muscle-tendon junction tear is caused by poor calf muscle flexibility. For this reason, it is most common to see this injury in the so-called weekend warrior, who is only intermittently active. These athletes often have maintained a fair amount of the muscle mass in their calf without maintaining adequate flexibility. This relatively larger muscle, compared with a totally inactive person, without corresponding flexibility is thus more susceptible to a partial or complete tear.

The tear often occurs as the result of an acute, forceful push-off with the foot, and has been coined "tennis leg" because of its prevalence in this sport. Although it does occur commonly in sports, it can occur in any activity, such as climbing a set of stairs.

Other contributing factors to this injury include unstretched muscles and prior injury that may have left fibrotic scar tissue. Such tissue absorbs force differently from normal tissue and is more likely to tear.

Diagnosis

The major symptom of a tear in the calf muscle is a sudden pain in the calf, accompanied by a popping noise one can actually hear. Sometimes a sensation like someone smacking the leg in the middle of the calf muscle is felt.

A complete history will often include a description of the moment the muscle was torn. Because the pain can be acute, athletes often know just when it happens and will recount the audible pop when the calf muscle tears. In addition, the patient will often complain of pain in the calf that radiates to the knee or the ankle. When the doctor performs range-of-motion exercise on the ankle, there is usually pain. Swelling of the leg and a change of color or bruising usually accompany this injury.

The physical exam will normally reveal swelling of the calf, sometimes spreading down to the ankle and foot. If the doctor is examining the patient after the swelling has resolved, the calf muscle will usually appear abnormal.

The entire calf is tender to the touch, but the point of the tear is extremely painful. The doctor will want to examine the Achilles tendon to rule out any tears there since the symptoms can be quite similar.

The doctor may exercise the ankle to test for pain with certain movements. This helps to ensure a proper diagnosis.

A torn calf muscle can normally be diagnosed without laboratory or imaging studies. Sometimes a doctor will order an X ray to rule out the possibility of an avulsion fracture in cases where the patient heard an audible pop with the injury.

Treatment

Initial treatment following a torn calf muscle is rest, ice, compression, elevation, and early weight-bearing as tolerated without pain. It is important to support the leg at all times in order to prevent further swelling. Crutches will help, as will a heel lift to take some of the strain off the calf. The patient should practice active foot and ankle range-of-motion exercises as long as there is no pain.

Doctors normally prescribe analgesics to manage the pain initially. It is important to be cautious about using nonsteroidal anti-inflammatory drugs immediately following the injury since they can increase bleeding and make the patient vulnerable to the development of hematomas.

Studies have also shown that bracing the ankle and foot in a position that allows for the greatest amount of flex in the calf without pain will help the muscle to heal better and faster.

The patient should perform exercises to maintain flexibility initially, increasing resistance as the pain in the calf resolves. This exercise is extremely important in avoiding complications as the muscle heals. Scar tissue formation can interfere with proper movement of the muscle and cause chronic pain or dysfunction.

In addition to exercise, ultrasound and massage may be useful for the muscles. The patient should begin walking with crutches as soon as possible, allowing the sole of the foot to have as much contact with the ground as possible. Strengthening and stretching of the injured leg should continue for several months.

The athlete is ready to return to sports when the pain is completely gone and there is full range of motion in the calf, ankle, and foot. Strength tests should be done to ensure that the athlete has regained at least 90 percent of the uninjured side's strength on the injured leg, taking leg dominance into account.

Prevention

The good news is that no matter what one's gender or sport, most calf muscle injuries are avoidable, if the basics of prevention are understood. Regular physical activity with maintenance of flexibility will help to reduce your chances of sustaining such injury. Appropriate stretching and warm-up techniques will also help in preventing these injuries since tight muscles tear more easily.

carbohydrate loading   Carbohydrate loading is a dietary technique used to increase performance in endurance athletes. Most often associated with long-distance runners who consume a large plate of pasta the night before a race, carbohydrate loading is actually a bit more involved than this image indicates.

How It Works

There are two types of carbohydrates—complex carbohydrates, also known as starches, and simple carbohydrates. Complex carbohydrates include grains, vegetables, and legumes, which are beans and peas. Simple carbohydrates are sugars and sweets, including fruit and dairy products.

Carbohydrates are the main fuel for muscles. When participating in an endurance activity, such as long-distance running, the body depends upon its stored carbohydrates, called glycogen, to keep it going. Muscles can store only small amounts of glycogen, and they can't borrow glycogen from other areas of the body where it is stored, so carbohydrate loading is designed to force the muscles to store more glycogen than they normally would so that they do not run out during the endurance activity. In addition, the extra carbohydrates will help the body to efficiently use its fat stores, which are its other source of fuel.

Carbohydrate loading is a two-step process. First, cut back on exercise just before a high-endurance event. Normally, the athlete would cut the amount of exercise in half during the week prior to the event. This will keep from using up the muscles' glycogen stores. It is important, however, not to stop exercising abruptly. Taper the exercise, cutting back a little more each day so as to rest completely for a day or two prior to the event.

The next step is to eat significantly more carbohydrates than normal for a short period of time prior to the event, so that the muscles are filled with excess glycogen that can be used as fuel during the endurance event. During the week prior to the event, consume about 70 percent of calories in carbohydrates. This does not mean to overeat; it is necessary to cut back on high-fat foods to compensate for the increase in carbohydrates during this period. Overall, consume about 10 to 15 percent of calories in protein, another 10 to 15 percent in fat, and the rest in carbohydrates. This should mean, roughly, eating about four to five grams of carbohydrates per pound of body weight every day. To carbo load properly, expect to gain two or three pounds in the week prior to the event.

Who Should Carbo Load

Carbohydrate loading is not for everyone. It is useful in endurance activities, those that require sustained hard effort for at least 60 to 90 minutes. Long-distance runners and swimmers, triathletes, and soccer players are among the athletes who might find carbohydrate loading helpful. Activities that last for shorter periods of times or are performed strictly on a recreational basis do not require this kind of preparation.

Side Effects

Weight gain, usually due to water retention, can result from carbo loading. In addition, if anyone who consumes high-fiber foods, such as beans, bran, and broccoli, might experience gassy cramps, bloating, and loose stools, so limit these foods in the days just prior to the event to avoid any discomfort during the event.

Be Aware

Carbo loading works best for those who have been on a carbohydrate-rich diet throughout training, because during that time the body learns to more effectively use carbohydrates. A daily diet containing about three grams of carbohydrates for every pound of weight should be sufficient. Good sources of carbohydrates are bread, pasta, vegetables, fruits, and cereals.

For those who have carbo loaded properly, expect to put on two to four pounds that week. Much of this weight is extra water because carbohydrates help the body store more water, but some may be the result of increased calorie intake.

carpal tunnel syndrome   The finger tendons pass through the wrist in a narrow, tunnel-like enclosure.

With chronic overuse or excessive twisting of the wrist, fluid builds up in the sheaths of the tendons, causing the tendons to become inflamed and swollen. In addition, the carpal ligament has a tendency to become thickened from overuse. Both of these conditions narrow the tunnel and pinch the main nerve that passes through the tunnel to the fingers. The result is the painful wrist condition known as carpal tunnel syndrome, named after the carpal ligament that goes across the top of this tunnel. The pain extends up into the forearm and down into the hand, and there may be numbness, tingling, and even loss of strength in the middle and ring fingers.

Also called repetitive motion injury, carpal tunnel syndrome is considered an occupational disease and occurs quite often in office workers who spend many hours typing on a keyboard, as well as in musicians, textile workers, meat cutters, and many other professions. Carpal tunnel syndrome can also be caused by certain athletic activities as well, especially sports that require gripping and swinging of a bat, club, or racket, such as baseball, golf, and tennis.

Causes

Most cases of carpal tunnel syndrome have no specific cause, although many factors may contribute to the development of the condition. Frequent, repetitive small movements of the hands, such as gripping a racket or grasping a ball, may help bring on carpal tunnel syndrome. WRIST INJURIES, such as sprains, strains, fractures, dislocations, and swelling that creates pressure on the median nerve may also make the wrist more vulnerable to developing this condition. Swelling can develop from many different conditions, such as arthritis, diabetes, hypothyroidism, and even pregnancy.

Diagnosis

Athletes with carpal tunnel syndrome will usually complain of pain, numbness, or tingling in the hand and wrist, especially in the thumb and index and middle fingers. Sometimes pain also radiates up into the forearm. The pain usually gets worse with use of the hand, such as when gripping an object or typing on a keyboard. There is also increased pain at night with carpal tunnel syndrome. A weak grip and a tendency to drop objects held in the hand are associated with carpal tunnel syndrome. Sensitivity to cold in the affected hand and muscle deterioration, especially in the thumb, are other symptoms of carpal tunnel syndrome.

In an examination, the doctor will take a medical history that focuses on the patient's use of his or her hands and the specific history of the symptoms. In the physical examination, the doctor will check for difficulty in making a fist, a burning or tingling sensation in the fingers, and a swollen feeling in the fingers. He or she may tap the inside middle of the wrist over the median nerve, which may cause pain or a sensation similar to an electric shock. The doctor may also want to test the response of nerves and muscles using electrical stimulation.

Treatment

Specific treatment depends upon the age, overall health, and medical history of the patient. Other factors that help determine treatment include the extent of the disease, the patient's tolerance for specific medications, procedures, or therapies, expectations for the course of the disease, and the patient's opinion or preference.

Treatment may include splinting of the hand to help prevent wrist movement and decrease the compression of the nerves inside the tunnel; oral or injected anti-inflammatory medications to reduce the swelling; surgery to relieve compression on the nerves in the carpal tunnel; and changing position of a computer keyboard, or making other ergonomic changes.

If surgery is recommended, it is normally performed in an outpatient setting under local or general anesthesia. The surgeon will make an incision in the wrist area, and the tissue that is pressing on the nerves will then be cut in order to decrease the pressure.

After the surgery, the wrist may be immobilized in a large dressing and wrist brace to help stabilize the area. The splint is usually worn continuously for the first two weeks after the surgery. Following this period, it is usually worn intermittently for the next month or so. There is a moderate degree of pain in the hand after the surgery, which is usually controlled with pain medications taken orally. The surgeon may also instruct that the affected hand be kept elevated during sleep.

The length of recovery varies for each individual. If the nerve has been compressed for a long period of time, recovery may take longer. Movement of the fingers and wrists are encouraged a few days following surgery to help prevent stiffness.

For patients who receive conservative treatment for carpal tunnel syndrome, it is helpful to take preventive measures so that the condition does not return. Elevating the arm with pillows when lying down is helpful. It is also advisable to avoid activities that overuse the hand and to find a different way to use the hand by using another tool or by trying to use the other hand. Patients should also avoid activities that require repetitive bending of the wrist.

The time it takes to heal will depend on how severe the damage was. Patients may return to their normal activities when they can painlessly grip objects like a tennis racket, bat, golf club, or bicycle handlebars. In sports such as gymnastics, it is important to be able to bear weight on the wrist without pain. There must also be a full range of motion and strength in the wrist.

Prevention

Athletes who perform repetitive work with their hands should make sure that the hands and wrists are comfortable when being used. It is important to take regular breaks from the repetitive motion and to avoid resting the wrists on hard or ridged surfaces for prolonged periods. In some cases, the cause is not known and carpal tunnel syndrome cannot be prevented.

cervical discogenic pain syndrome Cervical discogenic pain results from cervical intervertebral disk disease, which accounts for 36 percent of all spinal intervertebral disk disease. Lumbar disk disease is the most common spinal intervertebral disk disease, occurring in 62 percent of all cases. The most common sports injuries occurring to the cervical spine take place in soccer, football, wrestling, ice hockey, diving, and rugby. Trampoline jumping is also responsible for a fair number of injuries to the cervical spine. These injuries can include fractures, dislocation, slipped disks, disk degeneration, and ligament sprains. Although the incidence of

severe spinal injuries used to be high, better prevention strategies, such as education about the dangers of high-risk contact and about certain types of impact on the neck, as well as the improved shock absorption of contact surfaces have helped to reduce severe spinal cord injuries in contact sports.

Causes

Cervical intervertebral disk disease results from the degenerative changes that appear in the lower cervical spine as a result of injury and age. Discogenic pain syndrome develops when this degeneration occurs and the patient further stresses the spine through poor posture, sudden unexpected movements, or some other activity. Many times, the patient will develop pain even in the absence of these activities.

Diagnosis

It is crucial to obtain an accurate history of the patient when neck pain is a symptom. The following are warning signs of potentially serious spinal conditions that may interfere with treatment. The patient should be carefully assessed in the initial diagnosis for any presence of these warning signs:

- cancer/malignancy
- infection
- trauma with possible underlying fracture
- osteoporosis with possible underlying fracture
- conditions associated with spine instability, such as rheumatoid arthritis or Down syndrome
- significant or progressive neurological deficit, such as profound muscle weakness and/or reflex and loss, bowel and/or bladder incontinence or retention
- vertebral basilar artery insufficiency
- pregnancy

The doctor will need to obtain an accurate and specific description of the pain, including location, onset, duration, frequency, description, distribution, and aggravating and relieving factors. Cervical discogenic pain may be localized pain, referred pain, or radicular pain. It usually is worse in positions that involve prolonged sitting, especially in sitting positions with protruded head posture or prolonged flexing of the neck. Bending positions also provoke cervicogenic pain. Frequent changes of position provide relief. However, in cases of severe acute pain, a still position may be most comfortable. When the patient experiences worse pain immediately after waking, it is usually an indication that he or she is using an unsuitable pillow or inappropriate posture while sleeping.

The physical examination will include assessment for neurological deficits, including loss of balance, altered gait, weakness, and decreased sensation in the arms and hands, among other possible symptoms.

MAGNETIC RESONANCE IMAGING (MRI) is used most often in patients with suspected degenerative discogenic disease because it offers excellent soft tissue visualization, as well as information regarding the water content of the discs. In addition, cervical discography is essential when surgery is contemplated. The cervical discography allows the differentiation of symptomatic and nonsymptomatic discs.

Treatment

PHYSICAL THERAPY is the primary means of conservative treatment for cervical discogenic pain syndrome. It should include educating the patient about proper posture, proper body mechanics, and implementing a specific exercise program that uses patterns of movements and positions that decrease symptoms and help improve the range of motion. Treatment also may include use of anti-inflammatory medication, partial rest, and a short course of steroids on a tapering dose. Sometimes patients find the use of positive imaging techniques helpful in managing the pain during physical therapy.

Surgery is commonly recommended when there is persistent pain, motor weakness, progressive neurological deficits, or evidence of cord compression and no response to conservative treatment.

Initial treatment is aimed at eliminating the pain, normalizing the mechanics of the spine, and improving the muscular control of the spine. The goal is to achieve pain-free full range of motion and to strengthen the muscles to help prevent further injury and pain. The patient's sport-specific activities should be carefully reviewed to ensure that proper techniques are being used.

Prevention

Prevention of injuries to the cervical spine is best accomplished through use of proper body posture and sport techniques, appropriate conditioning, and use of safety measures, including the proper protective equipment for any sport and following the rules.

cervical radiculopathy   The nerves that control the shoulder, arm, and hand begin in the neck, within the spinal cord. If the roots of these nerves become inflamed or compressed, due to some sort of irritation or pinching, it is called cervical radiculopathy, and it results in pain from the neck down to the shoulder, arm, and hand. Although it is quite often associated with heavy manual labor, since those who routinely lift more than 25 pounds or operate heavy, vibrating equipment are at a greater risk of developing the injury, cervical radiculopathy is seen in athletes as well, under a variety of conditions.

Causes

A slipped disk and arthritic spurs in the neck are the most common causes of cervical radiculopathy. Injuries to the neck can also cause the disorder to develop, as can a spinal fracture which is normally indicated if there is persistent pain and or weakness in the arm following a neck injury.

Athletes can injure the nerve root through repetitive motions that involve extending the neck, lateral bending of the neck, or just rotating the neck, as in swimming. In athletes who already have some formation of arthritic spurs, the repetitive neck motion involved in swimming or tennis, for example, can aggravate the nerve further and result in cervical radiculopathy.

Diagnosis

If the patient describes pain in the neck that moves toward the shoulder, arm, or hand, cervical radiculopathy is definitely a possible diagnosis. The discomfort can range from a dull ache to severe burning pain, and the pain can radiate to the shoulder initially and then along the upper or lower arm and into the hand, depending on the nerve root that is involved. There may also be weakness in the arm. Occasionally, a patient will experience weakness without pain.

The doctor will take a detailed history of the patient and perform tests, including an X ray, to evaluate the bones. If the symptoms are severe, the doctor may also order an MAGNETIC RESONANCE IMAGING (MRI) scan in order to examine the nerves and disks in the neck.

For the patient's history, the doctor will want to determine the primary symptoms. It is helpful to know not just about the pain but also about any numbness and weakness that may be present. The doctor may test the patient's range of motion in the neck to determine which motions cause the symptoms to increase. Any previous experience of neck pain, and an exact description of when and how the current pain began, are important for diagnosis. If there was a prior injury, the doctor will want to know how it was treated. The doctor will also want to obtain information on the patient's occupation and sports participation history in order to understand any repetitive movements the neck may have been subjected to.

The physical examination will include observing the head and neck posture of the patient. Usually, the patient will tilt the head away from the side of the injury and hold the neck in a stiff position. The patient's range of motion is reduced, especially in extension, rotation, and bending to either side. Tenderness along the nerve roots and the muscles where the symptoms are experienced is common. There may even be spasms of these muscles. It is important that the doctor manually test the muscles for any subtle weakness, as well as for differences in reflex. The exact location of weakness will help the doctor diagnose which nerves are in trouble. Finally, a Spurling test will be performed. This involves extending the neck and rotating the head, then applying downward pressure on the head to see where the pain occurs. These tests are considered very specific in diagnosing acute radiculopathy.

X rays are always ordered to rule out fractures. Historically, COMPUTERIZED AXIAL TOMOGRAPHY (CAT) SCANS were often used as well, but the MRI is much more accurate in revealing soft tissue injuries, so it has largely replaced the CAT scan in diagnosing cervical spine injuries. The MRI shows the entire spinal cord and the nerve roots, as well as the skeleton. Finally, electrodiagnostic studies are important in identifying abnormalities of the nerve root and in ruling out other neurological causes for the athlete's complaints. Electromyography has been quite effective in diagnosing radiculopathy.

Treatment

Treatment normally begins with a conservative approach of rest, icing the injury, taking anti-inflammatory medication, and reducing the stress on the nerve roots by avoiding positions that increase symptoms. Sometimes a collar may be worn to help support the neck and increase the patient's comfort level. A cervical pillow at night keeps the neck in a neutral position and limits head positions that can pinch the nerves. If the initial pain is significant, the patient may also try electrical stimulation, which may help reduce the associated muscle pain and spasms that are often experienced with cervical radiculopathy. If all these measures fail to reduce the symptoms, cortisone injections may be considered. There has also been some success in managing radiculopathy pain through acupuncture treatments, which is a good alternative for patients who wish to avoid the cortisone injections.

In about 10 percent of patients, there is insufficient progress with the conservative approach, and surgery must be considered. In surgery, the approach is to remove the disk material or arthritic spurs that are compressing the nerves. Sometimes it is also advisable to fuse some of the neck spinal bones as well.

Once pain and inflammation are controlled, the patient's therapy should be progressed to restoration of full range of motion and flexibility of the neck and shoulder muscles. As range of motion and flexibility improve, cervical muscle strengthening should begin. It is important to strengthen the weakened muscles first before beginning activities that use multiple muscles. Various soft tissue mobilization techniques can be helpful. Stretching is best completed after a warm-up activity such as using an exercise bike or brisk walking, which is also helpful in maintain cardiovascular fitness throughout the rehabilitation period.

Athletes should not return to their sports until they are completely free of pain and have complete range of movement. Athletes at risk of reinjuring the neck, such as linebackers in football, should be fitted for a neck roll.

Prevention

Maintaining excellent strength, flexibility, and balance around the neck and shoulder may help prevent some forms of cervical radiculopathy.

Using good technique can prevent some injuries. Swimmers should take care to turn the body properly when breathing, and football players should use proper head positioning when tackling. Exercises that strengthen the neck and shoulder muscles may also be beneficial in preventing cervical radiculopathy.

clavicle injuries The clavicle is an S-shaped bone that connects the shoulder girdle to the trunk. It is a rigid structure that maintains the shoulder in a functional position in relationship to the skeleton and allows varied hand positions in sports. In addition to its structural function, the clavicle protects major underlying neurovascular structures. As a result, clavicle injuries can result in significant neurovascular injuries, although the incidence of this is quite rare.

The most common injuries to the clavicle and its associated joints are acromioclavicular (AC) and sternoclavicular (SC) dislocations, clavicle fractures, and osteolysis and degeneration of the clavicle. Clavicle fractures and dislocations occur quite commonly in a variety of sports, but especially those that involve heavy contact or use of a stick in play, such as football, ice hockey, and lacrosse.

Causes

Any significant trauma to the shoulder can result in an injury of the clavicle. Direct injuries associated with contact sports usually involve a direct blow to the clavicle, such as a hockey stick hitting the shoulder, which results in a fracture. Certain types of blows may cause shoulder separation or AC joint injury.

A fall onto an outstretched arm or the side of the shoulder is termed an indirect injury and may also cause a fracture. Falling on certain parts of the shoulder may cause injury to either the AC or SC joints or to the clavicle as well.

Diagnosis

Most injuries to the clavicle are readily visible. The clavicle lies just under the skin, and the deformity is usually apparent. In addition, patients can usually identity the specific location of the pain, and they hold the injured shoulder and arm close to the body, trying to support the arm.

Although the injury may be evident, the doctor will need to take a thorough history of the patient and conduct a good physical examination to rule out any associated injuries. Common injuries seen in conjunction with clavicle injuries include rib and other fractures, neck injuries, and vascular injuries.

The physical exam should begin with both the patients' shoulders exposed. Palpation can reveal tenderness at the AC or SC joints or the fracture site. Although pain will restrict the patient's active range of motion, there should be full passive range of motion unless there is an additional injury, such as shoulder dislocation or a muscle tear. Finally, the shoulder examination should include assessing the athlete's neurovascular status and cervical spine.

X rays are used to confirm the diagnosis. They will usually reveal any fracture in the clavicle complex as well as any trouble with the AC joint. They are not, however, very helpful in assessing SC joint injuries. A COMPUTERIZED AXIAL TOMOGRAPHY (CAT) SCAN is usually necessary to confirm diagnosis of an SC joint injury.

Treatment

Most clavicle injuries can be treated symptomatically and conservatively with rest, ice, anti-inflammatory medication, and a sling.

Clavicle fractures are classified by the location of the fracture and by the degree and angle of displacement. Those that do not require any realignment may usually be treated with a sling. Fractures where there is a greater degree of displacement require a figure 8 bandage to bring the fractured bones into better opposition.

Surgery is recommended in a number of fracture situations. These include fractures with severe displacement, those with neurovascular compromise, and those in patients who have sustained numerous fractures, among others. Complications of acute surgical treatment have been reported to be up to 20 percent and include infection, failure of fixation, prominent scarring, and nonunion of the fractures bones.

Rehabilitation is about the same regardless of the type of treatment the patient receives. Once the fracture pain has subsided and there is full range of movement without pain, the patient should perform strengthening exercises. The patient may return to noncontact sports only after the fracture is completely healed, there is full range of motion, and the patient has regained most of his or her strength in the shoulder. Contact sports should not be resumed for a minimum of six months, since it takes this long for the fracture union to become solid. Athletes who develop a prominent callus over the fracture site, may use a donut pad to prevent discomfort.

Prevention

Most of these injuries result from accidents, but use of proper protective gear when playing contact sports and maintenance of strong shoulder muscles will help to prevent injuries to the clavicle and associated joints.

compartment syndrome   A condition of the lower leg that results in excessive swelling or increased pressure in the muscles, compartment syndrome is seen most often in long-distance runners and is commonly misdiagnosed as shin splints or a stress fracture. When the leg swells, pressure builds on the blood vessels and nerve supply of the lower leg and foot, causing pain and sometimes loss of movement or weakness. Compartment syndrome varies in severity, from chronic conditions that are mild to acute conditions that threaten to do permanent damage to the leg.

Causes

The muscles of the lower leg are enclosed inside a fascia or "compartment" that is slightly flexible and allows the muscle to swell somewhat with exercise. Surrounded on three sides by bone, this fascia only allows limited swelling. If the muscles swell beyond the ability of the fascia to expand, pressure may be felt on the nerves and blood vessels. Loss of muscle strength and numbness occur if the

swelling continues to the point that blood flow to and from the muscle is shut off and the nerves are pinched.

Diagnosis

Patients with compartment syndrome normally describe pain toward the outside of the shin that is felt over a greater area than a stress fracture. Fascial hernias, tiny pouches that appear from under the skin on the shin, indicate compartment syndrome and help the doctor to distinguish between shin splints or stress fracture and compartment syndrome as the cause of pain.

The doctor will take a history of the patient's exercise and try to rule out the possibility of these other injuries. A physical examination will focus on detecting fascial hernias and testing for loss of muscle strength and numbness. If there is a history of an overuse injury, a muscle tear that causes bleeding, or some sort of impact trauma to the lower leg, the doctor may suspect acute compartment syndrome, which results in a serious disruption of blood flow that may lead to tissue death if not treated quickly once the symptoms appear.

Treatment

Treatment is conservative with chronic compartment syndrome. The patient should ice the injured leg but avoid wrapping the ice around the shin. Since there is already a problem with compression, it is important to not apply additional pressure to the area. In addition, the leg should be elevated above the level of the heart whenever possible and rested. Anti-inflammatories may be prescribed to help with the pain and swelling. Acute compartment syndrome may also be treated conservatively, depending upon the doctor's examination of tissue damage. If conservative treatment fails to reduce the problem, surgery may be the next option. In surgery for compartment syndrome, the goal is to release the myofascia at the front of the compartment, and sometimes the sides as well, to allow normal blood circulation to occur again.

Prevention

Long-distance runners and those who participate in sports that require a lot of running are at risk for compartment syndrome. Consequently, prevention includes wearing shoes that fit properly and provide ample cushion, running on soft surfaces, and cutting back on training whenever there are symptoms of excessive swelling, muscle weakness, or numbness in the lower leg. Athletes should also use strengthening exercises to address any muscle imbalances that may exist in the leg, and they should stretch to improve flexibility.

complex carbohydrates Carbohydrates is the name given to the large food group made up of sugars, starches, celluloses, and gums that contain carbon, hydrogen, and oxygen in similar proportions. There are two types of carbohydrates—complex carbohydrates and simple carbohydrates. Complex carbohydrates are found in grains, vegetables, and legumes, which are beans and peas. Simple carbohydrates are found in fruits, milk products, and vegetables. Complex carbohydrates are a good source of minerals, vitamins, and fiber. Although simple carbohydrates also contain vitamins and minerals, they are high in sugar and should be eaten in moderation. Simple carbohydrates derived from processed or refined sugars contain virtually no nutritional value. It is recommended that somewhere between 40 to 60 percent of our total calories come from carbohydrates, preferably from complex carbohydrates and naturally occurring sugars rather than from processed or refined sugars.

How They Work
The primary function of carbohydrates is to provide energy for the body, especially the brain and the nervous system. The body breaks down starches and sugars into a substance called glucose, which is used for energy by the body. The muscles store carbohydrates in the form of glycogen, which can be accessed by the body for fuel during exercise and physical work.

Side Effects
Excessive carbohydrates can cause an increase in the total caloric intake, causing obesity. Deficient carbohydrates can cause malnutrition or an excessive intake of fats to make up the calories.

Sources
Complex carbohydrates are found in breads, cereals, starchy vegetables, legumes, rice, and pastas.

Simple carbohydrates naturally occur in fruits, milk and milk products, and vegetables. They are also found in processed and refined sugars such as candy, table sugar, syrups (not including natural syrups such as maple), and carbonated sodas. These refined sugars provide calories but lack vitamins, minerals, and fiber.

Be Aware
It is important to limit intake of simple carbohydrates, especially those found in processed and refined sugars, since these contain calories without providing any significant nutritional benefits.

compulsive exercise Usually thought of as a subtle form of eating disorder, compulsive exercise is a condition that affects athletes who perform extreme amounts of exercise in order to control their weight and to expend excess calories. They tend to justify their behavior by believing that serious athletes can never work out too much. Consequently, many compulsive exercisers suffer from OVERTRAINING SYNDROME. Compulsive exercisers tend to cling rigidly to their regimens, claiming that cutting back on their training would negatively affect their performance. Sometimes they also claim that they gain weight if they fail to complete all their workouts.

Symptoms
Compulsive exercisers often do the following:

- force themselves to exercise even when they do not feel well
- work out at the same hard intensity every time instead of varying the intensity and duration of workouts
- feel very stressed out if they miss even one workout
- miss family obligations in order to exercise
- determine how much they will exercise based on how much they have eaten
- prefer exercise over socializing with friends
- have a hard time relaxing because it does not burn calories
- worry that not exercising for just one day will cause weight gain

Be Aware

As with eating disorders, compulsive exercise is dangerous and counterproductive. Since compulsive exercisers tend to participate in extreme forms of exercise and to eat erratically, the condition can result in numerous health problems, including a serious eating disorder, kidney failure, and heart attack.

Normally, people who exercise compulsively have a hard time seeing their problem. Because exercise is socially acceptable and highly rewarded among many, compulsive exercisers hide behind their illness, maintaining an illusion of good health, even feelings of superiority, when they are actually struggling with their compulsion, using exercise as an unhealthy means of control. It usually takes intervention from a coach or loved one and professional counseling to overcome the condition.

computerized axial tomography (CAT) scan

Also called computerized axial tomography or CT scan, the CAT scan is an imaging technique that uses a computer to organize the information from multiple X ray views to construct cross-sectional, or three-dimensional, images of areas inside the body. For some CAT scans, intravenous contrast material is inserted into the patient's body to enhance the scans and allow for evaluation of vascular structures, masses, and tumors.

CAT scans are often utilized in the trauma setting to evaluate the brain, chest, and abdomen. They can also be used to guide interventional procedures, such as biopsies and insertions of drainage tubes.

How It Works

CAT scan patients relax on a movable bed that slides into a doughnut-shaped scanner. Though this large equipment can be intimidating to patients, the procedure is quite safe and painless. Depending on the study being performed, the patient may need to lie on the stomach, back, or side. If contrast media (dye) is to be administered, an IV will be placed in a small vein of a hand or arm. The patient may initially feel a slight burning sensation within the injected arm, a metallic taste in the mouth, and a warm flushing of the body. These sensations are normal and usually diminish within a few seconds.

Once the patient is inside the scanner, a thin X ray beam rotates around the patient as small detectors measure the amount of X rays that make it through a particular area of the patient's body. Much like standard photographic cameras, movement causes blurred images on the CAT scan. Therefore, the technician operating the scanner and supervising the patient will instruct the patient through an intercom when it is especially important to hold the breath and not move. As the exam takes place, the bed will advance by small intervals through the scanner. Modern "spiral" scanners can perform the examination in one continuous motion of the bed. Generally, complete scans will take only a few minutes, however, contrast-enhanced or higher-resolution scans will add to the scan time. The newest multidetector scanners can image the entire body, head to toe, in less than 30 seconds.

By use of a complex algorithm, a computer analyzes the data to construct a cross-sectional image. These images can be stored, viewed on a monitor, or printed on film. In addition, stacking the individual images can create three-dimensional models of organs.

Risks

Risks associated with CAT scans are very low. CAT scans and other X rays are monitored and regulated to provide the minimum amount of radiation exposure needed to produce the image. They provide low levels of ionizing radiation, which has the potential to cause cancer and heritable defects. The risk associated with any individual scan is small; however, the risk increases as numerous additional studies are performed.

During pregnancy, CAT scans are usually not recommended, due to risk to the exposed fetus, including developmental malformations and childhood cancers. Patients who are or may be pregnant should speak with their health care provider in order to first take a pregnancy test or choose an appropriate alternative imaging modality without risk to the fetus, such as ultrasound.

Most complications with CAT scans arise from allergic reactions to the contrast material that is sometimes given to patients to make certain areas of the body stand out on the scans. A person who is allergic to iodine, such as those who have seafood allergies, may experience nausea, sneezing, vomiting, itching, or hives. When a patient has a history of allergic response to iodine, the doctor may choose to medicate the patient prior to administering the iodine with a short course of immune-suppressing steroids, or an alternative contrast material or imaging technique may be used.

In very rare cases, the contrast dye may cause a severe allergic reaction, called anaphylaxis, which usually creates swelling in the airways. Patients are instructed prior to scans to notify the technician immediately if they experience any difficulty breathing as this may be a sign of a serious allergic response. In the case of such a rare reaction, the CAT scan will be stopped immediately and the patient will be quickly treated with medication and monitored by the doctor.

Diabetic patients and those with kidney disease will require continuous hydration and special monitoring of the kidneys when they receive the contrast dye. Diabetics and real dialysis patients will need to consult with their doctors concerning stopping their medication prior to the scan and the appropriate scheduling of the scan in conjunction with dialysis.

History of the Procedure

The CAT scan was invented in 1972 by British engineer Godfrey Hounsfield of EMI Laboratories in England, and independently by South African–born physicist Allan Cormack of Tufts University, Massachusetts. Hounsfield was later awarded the Nobel Peace Prize and honored with knighthood in England for his contributions to medicine and science.

The original scanners could be used to image only the head. A single slice acquisition took four minutes. In 1976 whole body scanners became available, and by the early 1980s, the technology was being widely used.

The technology has grown substantially in its relatively short history. Scanners are faster, and more anatomy can be scanned in a shorter time. Scanners today can take images in less than half a second. A complete body scan can be acquired in a matter of seconds. The units are comfortable for the patient, and software development has permitted imaging techniques that were not available just a few short years ago.

concussion A concussion is a condition of temporary altered mental status as a result of head trauma. Most mild to moderately severe traumatic injuries of the brain can be classified as a concussion, and they occur at alarming frequency in many sports, but especially in football, hockey, and rugby. Overall, it is estimated that 300,000 sports-related traumatic brain injuries occur each year in the United States. Though not always visible and sometimes seemingly minor, head injury is complex. It can cause physical, cognitive, social, and vocational changes. In many cases recovery becomes a lifelong process of adjustments and accommodations for the individual and the family.

While singular concussion can be mild and have no lasting effect, repeated mild concussions occurring over months or years can result in cumulative neurological and cognitive deficits, and repeated mild concussions occurring within a short period of time, such as a few hours, days, or weeks, can be fatal. This latter situation is called second impact syndrome. Neurologists who treat brain injuries say that once a person suffers a concussion, he or she is as much as four times more likely to sustain a second concussion. In addition, after one concussion occurs, it takes less of an impact to cause injury and more time to recover. Second impact syndrome occurs when a second concussion occurs before complete recovery from a previous concussion. In such cases, brain swelling that occurs with the second concussion causes vascular congestion and increased pressure within the cranium, or skull, which can be difficult or impossible to control.

Causes

A concussion is typically caused by a severe head trauma that causes the brain to move violently within the skull. When this happens, the brain cells all fire at once, as in a seizure, which usually results in loss of consciousness, the length of which may relate to the severity of the concussion. There is usually loss of memory associated with a concussion, with patients being unable to recall events preceding the injury, as well as those immediately after they regain consciousness.

Many different types of impact can cause a concussion. A fall in which the head strikes an object, or a moving object striking the head, can cause concussion. Bleeding into the brain can occur with any type of blow to the head and may or may not cause unconsciousness.

Diagnosis

Symptoms of a concussion include repetitive vomiting, unequal pupils, clear or reddish fluid draining from the nose, mouth, or ears, confused mental state or varying levels of consciousness, seizurelike activity, and the inability to wake up (coma). Vacant stares, slowness in answering questions or following instructions, inability to focus attention, disorientation, slurred or incoherent speech, lack of normal coordination, emotions out of proportion to circumstances, and memory loss are all commonly associated with concussion. If any of these signs are present, especially following a known blow to the head, the patient should be taken immediately to the doctor.

Concussions are diagnosed based on the presence of some or all of these symptoms.

Treatment

An initial "baseline" neurological evaluation by a doctor determines treatment for an uncomplicated concussion. After the evaluation, the patient should be kept quiet. Concussion complicated by bleeding or brain damage must be treated in a hospital. Athletes must exhibit no symptoms, either at rest or with exertion, before returning to play. The period of time in which the athlete must remain symptom-free before returning to play varies depending on the severity of the concussion and is determined by the individual's doctor.

Impairments caused by concussions vary depending on the severity and location of the injury. Although the patient may have experienced only mild injuries, the long-term effects may be profound. Common problems associated with concussion include difficulties with memory, mood, and concentration. Others include significant deficits in organizational and reasoning skills and in learning, cognitive, and executive functions. In addition, changes in memory and organizational skills after a brain injury make it difficult to function in complex environments.

Recovery from a concussion may be inconsistent and thus frustrating to both the patient and family members. Sometimes the patient will improve only to experience a setback or a plateau, during which time no progress occurs, but plateaus are quite often followed by more progress.

Prevention

Attention to safety, including the use of appropriate athletic gear such as bike helmets and seat belts, reduces the risk of head injury. Anyone who has ever experienced a concussion of any severity should give special attention to avoiding a second injury since the risk of long-term damage increases significantly with subsequent injury.

congestive heart failure and exercise Congestive heart failure is a deteriorating illness that often occurs following a heart attack. More than 4 million Americans suffer from the disorder, which is broadly defined as an inability of the heart to pump enough blood to meet the body's metabolic needs. Often times the condition is caused when damaged heart tissue from a heart attack begins to heal, leaving behind scars that can cause stretching, thinning, or enlargement of the heart. This process is called remodeling, and it is associated with eventual heart failure. In the past, doctors thought that exercise might worsen the incidence of remodeling in patients with congestive heart failure, so these patients were often told not to exercise. Studies have now shown, however, that this thinking was incorrect. Regular physical activity improves the condition of the heart and may help prevent or delay the progression of disabling symptoms such as fatigue and breathlessness.

Exercise Intolerance

Exercise intolerance in patients with congestive heart failure is a result of the heart's impaired pumping efficiency, which causes decreased blood flow to the muscles. There is also pulmonary congestion involved, which reduces the amount of oxygen that is available for delivery to the muscles. When the respiratory muscles are weakened, this also impairs breathing. Another condition associated with congestive heart failure further reduces the amount of oxygen available to the muscles.

This is an elevated level of catecholamines, which increases vascular resistance, making it harder for oxygen to be transported to the muscles. Finally, and perhaps most important, the muscle atrophy that often occurs early in the disease contributes greatly to exercise intolerance. When patients first become sick, their decreased level of activity and reduced blood flow lead to atrophied muscles. In addition, the percentage of fast-twitch muscle fibers, in comparison with slow twitch fibers, increases following this. These fast-twitch fibers mean that the muscles produce more lactate with less work, resulting in quicker muscle fatigue.

Benefits of Exercise
with Congestive Heart Failure

Regular exercise can increase exercise tolerance—a major issue for most people with congestive heart failure—decrease fatigue, reduce the risk of arrhythmias, and improve general quality of life. Regular exercise may even reduce the risk of death for patients with congestive heart failure as it does for patients with coronary artery disease. Patients will probably need to start aerobic exercise with interval training and progress slowly as they build endurance. Strength exercises are also useful, but aerobic exercises, such as walking and cycling, will produce the most positive effects.

Be Aware

It is especially important that patients check with their doctor before beginning any exercise program. It is likely that the doctor will request some initial stress testing to assess the patient's beginning tolerance for exercise and determine the target heart rate in the new exercise program.

corneal abrasion   A corneal abrasion is a scratch on the outer layer of the cornea, which is the clear outer layer on the front of the eye. Corneal abrasion injuries are most often extremely painful.

Causes

Corneal abrasions can be caused by a number of different things. In athletics, they commonly occur in sports such as basketball or football when a player gets poked in the eye, or in tennis or racquetball when a player gets hit in the eye with the ball. A corneal abrasion can also occur while play-ing sports from something not directly related to the sport. For example, if running or hiking in the woods, it is possible for the cornea to be scratched by a tree branch or even by one's own fingernail. In addition, improper use of contact lenses can cause corneal abrasions.

Diagnosis

Symptoms of a corneal abrasion may include pain, redness, tearing, the feeling that something is in the eye, a scratchy feeling, sensitivity to light, and blurry vision.

The doctor will take a medical history to learn the nature of all the symptoms and to try to determine how the eye was scratched. The doctor will want to rule out the possibility of disease, so trying to determine the cause of injury is helpful. A physical exam is also necessary so that the doctor can see the severity of the abrasion. The doctor will use a light and special eye drops to look into the eye. The eye drops are painless but will make the vision yellow for a few minutes. This physical exam will also allow the doctor to make sure that there is not an object in the eye that is continuing to scratch the cornea.

Treatment

The first step in treatment is to remove anything foreign from the eye if that has not already occurred. This is done by flushing the eye with water or by using a swab or needle. If a needle is used, the eye will be numbed with a drop of anesthetic first.

Other treatment may include use of antibiotic drops or ointment for several days, as well as use of a medicine that dilates the eyes, helps relieve the pain, and promotes healing. The doctor may want the patient to wear an eye patch that keeps the eyelid shut during the early recovery period. This helps the cornea heal, and it also helps relieve pain. The doctor may also have the patient place a contact lens over the cornea to act as a bandage. The contact helps to speed up healing and reduce eye pain. Until the eye is healed, the doctor will most likely want to check the eye daily.

Corneal abrasions, although quite painful and disruptive, do heal quickly, usually within one or two days. Symptoms that last much longer may indicate a more serious problem. Once the cornea has healed, the patient can usually resume normal sports activities immediately.

Prevention

Corneal abrasions from sports injuries are best prevented by wearing protective eyeglasses, sports goggles, or eye shields that attach to the face mask of helmets. Sunglasses worn in sports that do not require protective eyewear can help to keep small debris from the eyes, especially on windy days. Prevention is also accomplished by proper use and cleaning of contact lenses, since some corneal abrasions occur as a result of wearing lenses for too long or wearing them when they have not been properly cleaned.

cortisone   A substance very similar to a steroid that is produced naturally in the body, cortisone improves the body's ability to reduce pain, heat, redness, and swelling of the joints. A member of a family of medications called corticosteroids, which are strong anti-inflammatory drugs, cortisone is used in the treatment of many conditions. It is most commonly taken in the form of an injection, although it can be taken orally, in a cream, or with an inhaler.

It is important to point out the difference between cortisone and anabolic steroids, since these are often confused. Anabolic steroids are a group of drugs that increase muscle mass and strength but have many negative side effects and are sometimes used illegally by athletes.

How It Works

A cortisone shot is often used to reduce swelling and pain in a bursa, joint, or tendon in a specific area of the body, such as the knee, elbow, or shoulder. Reducing the swelling helps relieve pain and discomfort and can speed up recovery from an injury.

Cortisone may also be used in the treatment of conditions such as rheumatoid arthritis or a severe allergic reaction to something that causes swelling over the entire body.

Cortisone is usually mixed with an anesthetic and then injected into the affected area of the body. The shot may be uncomfortable at first, but the anesthetic usually helps quickly with the discomfort. As with most injections, the area where the shot is administered will often be quite sore once the anesthetic wears off. Icing the site of the injec-tion for 20 to 30 minutes every three to four hours and taking an anti-inflammatory medication will help to ease the discomfort. It normally takes two to three days for the cortisone to begin working in the body so that a reduction in both inflammation and swelling is noticed. The duration of the relief from symptoms varies greatly. Sometimes an injection will permanently relieve the symptoms; in other cases, the relief may last from several weeks to several years. Inflammation caused by overuse, such as tendonitis, will likely return if the patient continues to overuse the injured area. In such cases, the effects of the cortisone shot will be quite limited.

Sources

Cortisone is derived from cow liver.

Side Effects

There are few common side effects associated with cortisone shots, but possible side effects include the following:

- slight discoloration of the skin
- shrinkage of the fatty tissue beneath where the shot was given
- pain
- infection
- weakening of the tendons or tendon rupture
- loss of bone calcification in a bone or joint (osteoporosis or vascular necrosis)
- increase in blood sugar among diabetics
- weakening of the immune system

Most of these side effects are quite uncommon, especially the loss of bone calcification, which would occur only after having many cortisone shots.

Be Aware

A temporary weakening of the immune system is a more common side effect of cortisone injection. Patients should avoid contact with people who have chicken pox or measles if they have never had these illnesses before.

creatine   Creatine monohydrate is a dietary supplement used for increasing muscle mass and improving performance in short-duration, high-intensity exercise. It is popular with many athletes, especially weight lifters, body builders, and others whose sports emphasize strength. Creatine is also an amino acid compound found naturally in the body in the skeletal muscle, heart, brain, testes, retina, and other tissues, and also in red meat. When taken as a supplement, it usually comes in the form of a powder or tablet.

Although there is evidence that oral creatine supplementation enhances performance in repeated short bouts of stationary cycling in a laboratory setting, the data on using creatine supplements for single athletic efforts of any kind, as opposed to repeated bursts of effort, do not support any beneficial effect. In addition, there is evidence that creatine supplementation may actually hinder runners and swimmers because of the weight gain it causes due to water retention. The argument can be made that athletes in sports such as football, which involves repeated bursts of maximal exercise, may gain a positive effect from creatine supplementation and may actually benefit from this weight gain.

There are negative side effects associated with creatine use and the effect of creatine use on the various organs of the body that already make creatine has not been sufficiently studied.

How It Works

When muscles contract, they use a substance called adenosine triphosphate (ATP), which is broken down into adenosine diphosphate (ADP). Creatine helps turn ADP back into ATP for the working muscles, giving them a greater energy source for short bursts of exercise such as sprinting. The creatine also enhances recovery from these efforts, making it especially useful for athletes who perform repeated bursts of exercise at maximal effort.

Studies show that creatine increases the amount of water stored in muscle and increases muscle volume, making athletes bigger though not necessarily more skillful or agile. Most athletes taking creatine will gain between two and 10 pounds over four to 10 weeks.

Supplementation with creatine must begin with a loading phase, which includes eating lots of carbohydrates because this will aid the body in bringing the creatine into the muscles and reducing excretion of the creatine through the urine. Creatine loading should be done in the preseason or several weeks before an important athletic event. Most sports medicine experts believe that athletes should not take creatine for longer than two months, since there have been no indications of a benefit derived from taking it for longer periods. Athletes often take creatine in cycles, going on it for a couple of months and then off for a couple of months. It is important to remember that there have been no studies about the side effects of long-term use, so no one knows how long it is safe to take it.

Side Effects

In the United States, creatine is considered a dietary supplement. Therefore, in accordance with the Dietary Supplement Health and Education Act of 1994, claims regarding performance and safety do not need to be substantiated by the U.S. Food and Drug Administration (FDA).

Reported side effects of short-term use are minimal. Commonly reported side effects include muscle cramping, which may be due to dehydration. To avoid dehydration and possible muscle cramping, drink lots of fluids while taking creatine.

Gastrointestinal disturbances including diarrhea and stomach pain have also been reported. Since the average diet includes one to two grams of creatine daily, it may be reasonable to assume that the loading dose, which is often 20 grams daily for five days, is excessive for some people's digestive systems.

Renal dysfunction has been reported in several cases, and there is concern about the effects of creatine on the kidneys, but this has not been adequately studied, and some health care providers believe creatine supplementation could lead to kidney disease in some athletes. People with renal disease or the potential for renal dysfunction (diabetics, for example) should not use creatine. In addition, effects on the heart, brain, reproductive organs, and other organs have yet to be determined. Comprehensive studies with larger samples and crossover design are needed.

Unstudied potential side effects could involve the heart, brain, and testicles. It is unknown what effect creatine supplementation has on the creatine concentration in the heart, brain, and reproductive organs. It is known that creatine supplementation results in the suppression of creatine synthesis in the liver, but the long-term effects of this have not been studied.

Sources
Creatine can be found in powder or tablet form at most health food and vitamin stores.

Be Aware
- The long-terms risks of using creatine are not known.
- If patients decide to take oral creatine, which is not banned by the International Olympic Committee or other sports regulatory organizations, physicians need to provide guidance for proper dosing as well as education about potential harmful effects.
- Three sports neurologists have proposed that creatine and ephedrine use may be responsible for the marked increase in heatstroke deaths among football players since 1995. They note that creatine has been shown to shift body water into muscle cells, increasing the risk of heatstroke.
- There are two common misconceptions about creatine's potential benefits.
  - The first is a gross generalization that creatine supplementation is beneficial for all types of "sprinting," including running, swimming, and cycling. The fact is, the literature has shown reasonable support for benefits only in repeated bouts of stationary cycling sprints in a laboratory setting.
  - The second common misconception is that creatine supplementation is beneficial in a single timed event, such as a single sprint. The fact is that, even with stationary cycling, creatine has not been shown to enhance single-event performance. Again, the strongest support for the potential benefits of creatine supplementation is in *repeated* maximal bursts of activity.

cryotherapy   The use of cryotherapy, or the application of cold for the treatment of injury or disease, is widespread in sports medicine today. It is used for ailments such as bruises, chronic joint and soft tissue inflammation, and numerous acute sports injuries. It is most effective in the following situations: when motion is limited by pain; during acute stages of inflammation; before range-of-motion exercises are begun; and following physical activity and rehabilitation.

Cryotherapy minimizes swelling and bleeding and is also used to reduce the recovery time as part of the rehabilitation program both after acute injuries and in the treatment of chronic injuries. Cryotherapy has also been shown to reduce pain effectively in the postoperative period following reconstructive surgery of the joints. Both superficial and deep temperature changes depend on the method of application, the initial temperature of the injured area, and duration of the application. Generally speaking, the therapeutic temperature range for cold therapy is from 32°F to 65°F.

How It Works
Cold reduces the flow of blood to the treatment area and acts as a painkiller because it reduces nerve-conduction velocity. Reduced local tissue metabolism and decreased blood supply offer relief from muscle spasm and pain. Patients receiving cryotherapy usually experience four natural stages of sensation—discomfort caused by the cold, stinging, burning or aching, and finally numbness.

Cold therapy appears to be effective and harmless. Few complications or side effects after the use of cold therapy are reported. Prolonged application at very low temperatures should, however, be avoided as this may cause serious side effects, such as frostbite and nerve injuries.

Cryotherapy is most effective in acute stages of the healing process immediately following injury when cooling of the injured tissue is the main goal. Cryotherapy most often involves the application of ice bags or frozen gel packs applied to the injured area.

History of the Procedure
Cold drinks and baths and natural ice and snow were used before the introduction of artificial ice in 1755 as the first forms of cold therapy. While ice is still commonly used today, instant chemical and freezable gel packs offer convenience and ease of use.

dehydration and replacement fluids Dehydration is the loss of water and important blood salts such as potassium and sodium, a condition that makes it impossible for the body to function at an optimal level. The body's vital organs, such as the kidneys, brain, and heart, cannot function without a certain amount of water and salt. Fluid replacement is probably the most important nutritional concern for athletes. Approximately 60 percent of body weight is water. With exercise, fluid is lost through the skin as sweat and through the lungs with breathing. If this fluid is not replaced at regular intervals during exercise, the athlete can become dehydrated. When dehydrated, the athlete has a smaller volume of blood circulating through the body. Consequently, the amount of blood the heart pumps with each beat decreases and exercising muscles do not receive enough oxygen from the blood. Soon exhaustion sets in, and athletic performance suffers. A loss of just 2 percent of an athlete's body weight during competition can adversely affect performance. Thus, proper fluid replacement is the key to successfully competing in the heat as well as for preventing dehydration and reducing the risk of heat injury during training and competition.

Causes
Dehydration can be caused by inadequate intake of fluids, which is often the case with athletes, or by fluid loss as a result of vomiting, diarrhea, excessive urination, excessive sweating or fever, or it can be caused by a combination of both.

Because of their smaller body weights and higher turnover rates for water and electrolytes, infants and children are more susceptible to dehydration than adults. In infants and children, the most common cause of dehydration is gastroen-teritis, which causes vomiting and diarrhea. Often, there is an accompanying fever, so that fluid loss occurs as a result of excess sweating as well.

Diagnosis
Dehydration is classified as mild, moderate, or severe based on the percentage of body weight lost during the acute illness. The following definitions show a range to represent difference depending on age.

- Mild dehydration is a loss of between 3 and 5 percent of body weight.
- Moderate dehydration is a loss of between 6 and 10 percent of body weight.
- Severe dehydration is a loss of more than 9 to 15 percent of body weight.

Symptoms of the three stages of dehydration are as follows:

- Mild dehydration is characterized by thirst, dry lips, and slightly dry mouth membranes.
- Moderate dehydration is characterized by very dry mouth membranes, sunken eyes, sunken fontanelle (the soft spot on an infant's head), and skin that is not resilient when pinched.
- Severe dehydration is characterized by all the signs of moderate dehydration plus a rapid, weak pulse, cold hands and feet, rapid breathing, blue lips, confusion, and lethargy.

Other symptoms that may be present include decreased or absent urination and decreased tears.

Treatment
Treatment for mild dehydration normally consists of drinking frequent, small amounts of fluid. With

an infant or child, it may be helpful to use a syringe or spoon, rather than trying to force a large amount of fluid at one time. All cases of mild dehydration can be safely treated at home as long as the dehydration does not worsen.

Teenagers and adults with moderate dehydration may often be effectively treated at home, but it is still recommended that a doctor be consulted by phone if not in person. Children under age 10 should see a doctor if moderately dehydrated. In some cases, moderate dehydration may require intravenous fluids and hospitalization to monitor the patient's condition.

Severe dehydration is a medical emergency and requires hospitalization and intravenous fluids in order to reverse the condition. Untreated severe dehydration may result in seizures, permanent brain damage, or death.

When dehydration is recognized and treated promptly, the outcome is generally good. It is important that the underlying causes of the dehydration be properly diagnosed and treated as well in order to ensure that the dehydration does not recur.

In order to properly treat dehydration, it is necessary to determine what has caused the patient to become dehydrated. Fever, vomiting, and diarrhea will each require their own special treatment, but while treatment is being administered for the underlying problem, the patient should start taking small amounts of an oral rehydrating solution. These drinks are not sports drinks, but are designed especially for sick people and formulated to replace blood salts and water in balanced amounts. They allow the intestines to absorb maximum amounts of water along with small amounts of salts. Sports drinks, on the other hand, are designed for concentrated energy and salt replacement in healthy, high-performance athletes. These drinks can actually aggravate vomiting and diarrhea and are so concentrated they can limit intestinal water absorption.

If the patient sees a doctor, the doctor will perform a medical history to determine the cause of the dehydration. A physical examination will also be done to identify exactly what types of stress the body is undergoing. The physical exam may reveal signs such as low blood pressure, rapid heart rate, and even shock in cases of severe dehydration.

The doctor may want to order a number of different tests, depending on the underlying causes of the dehydration and its severity. Possible tests include the following:

- blood chemistry tests to check the levels of electrolytes in the blood
- urine specific gravity test
- BUN test to check blood urea nitrogen
- creatinine test
- complete blood count (CBC) to check for any signs of concentrated blood
- blood sugar if diabetes is suspected as an underlying factor

Prevention

For athletes, the best way to prevent dehydration is to maintain body fluid levels by drinking plenty of fluids before, during, and after a workout or race. Often athletes are not aware that they are losing body fluid or that their performance is being affected by dehydration.

When uncertain how much fluid to drink, monitor hydration using one of these methods.

1. *Weight.* Weigh yourself before practice and again after practice. For every pound lost during the workout you will need to drink two cups of fluid to rehydrate your body.

2. *Urine color.* Check the color of your urine. If it is a dark gold color like apple juice, you are dehydrated. If you are well hydrated, the color of your urine will look like pale lemonade.

Thirst is not an accurate indicator of how much fluid was lost. If you wait until you are thirsty to replenish body fluids, then you are already dehydrated. Most people do not become thirsty until they have lost more than 2 percent of their body weight. And if you drink only enough to quench your thirst, you may still be dehydrated.

Keep a water bottle available when working out and drink as often as you want, ideally every 15 to 30 minutes. High school and junior high school athletes can bring a water bottle to school and drink between classes and during breaks so they show up at workouts hydrated.

Researchers have found that sports drinks containing between 6 percent and 8 percent carbohydrate (sugars) are absorbed into the body as rapidly as water and can provide energy to working muscles that water cannot. This extra energy can delay fatigue and possibly improve performance, particularly if the sport lasts longer than one hour. A sports drink can maintain the blood sugar level even when the sugar stored in muscles (glycogen) is running low. This allows the body to continue to produce energy at a high rate.

Drinks containing less than 5 percent carbohydrate do not provide enough energy to improve performance. So, athletes who dilute sports drink are most likely not getting enough energy from their drink to maintain a good blood sugar level. Drinking beverages that exceed a 10 percent carbohydrate level (most soda pop and some fruit juices) often have negative side effects such as abdominal cramps, nausea, and diarrhea and can hurt performance.

Sodium is an electrolyte needed to help maintain proper fluid balance in the body. Sodium helps the body absorb and retain more water. Researchers have found that the fluid from an eight-ounce serving of a sports drink with 6 percent carbohydrates (sugars) and about 110 mg of sodium absorbs into the body faster than plain water.

Some parents, coaches, and athletes are concerned that sports drinks may contain too much sodium. However, most sports drinks are actually low in sodium. An eight-ounce serving of Gatorade has a sodium content similar to a cup of 2 percent milk. Most Americans do get too much sodium, but usually from eating convenience-type foods, not from sports drinks.

Following are guidelines for fluid replacement for athletes:

- Drink a sports drink containing 6 percent to 8 percent carbohydrate to help give more energy during intense training and long workouts.

- Drink a beverage that contains a small amount of sodium and other electrolytes (like potassium and chloride).

- Find a beverage that tastes good; something cold and sweet is easier to drink.

- Drink 10 to 16 ounces of cold fluid about 15 to 30 minutes before workouts. Drinking a sports drink with a 6 percent to 8 percent carbohydrate level is useful to help build up energy stores in muscles.

- Drink four to eight ounces of cold fluid during exercise at 10 to 15 minute intervals.

- Start drinking early in your workout because you will not feel thirsty until you have already lost 2 percent of your body weight; by that time your performance may have begun to decline.

- Avoid carbonated drinks, which can cause gastrointestinal distress and may decrease the fluid volume.

- Avoid beverages containing caffeine and alcohol due to their diuretic effect.

- Practice drinking fluids while training. Athletes who have never used a sports drink should not start during a meet or on race day. Use a trial-and-error approach to find the drink that works.

For children and infants who are spending time in the heat or exercising vigorously, it is important to carefully monitor hydration status. If dehydration appears to be developing, consult a health care provider before the child becomes moderately or severely dehydrated. A few simple measures may prevent the development of severe dehydration.

In situations where illness is a factor in dehydration, always encourage fluids and remember that fluid needs are increased with fever, vomiting, and diarrhea. The easiest signs to monitor are urine output, saliva in the mouth, and tears with crying. In infants, it is best to avoid using water as the primary replacement fluid. Specific solutions are available for infants and children that provide the right amount of electrolytes to prevent electrolyte abnormalities.

ephedrine Ephedrine is a drug derived from the plant *Ephedra equisetina* that has been touted for its ability to assist in weight loss, improve athletic performance, and enhance concentration. It has been used for hundreds of years as a central nervous system stimulant and a decongestant. Ephedrine, otherwise known as ma huang, is a stimulant similar to the active ingredients in Sudafed. Pseudo-epinephrine in such over-the-counter drugs increases blood pressure and heart rate and decreases appetite. Ephedrine does the same thing. It increases alertness and energy and gives athletes a caffeinelike high. The difference, however, is in the way it is used. When physicians prescribe Sudafed to treat a cold, it is for short-term use, which is safe. Athletes who take ephedrine for performance enhancement, on the other hand, are using the supplement for a long period of time. Consumed on a daily basis for weeks at a time, ephedrine may cause hypertension, seizures, headaches, dizziness, mania, insomnia, and even death. The long-terms risks of taking ephedrine or ephedra are unknown.

How It Works
Structurally similar to amphetamines, ephedrine increases blood pressure and heart rate. The mechanisms behind ephedrine's effect on weight loss appear to be those of increasing energy expenditure through increased lipolysis, which is the process of breaking fat down into free fatty acids and glycerol so that it can be burned for energy; increasing basal metabolic rate through thyroxine; and decreasing food intake by suppressing appetite. Research, however, has found no effect of ephedrine on strength, endurance, reaction time, anaerobic capacity, or recovery time after prolonged exercise.

Athletes who choose to take ephedra or ephedrine should consume it according to national industry standards.

Side Effects
Side effects include:

- irregular heart rate
- elevated blood pressure
- dizziness
- headache
- heart attack
- stroke
- seizure
- psychosis
- death

Sources
Ephedrine is derived from the plant Ephedra equisetina. An herbal form of ephedrine called ephedra is sometimes sold under the name "ma huang," and can be found in many herbal products available in health food stores, often in combination with chromium.

Be Aware
- Ephedrine products have been found to contain from 0 percent to 100 percent of the amount listed on the label.
- Side effects vary and do not correlate with the amount consumed.
- Caffeine increases the effect of ephedrine and the combination can be dangerous.
- Ephedrine is banned by the National College Athletic Association and the International Olympic Committee.

- The FDA has documented 40 deaths and more than 800 side effects linked to ephedrine use.

- Ma huang, or ephedra, has been blamed for the deaths of several high school students who used it as a stimulant or aphrodisiac; the deaths presumably resulted from central nervous system bleeding or cardiac arrhythmia.

- Three sports neurologists have proposed that ephedrine and creatine use may be responsible for the marked increase in heatstroke deaths among football players since 1995.

exercise during pregnancy Exercise plays an important role in promoting health and well-being for pregnant women. Women who exercise during pregnancy experience reduced weight gain, more rapid weight loss after pregnancy, improved mood, and improved sleep patterns. Some studies have also shown faster labors and less need for induction of labor in women who exercise regularly during pregnancy. Others have demonstrated that women who regularly exercise are less likely to require epidurals and have fewer cesarean births. These positive benefits occur because exercise strengthens muscles needed for labor and delivery; helps reduce backaches, constipation, bloating, and swelling; improves posture; and improves mood and energy level.

Pregnancy, however, is a highly complex physiologic state, and precautions are needed during pregnancy to ensure that an exercise program does not cause complications.

General Guidelines

1. Those following a regular exercise program prior to pregnancy should be able to maintain that program to some degree throughout the pregnancy. Exercise does not increase the risk for miscarriage.

2. Those just starting an exercise program as a way of improving health during pregnancy should start very slowly and be careful to avoid overexertion.

3. Listen to the body. It will naturally give signals that it is time to reduce the level of exercise.

4. Never exercise to the point of exhaustion or breathlessness. This is a sign that the baby and body cannot get the oxygen supply they need.

5. Wear comfortable exercise footwear that provides strong ankle and arch support.

6. Take frequent breaks and drink plenty of fluids during exercise.

7. Avoid exercise in extremely hot weather.

8. Avoid rocky terrain or unstable ground when running or cycling. Joints are looser during pregnancy, which makes pregnant women more vulnerable to ankle sprains and other joint injuries.

9. Contact sports should be avoided during pregnancy.

10. WEIGHT TRAINING should emphasize improving tone, especially in the upper body and abdominal area. Avoid lifting weights overhead and using weights that strain the lower back muscles.

11. During the second and third trimesters, avoid exercise that involves lying flat on the back as this decreases blood flow to the womb.

12. Include relaxation and stretching both before and after the exercise program.

13. Eat a healthy diet that includes plenty of fruits, vegetables, and complex carbohydrates.

Which Muscles to Exercise

In addition to the heart, the three muscle groups to concentrate on during pregnancy are the muscles of the back, pelvis, and abdomen.

- Strengthening abdominal muscles will make it easier to support the increasing weight of the baby. It will also make it possible to push with more strength and more effectively during the last phase of delivering the baby.

- Strengthening pelvic muscles will permit the vagina to widen more easily during childbirth. This will help prevent urinary problems, such as leaking urine when coughing or sneezing, after delivery.

- Strengthening back muscles and doing exercises to improve posture will minimize the strain of pregnancy on the lower back. It will also help prevent discomfort caused by poor posture.

Recommended Exercises for Pregnancy

Many old ideas about strenuous exercise during pregnancy have been disproved in recent years. The type and intensity of sports and exercise one participates in during pregnancy depend on one's health and activity prior to becoming pregnant. This is probably not a good time to take up a new strenuous sport. Those who were active before becoming pregnant, however, can continue within reason.

- *Walking.* For those who did no exercise before becoming pregnant, walking is a good way to begin an exercise program.

- *Tennis.* Active players can probably continue to play unless they have special problems or feel unusually tired, but they should be aware of their change in balance and how it affects rapid movement.

- *Jogging.* Joggers can continue as long as they feel comfortable doing it. Avoid becoming overheated and stop when uncomfortable or unusually tired. Remember to drink plenty of water.

- *Swimming.* Swimmers can continue to swim. Swimming is an excellent form of exercise. The water supports the body's weight while swimming tones and strengthens many different muscles. Scuba diving is not advised.

- *Golf and bowling.* Both of these sports are good forms of recreation. Those who participate in them will have to adjust to an enlarged abdomen and be careful not to lose their balance.

- *Snow skiing, water skiing, and surfing.* These sports can be dangerous because athletes can hit the ground or water with great force. Falling while traveling at such fast speeds could harm the unborn baby. Participation in these activities should be discussed ahead of time with a health care provider.

- *Climbing, hiking, and skiing above 10,000 feet.* Elevations above 10,000 feet can deprive the athlete and the baby of oxygen. This can cause premature labor. Strenuous exercise at this altitude should be avoided, especially by those who normally live close to sea level.

Warning Signs

Those who experience any of the following warning signs should stop immediately and contact a doctor if the symptoms persist:

- pain, including pelvic pain, uterine contractions, or chest pain
- trouble walking
- bleeding or fluid leaking from the vagina
- faintness or dizziness
- a pronounced increase in shortness of breath
- irregular heartbeat (skipped beats or very rapid beats)

Physical Changes During Pregnancy That May Affect Exercise Ability

Lungs and breathing In pregnancy the respiratory rate is naturally increased. Because of this, the body works harder to give enough oxygen to the developing fetus. This can reduce the amount of oxygen available for exercise and can cause decreased endurance and a sense of breathlessness.

Musculoskeletal Because of the enlarging womb, the lower back develops more curvature and the body's center of gravity shifts. This can cause changes in sense of balance and requires adjustments in posture to prevent injury. Usually women find that they naturally alter their exercise program to accommodate these changes, especially in the last trimester of pregnancy.

The joints also undergo changes during pregnancy. The body releases a hormone called relaxin, which loosens up the joints of the pelvis to make room for the birth of the child. Because all of the joints in the body are more lax, there is a greater chance of spraining or straining muscles and joints during pregnancy.

Metabolism During pregnancy, the body uses carbohydrates more quickly. Exercise also increases the metabolism of carbohydrates. These two factors can lead to low blood sugar reactions during exercise. Increasing caloric intake to shift carbohydrate balance is very important for pregnant athletes.

Cardiovascular The body increases its blood volume by 40 percent in pregnancy, and the heart rate increases by about 15 beats per minute. This allows nutrients and oxygen to be transported to the fetus more efficiently. However, with the growth of the womb, the flow of blood in the body can be disrupted and light-headedness can occur.

Effects of Exercise on Pregnancy

Cardiovascular While exercising, blood flow shifts away from the body's internal organs so that the muscles, lungs, and heart get a larger share of oxygen. Extreme exercise can cause too large of a shift of oxygen away from the uterus. That's why reducing the length of time that one exercises strenuously and monitoring the heart rate may prevent problems with the pregnancy.

Neurotransmitter release During exercise, the brain releases more norepinephrine, a neurotransmitter that can reduce depression and influence blood flow to the heart and kidneys. Norepinephrine also increases smooth muscle contraction and can cause increased uterine activity in the form of painless contractions. These contractions have not been shown to cause labor, but because of the possible influence on contractions, women who have risks for preterm labor should limit their exercise programs to avoid bringing on contractions.

Elevated body temperature Exercise causes an increase in core body temperature. Some studies have shown that high fevers during the first three months of pregnancy can affect the fetus's development while other studies have not confirmed these findings. However, women who are extremely fit actually have improved body temperature regulation and have decreased core body temperature during pregnancy. Because of the conflicting data available, general guidelines would include caution when exercising in very hot weather and attention to adequate fluid intake during exercise.

Effects of Pregnancy on Exercise

Anemia Anemia, or a low blood count, results in lower oxygen carrying capacity of the blood. This has a big impact on endurance and may result in a marked decrease in exercise capability because of breathlessness, dizziness, and fatigue. Women with anemia who want to continue their exercise program should eat an iron-rich diet, take extra vitamin C with meals to increase iron absorption, and should take iron supplements if prescribed by the maternity care provider.

Contractions Some women experience preterm contractions throughout pregnancy. While preterm contractions do not always lead to preterm birth, they do increase a woman's risk of preterm labor significantly. If a woman has frequent contractions during pregnancy, strenuous exercise may lead to a higher rate of contractions. Exercise programs should be adjusted to include more nonweight-bearing exercises such as yoga, stretching, and swimming rather than speed walking or jogging.

Low back pain/sciatica Many women have episodes of LOW BACK PAIN or leg pain during pregnancy because of weight changes and changes in body posture. Weight-bearing exercise can increase pain levels and further stress the joints. Again, nonweight-bearing exercise may help with these symptoms. Swimming is particularly helpful.

Toxemia/high blood pressure Women who have high blood pressure can benefit from a regular exercise program. However, women who develop high blood pressure in pregnancy should stop their exercise program. Toxemia, or high blood pressure that develops during pregnancy, is thought to involve a severe problem with blood vessels throughout the body. Exercise can worsen toxemia and should not be continued.

Placenta previa/vaginal bleeding Placenta previa is a condition in which the placenta grows low in the uterus and actually covers the opening to the cervix. It can cause severe bleeding during pregnancy. Any women with placenta previa or with vaginal bleeding of an unknown cause should not participate in an exercise program.

Preterm labor risks Women who have delivered a baby before 36 weeks of pregnancy should be very cautious in participating in an exercise program during the second and third trimesters of pregnancy. Stretching, yoga, and walking are preferred forms of exercise, while weight-bearing exercise should be avoided. Also, women with preterm contractions should avoid exercise that increases uterine contractions, whether painful or painless.

Intrauterine growth retardation Intrauterine growth retardation (IUGR) is poor growth of the baby. This is diagnosed by a maternity care provider who measures the growth of the uterus and checks a fetal sonogram. If a baby has IUGR, it may mean that the baby is not getting an adequate oxygen supply from the placenta. There are many causes of IUGR including smoking, drug use, infections, and poor blood flow to the placenta. Because exercise shifts blood flow away from the placenta, a baby that is not growing well will not tolerate exercise by its mother.

Twin pregnancy Women who are pregnant with more than one fetus have a higher risk of complications in pregnancy including preterm labor. Exercise should be limited to nonweight-bearing activities and should focus on toning and stretching.

Heart disease Exercise increases the strain on the heart, as does pregnancy because of increased blood volume. Women with heart problems should exercise only under the supervision of their cardiologist and maternity care provider.

facet syndrome　Neck pain is a common ailment and has been estimated to occur among 35 percent of people in the general population. Chronic neck pain, defined as that lasting six months or more, is estimated to occur in approximately 14 percent of the general population. Facet syndrome is a condition involving the facet joints of the spine, which are located between and behind each vertebra. The facet joints allow limited movement between the vertebrae. Facet syndrome is a treatable condition characterized by pain in the neck and a decreased range of motion in the neck.

Causes

Facet syndrome is often diagnosed following a case of WHIPLASH and is, in fact, the most common cause of chronic neck pain following a whiplash injury. In these cases, the facets are jammed by some sort of trauma and become a source of chronic pain. The condition is also associated with degenerative disk disease, but it is difficult to determine which condition precipitates the other. Otherwise, the facet syndrome arises from the stresses of daily living. Poor posture and muscle tone, sometimes associated with a protruding abdomen, may cause facet syndrome.

Diagnosis

Patients with facet syndrome will often, though not always, complain of tenderness over the facet joints when touched and pain with extension or rotation of the spine. They usually have neck pain, headaches, and decreased range of motion in the neck. Patients usually describe the pain as a dull aching discomfort in the back of the neck that sometimes radiates downward to the shoulders and even mid back. A history of whiplash is often indicative of facet syndrome. Numbness, tingling, muscle weakness, and other nerve deficits should not be present in facet syndrome.

Except when needed to rule out other possible injuries, such as fractures or tumors, imaging studies are not helpful in diagnosing this injury. The diagnosis can be confirmed by the injection of local anesthetics or anti-inflammatory medication in the joints.

Treatment

In treating soft tissue injuries such as facet syndrome, the first goal is to reduce the pain and inflammation and increase the range of motion available to the patient without pain. Icing the injury, and using therapeutic techniques such as ultrasound, electrical stimulation, joint manipulation, soft tissue massage, and gentle muscle stretching may also help reduce the discomfort and the painful muscle spasms often associated with this injury. Range-of-motion exercises, first passive and then active, should be started initially as long as they do not cause pain, followed by strengthening exercises. Once patients are completely pain free, they should focus on exercises that balance strength and flexibility and increase their endurance in physical activity.

Surgical treatment, namely cervical fusion, should be considered only with great caution after aggressive nonsurgical care has failed. Surgical fusion as a treatment for facet syndrome is not particularly effective because cervical facet joint pain can still occur following fusion.

Prevention

Some approaches to treatment are also useful in preventing the condition. Exercises that improve muscle tone and posture are helpful for both. Using proper lifting techniques and sleep postures will contribute to a healthy spine, as will exercise and stretching of the back, which will strengthen the muscles and stabilize the facet joints. In addition, maintaining a healthy weight helps to reduce undue stress on the spine.

fatigue prevention While athletes should expect to be tired after an intense workout, they probably should not feel exhausted when they wake up, after a light workout, or several days following an intense workout. If they do, there may be cause for concern.

If one continually feels tired and cannot seem to recover normal energy levels, perhaps one of the following explanations is the reason. For each, there is a way to undo the damage.

Overtraining

A poorly conceived training program is generally regarded as the primary reason for overtraining in most athletes who experience this problem. The risk of overtraining occurs when there is a rapid increase in training volume or training intensity without adequate recovery time built into the program.

This can happen to athletes who compete frequently, take no rest days, eat a poor diet, experience environmental and psychological stress factors in their lives, or follow busy travel schedules.

Symptoms of overtraining include unusual muscle soreness, decreased performance, difficulty in completing normal training routines, an increased sense of effort while exercising, depression, insomnia, loss of appetite, and fatigue, which can be described as feeling tired at times when normally feeling ready for more training or competition.

Sports medicine professionals say that the best way to avoid the pitfalls of overtraining is to follow an organized training program. Training days should be grouped into heavy, moderate, and light exercise days, with scheduled rest days interspersed between the work days. Training programs should be individualized for each athlete to address their particular needs. In addition, it is most helpful to keep detailed records of training and competition performance to observe over time the effects of different strategies.

Nutritional Deficiencies

Athletes attempting to lose weight put themselves at great risk of developing nutritional deficiencies that can ultimately lead to fatigue. Specific calorie needs are very individual. They are affected by age, gender, weight, and exercise habits, among other things, so it is impossible to give general guidelines for calorie consumption. Most sports medicine professionals agree, however, that athletes need to consume about 23 calories per pound to maintain their weight.

What type of calories the athlete consumes, in addition to how many, plays a significant role in determining how much energy he or she has. Carbohydrates are extremely important for athletes who train hard day after day and want to maintain high levels of energy. Some sports nutritionists suggest that athletes should consume as much as 60 to 70 percent of their total calories in carbohydrates, although there is some debate about this number.

Dietary protein also plays an important role in maintaining energy levels. When an athlete burns through his or her carbohydrate stores, the body then turns to protein in search of energy. The amount of protein needed is again determined by the level of activity and the individual's specific needs, but a guideline for dietary protein is between .5 and .9 grams per pound of bodyweight, with the more active athlete consuming more than the recreational athlete.

Iron deficiency has been directly tied to fatigue. Anemia, or low iron levels, is a fairly common problem among female athletes, especially marathon runners, endurance athletes, female teenage athletes, and those who do not eat red meat.

The Recommended Dietary Allowances (RDA) for iron varies by age, gender, and medical condition. Men need 10 mg per day. Women up to age 51 need 15 mg per day, and some dieticians suggest as much as 18 mg daily. But the RDA drops to 10 mg per day after age 51. Pregnant women should take in 30 mg of iron every day.

One final nutritional concern is DEHYDRATION, which can cause a feeling of fatigue and adversely affect athletic performance. A general rule for preventing dehydration is to consume one quart of water or other fluid for every 1,000 calories expended.

Chronic Lack of Sleep

Loss of sleep over an extended period of time is definitely going to impair energy levels and athletic performance. Researchers in the field of sleep medicine have shown a number of negative responses, including chronic fatigue, that are associated with sleep loss.

Post-Viral Fatigue

Athletes who are just recovering from a cold or the flu may be quite susceptible to fatigue. The immune system may still be suppressed when the athlete returns to moderate or intense training levels, which can result in prolonged fatigue. Symptoms of this are a sore throat, fever, and aches throughout the body. It is probably advisable for athletes to eat well, drink adequate fluids, and wait for full recovery to take place before resuming training in order to avoid an even longer period of fatigue.

female athlete triad Female athlete triad is a serious medical illness that involves disordered eating, amenorrhea (failure to menstruate, see ATHLETIC AMENORRHEA), and osteoporosis (loss of bone mass), three distinct but interrelated conditions. Disordered eating is a range of poor nutritional behaviors that includes ANOREXIA, BULIMIA, or a combination of the two. Amenorrhea refers to irregular or absent menstrual periods, and osteoporosis refers to low bone mass, which leads to bone fragility and risk of stress fracture. Affecting girls and women in a number of different sports, it is often associated with gymnastics, figure skating, ballet, and running. It is important to remember that it may affect any girl or woman participating at any level in any sport. The common thread among women with female athlete triad is that they are extremely driven to excel in their sports. Although the illness can be difficult to detect and treat, it is essential that parents, coaches, and athletes understand the severe nature of female athlete triad, which can cause irreversible bone loss and even death in severe cases. If anorexia or bulimia goes untreated, individuals are at risk of premature death from heart problems, blood electrolyte disorders, suicide, or health problems.

Causes

Although there are numerous factors involved in the development of female athlete triad, it is believed that external social pressure and internal pressure to conform to expectations for thinness play a significant role. Some researchers also believe that eating disorders may be related to problems with the chemicals in the brain that regulate mood and appetite. In either case, girls and women who are determined to achieve a lean appearance and who believe their athletic success is tied to this achievement may try to reach this goal through excessive exercise and dieting. Such an approach may eventually lead to development of the female athlete triad. In addition, a tendency toward perfectionism, compulsive behavior, and being extremely goal-oriented make an athlete more susceptible to the illness.

Diagnosis

Warning signs for female athlete triad include the following:

- eating alone
- trips to the bathroom during or after meals
- use of laxatives
- fatigue
- anemia
- depression
- intolerance to cold
- lanugo (body hair)
- eroded tooth enamel from vomiting
- amenorrhea
- stress fractures

Disordered eating Recognizing and diagnosing female athlete triad may be difficult, but awareness of the symptoms is the first step in recognizing the illness and getting help. If the athlete sees a doctor, some symptoms may be revealed in a routine history of the patient. The occurrence of stress fractures, especially those that occur in unusual places such as femurs, ribs, or pelvis due to minimal

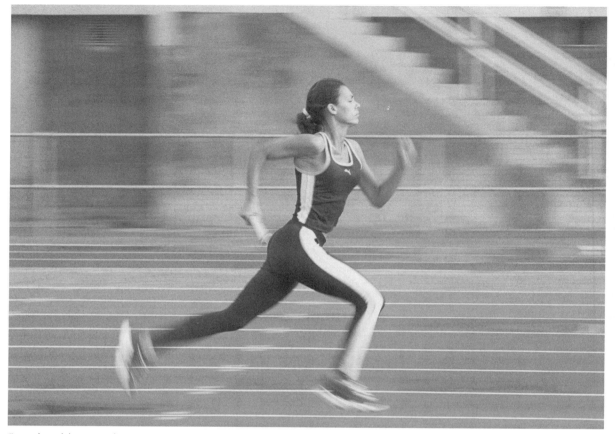

Female athlete triad is a serious condition that involves a combination of disordered eating, failure to menstruate, and osteoporosis. It often affects very young female athletes and can result in permanent bone loss, as well as other long-term damage. *(Fogstock, LLC)*

trauma, may indicate the possibility of osteoporosis. The physical exam may also reveal erosion of tooth enamel from frequent vomiting and enlarged parotid glands.

Symptoms of anorexia include morbid fear of fatness, distorted body image, refusal to maintain a weight at least 85 percent of that expected for height and age, and amenorrhea. There are two types of anorexia: restrictive anorexia does not involve any regular bingeing and purging; bingeing-purging anorexia involves regular use of this behavior during an anorexic episode.

Symptoms of bulimia include recurrent episodes of binge eating, with a sense of a lack of control over eating. There are two types of bulimia: purging and nonpurging. Patients with purging bulimia may purge by vomiting or using laxatives or diuretics. Those with nonpurging bulimia may fast or exercise excessively following the binge eating.

The consequences of untreated eating disorders are serious. They include the possibility of irreversible bone loss, disturbances of the cardiovascular, endocrine, and gastrointestinal systems, disruption of temperature regulation, and death.

Amenorrhea Primary amenorrhea is defined as the failure to begin menstruation before reaching the age of 16 or going two years beyond puberty without menstruating. Secondary amenorrhea is defined in many different ways, but is generally the failure to menstruate more than six to nine times in a year by a woman who has previously had normal menstrual cycles.

A history of the patient's menstruation will reveal a case of amenorrhea, which is associated with a decrease in estrogen levels. This leads to decreased bone mass and may raise the risk of heart problems.

Osteoporosis Generally defined as a decrease in bone mass, osteoporosis may result from one of two different conditions. The first is that bone may have been inadequately acquired during adolescence. The second is that a woman with normal bone mineral content may have lost it prematurely. Osteoporosis has been directly correlated in some studies with amenorrhea in female runners, but other studies have not supported these findings. Athletes who fail to menstruate normally may be at risk for developing osteoporosis.

Treatment

The treatment of female athlete triad involves a multidisciplinary approach that includes helping the patient to determine the factors contributing to her illness, educating her about the risks involved with the illness, restoring adequate nutrition, and prescribing estrogen therapy when appropriate.

Treatment will usually have to combat certain myths that are commonly held by athletes. These include believing that the loss of menstrual periods is a sign of adequate training as opposed to an unhealthy condition that puts the athlete at risk for many possible health complications. Another myth is that extremely low body fat contributes to athletic performance. Athletes often need help in understanding that the optimal weight for appearance is not necessarily the optimal weight for athletic performance. In fact, neither of these may be the optimal weight for general good health.

Another barrier to treating individuals with female athlete triad is that they are often reluctant to seek care and may deny that they have any nutritional or health problems. Quite often, it takes a team of professionals and friends to get the athlete the help she needs. A physician, nutritionist, and psychologist may each be helpful, in addition to friends, parents, and coaches. An individual who needs help may be more open to it if the risks of her illness are explained in a nonjudgmental way and if she is convinced that treatment would probably help her athletic performance. This type of intervention is often more successful in the early stages of the illness than it is later on.

A treatment plan for female athlete triad may include nutritional monitoring, hormone replacement, and reduced training.

When discussing the athlete's diet, it is helpful to emphasize increasing lean-body mass and sustaining the lean-body mass by eating a well-rounded, high-carbohydrate diet. The patient should understand that she needs sufficient calories to meet both her routine daily needs and her sport needs. It is likely that the physician or nutritionist will recommend taking supplemental calcium to provide some protective effect for the bones. Sufficient vitamin D is also important.

Hormone replacement therapy (HRT) should be prescribed for most patients with female athlete triad since these patients suffer from estrogen deficiency. This therapy may include separate estrogen and progestogen or a combination oral contraceptive pill. HRT with separate hormones will provide enough estrogen to protect the bones and to induce menstruation, but it will not be sufficient to ensure contraception. Thus, athletes who desire contraceptive benefits should choose to take the pill.

Prevention

Although the social pressures on women, and athletes in particular, to be thin will not likely change soon, parents, coaches, teachers, and friends can have a mitigating effect by refraining from focusing on the athlete's weight or from suggesting that she lose weight for any reason. In addition, alertness to symptoms will help interested parties intervene early, which increases the chances for successful treatment.

femoral neck fractures Femoral neck fractures in athletes are most often stress fractures to the hip, specifically to the femoral neck, or part of the hip where the femur and hip connect, that occur primarily in two distinct groups of people—young, active individuals who participate in a new strenuous activity or undergo changes in the level of their activity, and elderly individuals with osteoporosis.

A stress fracture is the result of a dynamic process over time unlike an acute fracture, which usually is a result of a single traumatic event. Although stress fractures of the femoral neck are uncommon, they can have serious consequences, and certain populations of athletes should be aware of the risk factors involved with this injury. Long-distance runners who change or add activities to their workout seem to experience this type of stress fracture more frequently than others.

Causes

Training errors are the most common risk factors, including a sudden increase in the quantity or intensity of training, and the introduction of a new activity.

Muscle fatigue has been implicated as a contributing factor in the development of stress fractures. Muscle imbalance leads to changes in the application of stress across the femoral neck that may exceed the bone's capability to respond appropriately to stress. Muscle fatigue secondary to repetitive activity can decrease its shock-absorbing capacity so that higher peak stresses occur in the femoral neck. This can lead to gait abnormalities, which, in turn, can alter the body's center of gravity and change the patterns of stress placed on the femoral neck.

Leg-length discrepancy also may predispose individuals to injuries by creating an unequal distribution of stress and tension across the hip joint.

Women experience stress fractures more commonly than men. This may be due to actual physical differences, as well as to exercise-induced hormonal differences that result in amenorrhea or nutritional deficiencies, which can lead to bone demineralization and place these women athletes at risk for various overuse injuries. Studies have shown that certain stress fractures are associated with a decrease in bone mineral content, which can occur from a decrease in circulating estrogen in the body. Lack of protective estrogen leads to a decrease in bone mass. Women with the FEMALE ATHLETE TRIAD of amenorrhea (see ATHLETIC AMENORRHEA), osteoporosis, and disordered eating are most certainly at greater risk for stress fractures.

Other factors that have been implicated in femoral neck fractures include low bone density, abnormal body composition, dietary deficiencies, biomechanical abnormalities, and menstrual irregularities.

Diagnosis

Patients with a stress fracture of the femoral neck will usually describe groin or hip pain associated with walking. A doctor will take a complete medical history and conduct a physical examination in order to establish a diagnosis. Combining the findings of the history and physical examinations should increase the overall predictive value of the evaluation process.

The basic history should include a thorough account of the patient's symptoms, including a timeline of when symptoms developed, a complete description of the patient's symptoms. The doctor will want to know if the symptoms are associated with any specific sport or activity. Particular attention should be given to any changes in activity level, intensity level, workout regimen, equipment, and technique.

Most athletes describe an insidious onset of pain over two or three weeks, which corresponds with a recent change in training or equipment. Typically, runners have recently increased their mileage or intensity, changed their terrain, or switched running shoes. The physician should inquire about the individual's training log and mileage.

Features common to all stress fractures include the following:

- participation in repetitive cyclic activity
- insidious onset of pain
- recent change in activity or equipment
- atraumatic history
- pain with weight bearing
- relief of pain with rest
- menstrual irregularities

The doctor should question the patient about previous experience of these symptoms and how they were treated. If there was a previous treatment plan, the doctor should attempt to understand the plan and the affects it had on the symptoms.

In addition, if the patient is female, a menstrual history should be taken. The absence of menstruation is a warning sign for the presence of female athlete triad, a serious illness that includes disordered eating, osteoporosis, and amenorrhea (absence of menstruation) and can lead to disturbances of the endocrine, cardiovascular, and gastrointestinal systems, as well as irreversible bone loss.

Symptoms and signs of female athlete triad include but are not limited to the following:

- depression
- intolerance to cold
- disordered eating habits
- obsessive exercise habits
- lack of appropriate body image
- lanugo
- eroded tooth enamel

The physical examination of the hip should include an in-depth evaluation of the neurological and musculoskeletal systems. The doctor's initial inspection of the patient should include noting any grimacing when the patient moves and observing any abnormal gait patterns. If the patient has a displaced femoral neck fracture, he or she will usually be unable to stand or walk. The doctor will want to look for any indication of leg-length discrepancy as well as any appearance of muscle atrophy or asymmetry.

When the doctor palpates the injury site, he or she will be looking for any tender points in the groin and hip regions. There is usually local bony tenderness with a stress fracture; however, the femoral neck is fairly deep and thus this type of tenderness may be absent.

The doctor will also want to determine range of motion for the hip and knee by performing certain basic passive movement exercises on the patient. It will be important to examine range of motion in the iliotibial band, as well as in the spine and lower back. Pain patterns may be confusing when there is an injury at the hip. The pain of a hip injury may be felt primarily in the thigh and knee, for example.

Determining a baseline for muscle strength will also help the doctor diagnose any nerve injuries that may exist. Abnormal reflexes can indicate nerve root abnormality. The asymmetry of reflexes

is most significant; therefore, a patient's reflexes must be compared with the opposite side of the body. Finally, a decrease or loss of sensation can suggest or eliminate any specific nerve damage.

For 70 percent of patients with a stress fracture of the femur, hopping on the injured leg will reproduce the pain associated with the injury, so the hop test may also be performed.

Femoral neck fractures are divided into the following four grades on the basis of the degree of displacement of the fracture fragment:

- Grade I is an incomplete or valgus-impacted fracture.
- Grade II is a complete fracture without bone displacement.
- Grade III is a complete fracture with partial displacement of the fracture fragments.
- Grade IV is a complete fracture with total displacement of the fracture fragments.

It is quite difficult to differentiate between these four types of fractures, but the most important classification is to distinguish between nondisplaced and displaced fractures.

Laboratory studies are generally not necessary in the diagnosis of femoral neck fractures. Basic X rays traditionally have been ordered as the initial step in the workup of hip fractures. The main purpose of X rays is to rule out any obvious fractures and to determine the site and extent of the fracture, but plain X rays have poor sensitivity. Bone scans are much more sensitive to showing bone stress but less specific in revealing the exact location. Although expensive, MAGNETIC RESONANCE IMAGING (MRI) is highly accurate and specific in identifying femoral neck fractures and often the study of choice.

Treatment

The goals of treatment are to promote healing, prevent complications, and return normal function to the hip. The primary goal of fracture management is to return the patient to his or her pre-injury level of function. This is completed either with surgical or nonsurgical treatment. Several factors must be considered before a treatment plan is recommended.

The decision for operative or nonoperative treatment and the decision of the type of surgical intervention are based on many factors. Compression fractures are more stable than tension-type fractures, and can be treated without surgery.

Treatment for nondisplaced fractures is bed rest and/or the use of crutches until passive hip movement is pain free and X rays show evidence of a callus formation. Patients should be monitored closely with serial X rays since there is a high risk of displacement of the fracture. Immediate open reduction and internal fixation (ORIF) is indicated if the fracture widens.

A physical therapist may be useful for reinforcing the physician's instructions for rest and helping the patient modify a training program to allow healing to take place. The athlete can maintain physical fitness and mobility by exercising the remaining extremities and performing nonweight-bearing strengthening activities that do not cause strain on the affected hip joint. The physical therapist can evaluate the patient for any gait and/or anatomic abnormalities that may have predisposed the patient to development of the fracture. Some patients may need orthotics to prevent excessive pronation, which causes increased stress on the femoral neck. The physical therapist completes patient education throughout the rehabilitation process, whether surgical or nonsurgical treatment is rendered. Once the painful symptoms of a stable fracture are controlled during the acute phase of treatment, strengthening exercises for the hip stabilizers and associated muscles can be initiated. The main objectives are to improve and restore range of motion (ROM) of the hip. Once the patient is pain-free, weight bearing can be progressed. When patients are able to tolerate partial weight-bearing ambulation, general conditioning workouts including swimming and cycling are permitted. Serial X rays are obtained at weekly intervals until the patient can ambulate with full weight bearing and no pain. Running is gradually reintroduced and progression of distance is slow. If pain occurs, a couple of days of rest are recommended and mileage is reduced, and then progressed again depending upon the individual's symptoms.

For patients with overt fractures or displacement on the tension side, surgery is indicated. Usu-ally fixation with a plate and screws is used. Following the surgery, the patient rests until pain resolves and then progresses to full activity as healing occurs. Once the plate is removed, further rehabilitation is needed. Removal of the plate depends upon the age and activity level of the patient. Some patients prefer weight bearing with crutches. Patients usually are allowed to return to running; however, contact sports are limited.

Maintaining aerobic conditioning throughout the rehabilitation process is important. If walking with crutches is necessary, then upper body exercise such as an upper body ergometer can be used. Once the patient begins to bear his or her own weight again, aquatic training may be used, such as swimming or deep water running.

The maintenance phase of rehabilitation includes muscle-strengthening exercises and sport-specific training.

The athlete can return to play when there is an absence of signs or symptoms of the original injury, full range of motion, normal strength and flexibility, and normal sport-specific mechanics. Athletes must be aware of their own limitations, which is particularly important for the individual gradually returning to a competitive level of activity after injury. Complications include recurrent stress fractures. There is also the possibility that the patient may not return to pre-injury functioning. A displaced femoral neck fracture may end the career of an elite athlete even if properly treated.

Prevention

Patient education is an important factor in the prevention of stress fractures. Female athletes should decrease their risk of recurrent fractures by maintaining adequate muscle mass and bone density.

Maintaining proper flexibility also is thought to play a significant role in the prevention of sports-related injuries. Additionally, improvement in aerobic fitness can increase blood flow and oxygenation to all tissues, including the muscles and bones, and it would be a reasonable addition to any rehabilitation and prevention program. Seasonal athletes should be encouraged to cross-train year round or at least undergo preconditioning before participating in their particular sport so that they are less vulnerable to stress fracture injuries when they return to intense workouts in their sport.

femur injuries and fractures A structure designed specifically for standing and walking, the femur is the strongest, longest, and heaviest bone in the body. It is subject to numerous forces during normal walking and running, but the femur is vulnerable to fracture in trauma-induced situations that involve high-speed force. In order for the femur to actually break, a significant amount of energy must be transferred to the limb. In sports, this type of energy is often generated in skiing, football, hockey, and motor sports. These high-energy fractures most often are associated with multiple system injury, as well as other bone injuries. Isolated fractures of the femur can also occur in situations with lesser velocity forces or with bone that is diseased.

Femur fractures can range from stress fractures with no displacement of the bone to complex fractures with severe displacement and associated soft tissue injury that sometimes require amputation. Since the femur is very vascular, fractures of the femur may result in significant blood loss.

Fractures of the femur occur most often in individuals under the age of 25 or over the age of 65, with males under the age of 30 experiencing the greatest incidence of this type of fracture. Among athletes, the most common form of femur fracture is the stress fracture. A stress fracture is defined as an exaggerated bone remodeling process in response to lower levels of repetitive stress placed on the bone. A stress fracture may also occur if there is a single dramatic increase in the muscle forces at the point of insertion with the bone. This is called a microfracture. Runners, baseball players, and basketball players experience the highest rate of stress fractures.

Causes

Trauma experienced in high-speed and contact sports, such as skiing, football, and hockey, accounts for a number of femur fractures. Other types of violent trauma, such as motorcycle or racecar accidents, mountain climbing falls, pole vaulting falls, and gunshot wounds to the leg cause fractures of the femur. Stress fractures are usually caused by running and jogging, either alone or in team sports such as basketball, baseball, and soccer. Shoes that do not fit properly and improper training techniques are sometimes responsible for stress fractures in athletes who run a lot. In female athletes, amenorrhea (see ATHLETIC AMENORRHEA) and its associated lower bone density can make an athlete, especially a runner, more susceptible to stress fractures of the femur.

In addition to sports-related causes of femur fractures, plane crashes, tumors, and metabolic bone disease can often be the cause of a femur fracture.

Diagnosis

Most often the result of high-energy trauma, femoral shaft fractures are not subtle injuries. The first priority when diagnosing the injury is to stabilize the patient and rule out other life-threatening injuries. In a traumatic injury of the femur, the history of the patient will reveal a high-velocity impact that results in significant pain and the inability to bear weight on the leg. With stress fractures of the femur, the patient will often be a runner or jogger who describes a sudden increase in mileage, intensity of workouts, and/or frequency of training. Other characteristics commonly seen in stress fractures of the femur include a change in terrain or running surface and use of improper footwear. The patient will often complain of a gradual onset of symptoms, though the symptoms may be severe by the time the patient sees the doctor. There may be pain in the groin or thigh, and all symptoms are aggravated by activity and relieved by rest. In female athletes, it is important to take a menstrual history to determine the possibility of what effects amenorrhea may be having on the strength of the bones.

In traumatic injuries, the physical examination will first address the most serious injuries. The physician will examine the patient from head to toe, including thorough evaluations on the pelvis, hip, and knee and assessments of vascular and neurological functioning to ensure that there is no damage to the blood vessels and nerves.

In stress fractures, there are usually very few physical findings in an examination. The physician will palpate the site of the symptoms and test for range of motion in the leg. Usually there is limited range of motion and there may be some swelling present.

In traumatic injuries, a number of laboratory studies are called for, including a chemistry panel and urinalysis. Other tests that may be needed include X rays of the chest, spine, pelvis, femur, hip, and knee. A COMPUTERIZED AXIAL TOMOGRAPHY (CAT) scan of the head may also be beneficial.

With stress fractures, doctors may call for X rays of the femur, but X rays will often not show any findings until two to six weeks following the onset of symptoms. For this reason, radionucleotide scanning is the standard in diagnosing stress fractures of the femur. It is more sensitive than other types of film and will show abnormalities up to three weeks earlier than plain X rays.

Treatment

In situations of traumatic injury that have caused a break in the femur, treatment usually involves surgical stabilization of the bone, performed by a trauma surgeon. Prior to surgery, acute management is designed to restore alignment in the leg. This usually involves applying traction and placing the limb in a splint that will help it to maintain proper alignment during transport to the hospital. The goals of surgery are to restore length, rotation, and alignment to the limb to ensure a full return of function.

Rehabilitation after surgery is designed initially to strengthen and improve range of motion in the hip and knee. The patient will progress to gait training, using crutches to avoid full weight bearing. Patients with simple fractures may be able to bear more weight immediately following surgery than will patients with more complex fracture patterns. Weight bearing is permitted once the bone has healed enough to be stable. The physician will want to monitor the patient's progress by continuing periodical X rays of the femur on an outpatient basis. The fracture should be completely healed in three months. Once the bone has fully united, treatment is focused on muscle rehabilitation and progressive strengthening of muscles in the lower leg. Sports-specific rehabilitation can begin once the patient has regained normal levels of strength in the injured leg. A return to pre-injury status should be achieved within one year of the injury. About 95 percent of all femur fractures heal completely with infection and nonunion of bone rates very low in this type of surgery, so the prognosis is extremely good.

For stress fractures of the femur, treatment usually includes the use of crutches to alleviate weight bearing on the affected leg for one to four weeks, until the symptoms begin to resolve. Once the pain is gone, the patient may begin full weight bearing, but running is not recommended for at least eight weeks and up to 16 weeks. Prior to resuming running, the patient should participate in a low-impact rehabilitation training program that includes cycling, swimming, and running in water. With the exception of stationary cycling, the patient should avoid most lower body exercise in favor of exercises that maintain upper body strength and cardiovascular fitness. As symptoms decrease, the patient may gradually increase lower extremity exercise and work on correcting any poor training habits that may have contributed to development of the injury. It usually requires a minimum of six weeks for the bone to heal before the patient is able to resume full activities. Resumption of activities should be gradual. If symptoms recur, the patient should return to the previous phase of treatment for a minimum of three weeks. Occasionally, stress fractures of the femur will recur again and again. In these cases, surgical stabilization is recommended.

Prevention

Proper training and appropriate footwear are the most important elements in preventing stress fractures. Traumatic fractures are harder to prevent, but following safe play practices in sports such as football and hockey will help athletes to avoid situations that can cause serious femur fractures.

fifth metatarsal fractures (avulsion fractures, mid-shaft fractures, jones fractures) The metatarsals are the long bones of the feet, and the fifth metatarsal is the outermost foot bone, connecting the little toe to the foot. A fifth metatarsal fracture is a break occurring in this outermost bone. There are three types of fractures associated with the fifth metatarsal. These include an avulsion fracture, a mid-shaft (or pseudo-Jones) fracture, and a Jones fracture (so-named after the physician who defined it). Distinguishing between these is an important step in determining the proper treatment.

Causes

Avulsion fractures often occur in conjunction with ankle sprains. When the ankle or foot rolls, a tendon that attaches a muscle to the fifth metatarsal can pull off a piece of the fifth metatarsal bone, creating the avulsion fracture.

When the foot gets violently twisted or impacted by a heavy object, a mid-shaft fracture can occur. In addition, repetitive cyclical stress on the foot may also cause a mid-shaft fracture.

Finally, the Jones fracture is usually a stress fracture that results from overuse. The bone actually wears out in the course of chronic overuse and often due to poor biomechanics. Eventually, it gets so thin that it breaks. This occurs most often in sports involving running and jumping. A Jones fracture can also occur with an acute inversion injury.

Diagnosis

A patient with a fifth metatarsal fracture will complain of pain, swelling, and tenderness on the outside of the foot, as well as difficulty walking. Although a history of activity and symptoms will help the doctor diagnose the problem, an X ray is necessary to specifically define the location of the break. In the case of a Jones fracture and other stress fractures, a bone scan may be necessary, as X rays sometimes fail to detect stress fractures.

Treatment

Treatment varies depending on the type of fracture, but immediately following the injury, it is helpful in all cases to keep the foot elevated above the level of the heart and to take anti-inflammatory medication or other pain medication as prescribed by the doctor.

Prior to casting, the patient should apply ice packs to the injured foot for 20 to 30 minutes every three to four hours for the first two or three days following the injury or until the pain subsides somewhat. Following those initial few days, the patient should ice the foot at least once a day until all the symptoms are gone.

Long-term treatment of avulsion fractures and mid-shaft fractures usually requires immobilization. The patient will wear a stiff-soled shoe or a removable cast boot for four to six weeks in the case of an avulsion fracture and six to eight weeks with the mid-shaft fracture. Following removal of the cast or shoe, the patient will normally be on crutches until he or she can walk without pain.

Jones fractures sometimes take longer to heal than the other fifth metatarsal fractures. They can also be treated with a removable cast boot or cast worn for six to eight weeks, but quite often the patient will need a more aggressive approach. In these cases, a surgeon places a screw in the bone to hold it together where it has broken. The patient will also be on crutches following the surgery until walking causes no pain.

Patients may begin the rehabilitation process when a follow-up X ray indicates that the fracture has healed. This recovery period consists of strengthening and range-of-motion exercises, as well as balance exercises. Manipulation can be used to reintroduce motion and joint play into the foot, especially after prolonged immobilization, which often occurs during the post surgical period or during fracture care. This manipulation can speed up return to play, which is the essential issue in athletic injuries. Most athletes with fractures, however, will rehabilitate around the injury, cross-training in sports that do not use the injured foot, in order to minimize joint restriction and to maintain fitness levels.

The patient may return to his or her sport when full range of motion and strength have been restored to the injured foot, and the patient can run, jump, and do figure-eights at half speed and full speed without any pain.

Prevention

Fifth metatarsal fractures are often the result of accidents that cannot be prevented, but runners can help prevent stress fractures by avoiding running on hard and uneven surfaces and by ensuring that their running shoes always provide adequate cushion and support.

flexibility   Flexibility is recognized as an important component of physical fitness, and flexibility conditioning should be part of any complete fitness program. Like other components of fitness, flexibility is more important in some sports than in others, but it is useful in all. For example, long-distance runners tend to be relatively inflexible because the activity of running does not require large deviations in joint motion. Sprinters and hurdlers, however, require excessive hip motion for the sprinting stride and to clear the hurdles. Consequently, sprinters are required to be relatively flexible in the hip region. Not only are flexibility requirements sport-specific, but they can also be joint-specific. In general, athletes must have sufficient musculoskeletal flexibility to meet the demands of their chosen sport, otherwise their performance will be hindered and their risk of injury will be increased.

Definition and Measurement

Flexibility can be measured using static or dynamic tests that involve either passive or active motion. Flexibility is typically understood to refer to the maximum available range of motion in a joint or series of joints. For example, the passive straight leg raise test measures hip flexion range of motion with the knee extended, and is thought to reflect hamstring flexibility. This is a measure of static flexibility, measured passively. Field tests of flexibility generally involve passive static measures. However, tests of maximum active motion, such as the sit and reach test, are also commonly used. More recently there has been increased interest in the measurements of dynamic flexibility whereby the passive or active stiffness of muscle is quantified. While these measurements are thought to better reflect the functional significance of flexibility, the measurement techniques are not conducive to testing large populations.

While the term *flexibility* is generally thought to refer to the extensibility of muscles, the measurements are also affected by the looseness of ligaments and joints. The most flexible athletes also tend to have looseness in their ligaments.

Developing Flexibility

An individual's flexibility is an inherent attribute with some potential for adaptation to habitual activity or with flexibility training. Flexibility training refers to the practice of stretching. There are many approaches to stretching musculoskeletal tissues, but typically stretching practices involve some type of static or ballistic stretches. Static stretches are thought to be safer because they involve a slow passive stretch to the targeted muscle. The muscle is held in a stretched position for a time period usually varying from 10 to 60 seconds, and this is repeated two to six times. Ballistic stretches are cyclic active movements intended to repeatedly stretch and release the target muscle group without a hold period. Five to ten repetitions or cyclic movements for up to 60 seconds are typical. There is some injury risk with ballistic stretching if the movement velocity is high.

Regardless of the type of stretch that is utilized, it is essential that the stretch sufficiently stresses the target muscle or joints in order to induce an adaptation. However, it is also important to avoid causing an injury by overstressing the target area. Therefore, the recommendation is to stretch to the point of mild discomfort but not to the point of pain. One of the first adaptations to a stretching program is an increased tolerance of stretch, whereby the perceived discomfort decreases for a given degree of stretch. This allows for an increase in joint range of motion. For long-term improvements in flexibility, stretching should be performed at least every other day for a minimum of six weeks. However, soon after training discontinues the gains in flexibility will start to reverse.

Flexibility and Injury Risk

The flexibility concerns of the athlete should be twofold: 1) Does the athlete have sufficient specific flexibility to adequately perform the activities required of his or her sport? 2) Is the athlete's overall flexibility sufficient so as not to place him or her at increased risk for injury? Too often, the emphasis is on overall flexibility rather than addressing the specific flexibility requirements of a given sport. The association between flexibility and injury risk is often overstated and interpreted simplistically. The inflexible or "tight" athlete may not be at increased risk for injury. It is probably those athletes at either extreme of the flexibility continuum that may be at increased risk. The key is to determine the flexibility patterns typical for individuals in a given sport and assess the athletes with inadequate flexibility so they can be encouraged to work on improving their flexibility by emphasizing that it is not within the accepted standards for their sport.

Warm-up and stretching prior to a sports activity are thought to protect against injury and prepare the athlete to adequately perform the given activity. It is important to consider warm-up and stretching prior to activity as distinct from flexibility. Flexibility is largely an inherent or intrinsic attribute while pre-activity warm-up and stretching are practices that the athlete chooses to perform. Warm-up and stretching are as important to the flexible athlete as the inflexible athlete. Warm up by lightly exercising the major muscle groups to be used in the given activity. This has the same effect as lightly stretching those muscles. Both activities decrease the passive tension in the muscles, thereby increasing available joint motion.

Flexibility and Aging

Flexibility is known to decrease with age, and the older athlete often complains of increased stiffness when trying to perform habitual sporting activities. The loss of flexibility parallels the age-associated loss of strength. The primary flexibility problem is that the functional range within which the muscles operate decreases as one gets older. Surprisingly, the muscle stiffness with this functional range is not significantly increased. The muscles are simply shorter and subsequently lose their ability to operate effectively at the extremes of motion. Although flexibility exercises are useful in improving mobility, maintaining muscle strength throughout the range of motion is probably more important for the elderly.

flexus hallucis longus (FHL) tenosynovitis Commonly seen in dancers who perform *en pointe,* FHL tenosynovitis also occurs in runners, especially sprinters, and soccer players. Tendons are the strong cords that connect muscle to bone throughout the body. The flexor hallucis longus (FHL) tendon in the foot serves to flex the great toe, elevate the arch, and assist with plantar flexion of the ankle. Tenosynovitis refers to inflammation of this tendon and the sheath in which the tendon is housed.

Causes

Although foot injuries can result from a variety of situations, FHL tenosynovitis commonly results from overuse, intense workouts, improper footwear, and exercising on hard surfaces. When dancers and sprinters work out, they repeatedly push off, rising onto the big toe and arching their feet. This motion, which places the foot in a plantar flexed position, stresses the FHL tendon, sometimes causing FHL tenosynovitis.

Diagnosis

Patients with FHL tenosynovitis will often complain of tightness in the first MTP joint, which is the joint where the big toe joins the foot. They often describe pain along the course of the tendon, which runs from the ankle under the arch to the big toe. The doctor may observe a clicking or locking of the FHL when the foot is flexed. There is usually no tenderness to the touch since the tendon is located deep within the foot, but patients usually report some pain and weakness when asked to flex the foot against resistance. The pain associated with FHL tenosynovitis improves with rest and worsens in sports that require pushing off or extended running.

A simple radiograph of the foot may help to diagnose this problem. If the doctor suspects a tear in the ligament, a MAGNETIC RESONANCE IMAGING (MRI) scan may be necessary.

Treatment

Conservative treatment for the FHL tenosynovitis includes immobilization of the foot, restricted activity, and use of nonsteroidal anti-inflammatories to reduce the swelling and help with the pain.

Following the immobilization, some PHYSICAL THERAPY is helpful in restoring full range of movement to the foot. Exercises that build strength and balance are also helpful in speeding the return to normal activity. When an athlete returns to his or her sport, it may be helpful initially to tape or brace the foot to provide additional support. But players should not resume normal activity until they have achieved a return of about 90 percent of the strength in the affected foot, their range of motion is fully restored, and they are essentially pain free.

Steroid agents are sometimes injected into the tendon sheath to treat chronic inflammation, but this treatment is normally reserved for injuries that do not respond to any other treatment. Surgery is rarely necessary unless there is a rupture in the ligament.

frostbite   Frostbite is an injury caused by freezing of the skin and underlying body tissues. The toes, feet, fingers, hands, nose, and ears are the body parts most vulnerable to frostbite.

Causes

Frostbite occurs when part of the body is exposed to temperatures or wind chills below freezing, causing the temperature of the body part to drop below freezing. The skin and body tissues just below the skin become frozen, and the blood flow decreases.

Diagnosis

Frostbitten skin may appear hard, pale (white or blue), and cold to the touch. There may be a tingling sensation or numbness. In severe cases of frostbite, the skin may blister or turn black. Examination by a doctor will include checking for appearance of these symptoms as well as a history of exposure to cold.

Treatment

If frostbite is suspected and medical help is unavailable, find shelter and begin rewarming the frostbitten skin. The following methods are the best way to do this:

- Place the hands under the armpits or the feet against a warm person's belly.
- Dry and cover the frostbitten area with warm clothes and then layers of blankets.
- Immerse the area in warm water (about 105°F, or 40°C).

Rewarming the frostbitten skin can be painful and often takes up to an hour. If needed, the patient may take acetaminophen, ibuprofen, or aspirin for pain relief. When the area is thawed, cover it with a clean cloth or bandage. It may blister. Continue to warm the body by drinking warm fluids such as coffee or tea. Never drink alcohol or smoke when suffering from frostbite. Also avoid putting snow or direct heat on the frostbitten area. It is important that the frostbitten skin not refreeze once it has thawed because the tissue damage will be worse the second time.

If the frostbitten areas do not look normal after thawing, go to an emergency medical facility at once. Treatment may include a shot of a strong pain reliever and hyperbaric oxygen, which is oxygen at greater than normal atmospheric pressure. It is administered in a special chamber to deliver high levels of oxygen to frostbitten tissues. Body parts that have suffered severe frostbite may need to be amputated if there is presence of gangrene.

In most cases, full recovery from frostbite is likely if only the skin and uppermost tissue layers were affected. However, the recovery process is slow, and it may take some time for frostbitten areas to regain full sensation and strength. In some cases, numbness at the tips of fingers or toes does not improve, and a body part that has been frostbitten will always be more sensitive to the cold than parts of the body that have not been frostbitten.

Since the recovery process is slow, the full extent of the injury may not be known for up to six weeks. Sometimes permanent damage occurs when blood vessels are injured. Tissues then die because of the lack of oxygen, and the dead tissue can become infected. Gangrene can be fatal, so the dead area may have to be amputated, but sometimes the blackened areas of severe frostbite heal if they are cared for properly under medical supervision.

Prevention

Frostbite is best prevented by being prepared for the cold and dressing appropriately. Be sure clothing provides protection for the head, ears, nose, hands, and feet. It is always preferable to wear several layers of clothing rather than a single, thick layer. The best materials for layering include polypropylene, polyester, and wool, all of which provide good insulation and keep moisture away from the skin. Wear an outer garment over the layers that is waterproof but will also "breathe," such as Gore-Tex.

frozen shoulder (adhesive capsulitis)   Frozen shoulder, or adhesive capsulitis, is a condition characterized by a loss of motion in the shoulder joint, as the name implies. It is frequently caused by injury that leads to lack of use due to pain. When this happens, intermittent periods of use may cause inflammation, and adhesions, or abnormal bands of tissue, may grow between the joint surfaces, restricting motion. This is also accompanied by a lack of synovial fluid, which normally lubricates the gap between the arm bone and socket to help the shoulder joint move. Adhesive capsulitis is distinguished from other less complicated stiff shoulders by the presence of this restricted space between the capsule and ball of the humerus. The condition rarely appears in people under 40 years old and is most common in people between the ages of 40 and 60. It is twice as common in women as in men.

Causes

The shoulder joint is a ball and socket joint. The ball is the top of the arm bone, or humeral head, and the socket is the glenoid. Together they form the glenohumeral joint. In the normal state, the shoulder joint has more range of motion than any other joint in the body. With frozen shoulder, however, the limits in motion can make this a functionally useless joint. These limitations may develop over time as a result of painful movement that gradually causes less and less shoulder use, restricting its usual range of motion. Sometimes, however, a frozen shoulder may occur for no known reason. In addition to injury that leads to lack of use, other risk factors for developing frozen shoulder include diabetes, stroke, accidents, lung disease, and heart disease.

Diagnosis

The diagnosis of frozen shoulder is often used for any painful shoulder condition associated with a loss of motion, but it is important to understand the cause of the symptoms in order for the appropriate treatment to be prescribed. Other conditions can also cause restricted motion and a stiff joint, but with frozen shoulder, the joint becomes so tight and stiff that it is nearly impossible to carry out simple movements, such as raising the arm. People complain that the stiffness and discomfort worsens at night. A doctor may suspect the patient has a frozen shoulder if a physical examination reveals limited shoulder movement. An arthrogram may confirm the diagnosis.

The condition is characterized by a decrease in motion, primarily lifting the arm and turning it inward. The shoulder will lose its normal ability to move in all directions. The patient may not be able to lift the arm above the head or be able to scratch the back. Movement of the shoulder may be very painful. The patient may feel grinding when moving the shoulder.

The doctor will take a thorough medical history and perform a physical examination. The history will focus on uncovering any recent trauma to the shoulder, as well as on establishing a timeline for the symptoms. The physical examination will focus on determining the range of motion available in the shoulder and the specific points where pain is felt. X rays may be necessary, including an arthrogram which is an X ray taken after dye is injected into the injured area of the body. A MAGNETIC RESONANCE IMAGING (MRI) scan may also be requested.

People usually experience pain as the first symptom of frozen shoulder, followed by the loss of motion and a decrease in pain. Normally a gradual return of motion will follow; however, the length of time for recovery from frozen shoulder can be prolonged, with an average duration of 18 months.

The necessary and sufficient criteria for the diagnosis of a frozen shoulder are:

• functionally significant restriction of shoulder motion
• absence of history of previous major shoulder injury or surgery
• limited glenohumeral motion in all directions
• no changes in cartilaginous joint space shown in X ray
• absence of pathological changes other than osteopenia, which is bone loss associated with aging and osteoporosis

Treatment

The doctor will most likely prescribe a program of physical therapy, including stretching exercises to be done at home. In addition, he or she may prescribe an anti-inflammatory medication as well as an injection of a corticosteroid medication into the shoulder joint. When the shoulder is painful, it is important to use ice packs on the shoulder for 20 to 30 minutes three or four times a day. In some cases, the doctor may also recommend a type of therapy called transcutaneous nerve stimulation (TENS), which uses a small battery-operated unit to reduce pain by blocking nerve impulses.

In cases that do not respond to therapy, the doctor may discuss doing what is called a "manipulation under anesthesia." In this procedure, the patient is put to sleep with a general anesthetic and the doctor moves the shoulder in various directions to break up the adhesions, or bands of scar tissue, that have formed in the shoulder capsule. The patient may also require arthroscopic surgery to see if there are other causes for frozen shoulder. Surgery to probe into the joint and cut the adhesions is necessary only in some cases.

The goal of rehabilitation is to return the patient to his or her sport or activity as soon as is safely possible. If the patient returns too soon, the condition may worsen, which could lead to permanent damage. Everyone recovers from injury at a different rate. Return to the activity will be determined by how soon the shoulder recovers, not by how many days or weeks it has been since the injury occurred. In general, the longer a patient has symptoms before starting treatment, the longer it will take to get better.

It is safe to return to normal activities when the following conditions are present:

• The injured shoulder has full range of motion without pain.

• The injured shoulder has regained normal strength compared to the uninjured shoulder.

In throwing sports, it is especially important not to overdo it at first. The patient must gradually rebuild tolerance to throwing. This means the patient should start with gentle tossing and gradually throw harder. In contact sports, the shoulder must not be tender to touch, and contact should progress from minimal contact to harder contact.

Prevention

Following a shoulder injury, it is important for the patient to begin working on restoring normal range of motion as soon as the doctor feels it is safe to do so. It is also important to do shoulder rehabilitation exercises as they have been prescribed. Patients should be careful about observing their progress and should consult with their doctor if they feel they are losing a range of motion.

gamekeeper's thumb Gamekeepers used to kill barnyard chickens by placing the bird's neck between the thumb and forefinger and snapping the neck of the bird. The thumb would sometimes suffer injury due to the extreme force placed on the knuckle joint, often causing a ligament to stretch or rupture. This would cause pain and weakness with the pinch grasp of the thumb. Now the injury is more commonly associated with skiers, who are vulnerable to the injury due to their use of ski poles. This is actually a more acute injury and usually occurs when a skier's hand lands on a ski pole, causing an extreme force on the thumb. This is often called "skier's thumb." The injury is fairly common and occurs regardless of the type of ski pole used. Gamekeeper's thumb is sometimes treated as a minor sprain, but it can seriously affect ability to pinch or grasp, so it should be treated by a sports medicine specialist or hand surgeon in order to ensure proper and full recovery.

Causes

Following are some of the most common causes of gamekeeper's thumb:

- skiing with poles
- falling on an outstretched arm with the thumb extended
- extreme force placed on the knuckle joint of the thumb
- rheumatoid arthritis
- generally stretched ligaments in the thumb

Diagnosis

A thorough medical history and a physical examination will be combined in the determination of a diagnosis. The history will focus on revealing any injury caused to the thumb. The most common history in patients diagnosed with gamekeeper's thumb is a fall on an outstretched arm with the thumb in an extended position, which commonly occurs when using a ski pole. The ski pole prevents the patient from drawing the thumb in when falling.

In the physical examination, the doctor will want to examine the uninjured thumb to determine a baseline for range of motion and stability. The injured thumb should be evaluated for swelling and pain. In many cases, bruising accompanies the injury. The doctor will want to check the ligaments to determine if the injury involves stretching of the ligament or a possible rupture. Another possibility is gamekeeper's fracture, a condition in which part of the bone is actually pulled away. Defining the exact type of injury is necessary in determining the appropriate treatment.

Lab tests are not necessary in diagnosing gamekeeper's thumb. X rays must be taken before any manipulation of the thumb occurs to ensure there are no fractures involved. Careful stress examination using anesthesia during the physical examination will usually be adequate to make the diagnosis concerning damage to the ligament. However, arthrography, ultrasound, and MAGNETIC RESONANCE IMAGING (MRI) have all been used effectively to identify ruptured, or completely torn, ligaments.

Treatment

Partial tears, or stretched ligaments may be successfully treated with immobilization of the thumb in a cast for four weeks. The cast needs to be well molded around the MP joint, which is the knuckle joint. These treatments have a high success rate.

Torn or ruptured ligaments require surgical intervention for repair, and this surgery is best done as soon as possible following the injury for best results. Surgeries that take place more than three weeks after the injury occurs have an increased chance of being unsuccessful, meaning there may be permanent weakness and pain associated with the pinch grasp if the surgery occurs outside the three-week window. In addition, arthritis is more likely to develop in the thumb's knuckle joint if the ligament is not repaired sooner.

Some torn ligaments are treated with bracing, but full stability may not be returned to the thumb with this approach, and thus it is only recommended in cases in which the patient cannot tolerate surgery.

If a patient undergoes surgery, the thumb will usually be placed in a cast following the operation for at least four weeks, at which time the cast and any pins placed in the thumb may be removed. Then the patient wears a hand-based splint to immobilize the knuckle joint for two more weeks. During these two weeks, the splint is removed for therapy, during which time active motion is reintroduced to the joint. After three months, unrestricted movement of the thumb is allowed.

Complications of surgical treatment for gamekeeper's thumb include nerve injury and stiffness of the knuckle joint in the injured thumb. Other complications are associated with failure to treat the injury in a timely manner and include chronic instability in the thumb. Treatment in the form of ligament reconstruction is sometimes the only way to address chronic instability.

Following a surgical repair and the period in which the thumb is immobilized, patients may begin to return to sports. This usually occurs about three months following the surgery. Premature return to full activity can stress the repair of the ligament and cause chronic joint instability, which is then very difficult to treat. Chronic pain and degeneration can then develop at the knuckle joint of the thumb.

If there has been an early diagnosis and the ligament has been repaired within three weeks of the injury, the prognosis for a complete recovery is good. When nonoperative treatment is chosen, the result will usually be a painless thumb with nearly normal motion. Pain and stiffness can be expected to be mild or absent, and pinch and grip strength should be nearly normal.

Prevention

Since gamekeeper's thumb occurs most often as a result of accidents involving extreme stress to the thumb, there is no known means of prevention. There are, however, ski gloves being designed to protect thumbs during falls, but these have not yet been proven effective.

glucosamine The nutritional supplement most commonly mentioned as a treatment for various forms of arthritis, glucosamine is naturally synthesized in the body and is an important component in the repair and maintenance of joint cartilage. It is a carbohydrate, or complex sugar, that the body makes from sugar in foods. The body uses the substance to form cartilage, the protective tissue in joints. It is important in providing nutrition for cartilage cells as well as in determining the mechanical properties of the cartilage.

How It Works

It is believed that the oral supplement provides the following benefits in the prevention and treatment of osteoarthritis:

- plays a role in maintenance and repair of cartilage
- stimulates cartilage cells to synthesize cartilage building blocks
- may have an anti-inflammatory action by interfering with cartilage breakdown

Damaged cartilage has difficulty repairing itself because it has such a poor blood supply. It is believed that taking oral supplements of glucosamine enhances the cartilage's ability to repair itself. Studies have shown that improvement of symptoms of osteoarthritis may occur when taking supplements of glucosamine, but no long-term protective effect for the cartilage has been shown.

Most medical professionals believe it is reasonable to try glucosamine for the relief of pain and the restoration of the cartilage. There are few side effects, and the medication is not overly expensive. Remember, however, that this is not a controlled medication and as a result there is great variation in the quality of the product available in stores. It would be wise to read all labels well and review all components present in the substance.

Sources

Glucosamine supplement, which is made from the shells of crabs and other shellfish, is available in pill form at most health food and vitamin stores.

Side Effects

Glucosamine generally has few side effects, though there have been some reports of stomach pain, heartburn, and diarrhea with its use.

Recent research suggests that glucosamine may increase blood sugar levels in people with diabetes. People with diabetes should consult the doctor if interested in using glucosamine. They may need extra monitoring when using this supplement.

Be Aware

- Glucosamine is most effective for early arthritis when cartilage is still present.

- Glucosamine is less effective for severe arthritis.

- Glucosamine appears safe; however, more long-term research is needed to determine effectiveness.

- Glucosamine is not regulated in the United States, so finding a trustworthy manufacturer can be difficult.

- Taking an oral supplement such as glucosamine is not the first step in addressing symptoms of osteoarthritis. Losing weight if overweight, exercising the muscles around the arthritic joints, and avoiding painful activities that place a lot of weight on the joints are all significant steps that should be taken to address painful joints.

gluteal strain The gluteal muscles are the muscles in the buttocks. A gluteal strain occurs when the muscle fibers of the gluteal muscles are stretched or torn.

Causes

A gluteal strain usually occurs with running or jumping. It is often seen in hurdlers and dancers.

Diagnosis

An athlete with a gluteal strain complains of pain in the buttocks. There may be pain when walking up or down stairs and pain when sitting. Moving the leg backward usually causes pain as well.

After taking a complete medical history and recording the symptoms experienced by the patient, the doctor will perform a physical exam that will focus on checking the hips, buttocks, and legs for tenderness around the gluteal muscles. This is the most significant indicator of gluteal strain.

Treatment

Initial treatment of a gluteal strain involves icing the injury for 20 to 30 minutes every three to four hours for two or three days or until the pain goes away. The doctor may also prescribe an anti-inflammatory medication and provide a set of rehabilitation exercises.

While recovering from the injury, it is important to change the sport or activity that aggravates or causes the injury. If running causes pain in the gluteal muscles, for example, the patient should switch to swimming.

Although the goal is to return to activities as quickly as possible, it is important not to return too soon because this may worsen the injury and lengthen the total recovery time required for the injury to heal. In general, an athlete can return to full activities when he or she has full range of motion and strength in the injured gluteal muscles compared to the uninjured muscles. The athlete should also be able to run, sprint, and jump without pain or limping.

Prevention

Gluteal strains are best prevented by warming up properly and doing stretching exercises before strenuous activity. Proper rest between workouts is also important for athletes who rely heavily on their gluteal muscles. This includes hurdlers, dancers, sprinters, pole vaulters, and gymnasts, among others.

golfer's elbow Golfer's elbow, also known as medial epicondylitis and as wrist flexor tendonitis, is a painful inflammation of the bony bump on the inner side of the elbow that usually results from a specific strain, overuse, or a direct traumatic blow.

The elbow joint is made up of the bone in the upper arm, the humerus, and one of the bones in the lower arm, the ulna. The bony bumps at the bottom of the humerus are called the epicondyles. The bump on the side closest to the body is called the medial epicondyle, and the bump on the outer side of the elbow is called the lateral epicondyle. The tendons of the muscles that work to bend the wrist attach at the medial epicondyle.

Golfer's elbow is quite similar in pathology to TENNIS ELBOW, which affects the opposite side of the elbow.

Causes

The funny bone on the inside of the elbow, the medial epicondyle, is where the muscles that are responsible for bending the wrist down begin. Forceful and repeated bending of the wrist and fingers cause tiny ruptures of the muscle and tendon to this area. Small tears in the muscle begin to heal but when re-injured by continued use, they become scarred and painful.

Although called golfer's elbow, medial epicondylitis is seen in a wide variety of people who are overusing their arm in some repetitive activity. It commonly occurs in throwing sports and in racket sports, as well as in golf. It also may happen in work activities such as carpentry or typing.

In the golf swing, the flexor muscles and tendons must tighten to hit the ball. Similar tasks that require repeated bending of the wrist, gripping, grasping, and turning the hand will also cause medial epicondylitis. The most common cause is overuse of the muscles that are attached to the bone at this part of the elbow, that is to say, the muscles that pull the palm of the hand toward the arm, the wrist flexors. All the flexor muscles of the hand attach to the inner elbow. If they are strained or overused, they become inflamed, which means they are swollen, painful, and tender to touch. Sometimes the inflammation is caused by a direct injury or bang. Sometimes, especially when the cause is direct injury or strain, the muscles are actually partially torn.

Rarely, the inflammation comes on without any definite cause, and this may be due to arthritis, rheumatism, or gout. Sometimes the problem is partly or completely due to a neck problem, which is causing pain in the elbow via the nerves from the neck.

Diagnosis

Patients with golfer's elbow tend to complain about pain and tenderness at the elbow. Movement of the elbow, and movements that involve lifting something with the hand underneath, palm turned upward, usually produce pain as well. The pain occurs on the inside of the elbow, the side closest to the body, and may extend down the entire inner side of the forearm when the wrist is in a bent position. Making a fist may also cause pain.

A doctor will take a complete medical history and conduct a physical examination in order to determine a diagnosis. A history of the symptoms, including any traumatic injury to the elbow, will be taken, and the doctor will test for tenderness at the elbow and pain with various movements, including flexing the wrist toward the arm against resistance. The doctor may also examine the neck since this may be the cause of the problem or part of the problem.

Treatment

Patients with golfer's elbow should apply ice packs to the elbow for 20 to 30 minutes every three to four hours for two or three days or until the pain goes away. If the elbow is swollen, the patient should elevate it by placing a pillow underneath it when lying down and by elevating it on the back of a chair or couch while sitting. Compression may also help, so the doctor may provide an elastic bandage to wrap around the elbow to keep it from swelling. Taking anti-inflammatory medications to reduce the swelling and help control the pain may also be recommended. A wrist splint holds the wrist in one position, limiting stresses at the elbow. Pain with activity is a sign that irritation is occurring. Try to avoid movements and activities that increase pain. As healing continues, different types of exercises are used. Physiotherapy treatments, which may include heat or ultrasound therapy, can be tried as well. Early on, isometric exercises help to maintain muscle mass without over stressing the tissue. Later, progressive resistive exercises are used to increase endurance and strength. The doctor may also prescribe a tennis elbow strap for the patient to wear just below the tender spot on the elbow. This will allow the forearm muscles to pull against the strap instead of against the painful epicondyle. A corticosteroid injection around the medial epicondyle may be given to reduce the inflammation.

Only very severe cases of medial epicondylitis require surgery. This happens generally when all other forms of treatment have been tried without success. In the surgery, the tendons that attach to the medial epicondyle are split to reveal the scar tissue so that this scar tissue can be removed. Following surgery, the patient will need about three weeks before resuming light activities and about three months before resuming heavy activities and sports.

During the recovery period, it is important not to do the sport or activity that caused the injury. Concentrate on activities that do not stress the wrist. The goal of rehabilitation is to return the patient to his or her sport or activity as soon as is safely possible. Returning too soon may worsen the injury, which could lead to permanent damage. When the patient is able to forcefully grip a tennis racket, bat, or golf club, or do activities such as working at a keyboard without pain in the elbow, it is safe to return to those activities. In sports such as gymnastics, it is important to be able to bear weight on the elbow without pain. There should also be no swelling around the injured elbow, and it should have regained its normal strength compared to the uninjured elbow. There must be full range of motion in order for the elbow to be considered healed.

Prevention

Since golfer's elbow occurs because of overuse to the muscles that bend the wrist, it is important to avoid this kind of repetitive overuse. At the earliest signs of pain on the inner side of the elbow, slow the activity and seek treatment. Wearing a tennis elbow strap and doing elbow stretching exercises will help prevent the condition from developing.

In addition, taking frequent breaks during work or play, improving overall arm muscle condition, and limiting heavy pushing, pulling, and grasping motions will also help.

groin strain   A strain is a stretch or tear of a muscle or tendon. People commonly call such an injury a "pulled" muscle. The muscles in the groin help bring the legs together. There are two muscles that may commonly become injured in a groin strain. These are the adductor magnus, which is the large muscle running down the inner side of the thigh, and the sartorius, which is a thinner muscle that starts on the outside of the hip, crosses the thigh, and attaches near the inside of the knee.

Causes

A groin strain most commonly occurs in sports that involve running or jumping, especially when there is a forced or abrupt push-off or cut. Football, basketball, soccer, hockey, and lacrosse can all present conditions that make athletes especially vulnerable to groin strains.

Diagnosis

Pain or tenderness along the inner side of the thigh or in the groin area signal a possible groin strain. The athlete usually has pain when bringing the legs together and sometimes when doing knee lifts.

The doctor will take a medical history to determine the possible cause of the injury and when the injury may have occurred. The physical examination will include close inspection of the thigh and hip, checking especially for tenderness and pain.

Treatment

Treatment often includes the application of ice initially for 20 to 30 minutes every three or four hours for the first three days following detection of the injury. Anti-inflammatory medication may be prescribed by the doctor. Often the doctor will also prescribe wearing a protective bandage called a thigh wrap or taping the thigh and groin to provide an extra support. Rehabilitation exercises are also part of the usual treatment approach.

During recovery, it is important that the athlete not participate in activities that aggravate the injury. This means switching from the sport that caused the injury to something that does not affect the groin as much. Once the pain is gone and the athlete has full range of motion and strength in the groin again, as well as the ability to run, sprint, and jump without pain or limping, it is safe to begin gradually returning to normal activities.

Prevention

A groin strain is best prevented by warming up properly and doing groin muscle stretching exercises prior to sports activities. This is especially important for athletes who participate in activities such as sprinting and jumping.

hamate fracture The wrist and hand are the most common sites for upper-extremity injuries in sports activities, and the wrist joint can be daunting in its complexity. As a result, physicians have often resorted to the vague diagnosis of wrist strain or sprain in patients injured during sports activity. This type of diagnosis has begun to change in recent years as a greater understanding of specific injuries has led to more specific diagnoses and better treatment of wrist injuries. As with any injury, a more accurate diagnosis and treatment leads to more complete recovery and shorter recovery time.

The hamate bone is the wrist bone in line with the fourth and fifth fingers of the hand. Fractures to the hamate are common in athletics and may be either isolated or associated with more widespread injury. Hamate fractures are most often seen in sports such as baseball, tennis, racquetball, squash, and golf, where the athlete uses a bat, racket, or club. Most of these injuries are not acute and patients do not show symptoms until days or weeks following the occurrence of the injury. Exceptions to this include traumatic injury of the wrist, such as with a crushing blow to the wrist that produces immediate symptoms and requires immediate attention.

Causes

Hamate fractures generally are associated with sports activities that use a racket, bat, or club. The hook of the hamate is fractured most often in one of two ways. Falling on an outstretched hand that affects the ulnar side of the wrist may fracture the hook as a result of direct trauma. More frequently, injury is incurred while the individual is engaged in a sport involving a racket, bat, or club. These fractures are the result of shear forces transmitted through ligamentous insertions, as the wrist is hyperextended forcibly while gripping an object. In these cases, the fracture usually occurs when a handle sharply strikes the palm of the hand.

In sports such as baseball, hockey, and golf, hamate fractures usually occur in the nondominant hand. Fractures to the dominant hand often occur in racket sports. More serious injuries are usually the result of direct force trauma or crush injuries.

Diagnosis

Patients with a hamate fracture often show symptoms days or even weeks after the injury has occurred. They normally complain of pain in the palm of the hand and decreased grip strength. More acute injuries sometimes occur following a hard swing of the bat, racket, or club or some sort of direct trauma to the wrist. Patients will present with symptoms immediately following such injury.

The hamate is made up of two parts—the hook and the body. Injury can occur to either or both of these. Fracture of the hook is commonly an isolated injury and is the most common hamate fracture. These fractures may occur during a fall on an outstretched wrist or, most often, while swinging a bat, racket, or golf club. Isolated fracture to the body of the hamate can occur, but it is fairly rare and requires some sort of direct force to the wrist.

During a physical examination, the physician will usually palpate the point of symptoms, and this reveals specific tenderness over the hook of the hamate. If there is significant swelling and no apparent damage to nerves or blood vessels, the hand and wrist can be rested for three days before further assessment of the injury. In cases of more severe injury, however, the physician will need to order basic X rays and then complete more detailed exploration under anesthesia. X rays should include multiple views of the wrist in order to be certain of revealing the damage. In cases where the physical examination suggests a hamate fracture but the X ray is questionable, COMPUTERIZED AXIAL TOMOGRAPHY (CAT) SCANS should be ordered to confirm the diagnosis. Lab studies are not normally required in the diagnosis of hamate fracture.

Treatment

Treatment ranges from immobilization to corticosteroid injections to surgical repair of a fracture or underlying cause. Hamate fractures are prone to nonunion and may result in secondary complications, thus their treatment is often complex.

Standard treatment of a hook fracture usually involves excision of the hook fragment and smoothing the base to prevent future tendon chafing, which can interfere with complete recovery.

In acute injuries, immobilization may be adequate for the fracture to heal. When there is swelling but no apparent neurovascular damage, the patient should apply ice to the area and keep the upper extremity elevated as much as possible for 72 hours before further treatment.

An orthopedic or hand surgery consultation is necessary for patients requiring surgical intervention. In injuries that require surgical repair, the wrist is usually immobilized in a cast if the treatment occurs shortly after the injury. In serious baseball players, the physician will often perform an excision of the bone fragment from the hook in order to avoid recurrent pain and injury and to return the player to the field as soon as possible.

Fractures to the body of the hamate are commonly associated with dislocation of the fourth and fifth fingers. Although reduction of the joints in these fingers can often repair the injury, internal fixation of the fractured bone in surgery is usually required because there is a high incidence of instability in these injuries in the hand.

During surgery, one possible complication is compression of the ulnar nerve, which is located close to the hook of the hamate. Care must be taken to prevent damage to the motor branch of the ulnar nerve, which turns around the hook of the hamate and travels deep into the surrounding musculature. Additionally, rupture of the tendons in the small finger and ring finger may sometimes occur as a result of the irregular edges of the fracture.

PHYSICAL THERAPY is not recommended until substantial healing or fracture consolidation has taken place and the patient is ready to regain range of motion of the wrist and hand. The stages of recovery include wound healing, recovery of motion, recovery of strength and power, and recovery of endurance. Early motion in the recovery of a hamate fracture is associated with better functioning following recovery. When new collagen is first forming following the injury, it has more elasticity and allows for greater movement. Over time, scarring of the collagen occurs, decreasing its range of movement. In most injuries, active range-of-motion exercises can be performed as soon as 48 to 72 hours following surgery. The application of heat will enhance the patient's ability to perform the exercises.

The return of muscle strength and power comes with exercising the hand and wrist. The more the patient exercises a group of muscles, the more endurance those muscles build. The exercises should be tailored to meet the demands of the patient's sport and occupation. During this period of physical therapy, every effort should be made to avoid swelling. Elevation, compression, and motion should all be used to move excess fluid away from the wound. This helps to limit the build-up of scar tissue, which can occur as a by-product of the swelling.

As the patient regains endurance, the exercises should focus more and more on specific sports-related or work-related activities. In typical injuries of the hamate, the fractures are unified within six to eight weeks, and the patient can return to full pre-injury activity. However, if the patient participates in contact sports, the hand and wrist should be given extra support in the form of a brace or other protection. Normally, muscle strength and flexibility will have returned to pre-injury levels within about 12 weeks of the injury if the patient is diligent in performing physical therapy exercises. If there is persistent pain, the injury should be reevaluated for a possible nonunion of the fracture of a fracture line that was not seen on the first examination.

The prognosis is excellent for patients with simple hamate fractures who are treated soon after the injury occurs and who are committed to their physical therapy program. Crush injuries of the hamate body with massive tissue loss are more complicated and may involve repeated attempts at repair.

Prevention

Athletes who maintain excellent strength and flexibility in their wrists have a better chance of avoiding wrist injuries. Those who rollerblade, ski, ice skate, or participate in other sports that routinely involve diving or falling should wear protective wrist guards to prevent injuries to the wrist and hand. Golfers, too, stand a greater risk of experiencing a fracture of the hook of the hamate as a result of the repetitive wrist extension involved in the swing. Using clubs that are the proper length will help to minimize the risk of this type of injury.

hammer toe   A hammer toe deformity is a condition that is most often caused by wearing shoes that are too tight. Sometimes, however, this condition can be genetic, and in these cases it is due to a nerve disorder in the foot. The hammer toe deformity occurs when the toes appear to be bent downward, grabbing the floor.

Causes

Wearing shoes that are too tight is the most common cause of hammer toe deformity. When shoes that are too short are worn, the toes are forced to curl under and remain compressed in this abnormal position. When this happens repeatedly, the toes remain in this position permanently. High-heeled shoes are especially notorious for causing this condition because they often have a toe box that is too narrow to hold the ball of the foot and toes. In addition, the toes are not only bunched up, but the weight of the body is pushing them forward even farther, causing them to curl under even more.

Diagnosis

A thorough medical history and physical exam by a physician is always necessary for the proper diagnosis of hammer toe and other foot conditions.

Because the condition involves a bone deformity, X rays can help to confirm the diagnosis.

A doctor will examine the toes in making a diagnosis and look for a deformity in the second, third, and fourth toes primarily. The big toe and little toe on either end of the foot are less likely to become deformed than the middle three toes. On the deformed toes, the main toe joint, in the middle of the toe, will be bent upward like a claw. The doctor will want to test the toes to determine if there is still flexibility in the toes or if they have become fixed. Flexible hammer toes are fairly easy to treat, but fixed toes require surgery. Often, there are calluses on the top of these middle joints where the toes have rubbed against the top of the shoe or on the tips of the toes where the toes have rubbed against the end of the shoe. In addition the patient may also feel pain in the toes or feet and have difficulty finding any shoes that are comfortable.

Treatment

Conservative treatment of hammer toe initially involves wearing more comfortable shoes. Patients must refrain from wearing any shoes that do not fit properly and that cause pain in the toes or feet. If this does not work to release the toes in a reasonable period of time, outpatient surgery with a local anesthetic will be needed to correct the problem. In this surgery, the toe joints will be loosened to allow them to realign properly. The actual procedure used will depend on the type and extent of the deformity. Following the surgery, there may be some stiffness, swelling, and redness, and the affected toes may be slightly longer or shorter than they were before.

Patients will be able to walk following surgery but should not plan to spend long periods of time on their feet until the toes have healed. It is best to keep the foot elevated above the level of the heart as much as possible to reduce the swelling.

Prevention

The most important step in preventing hammer toe is wearing shoes that fit properly. Shoes should be long enough that the toes do not touch the end of the shoe, and they should be roomy enough in width to accommodate the toes and ball of the foot without compressing the toes.

hamstring injury   The hamstrings derived their name from the butcher's practice of hanging the pig by this group of muscles located on the back of the upper leg. Injury to these muscles is common, especially among runners and those involved in contact sports such as football. Often the cause of chronic pain among athletes, hamstring injuries are classified according to the following grades:

Grade 1 is a mild strain with few muscle fibers being torn.
Grade 2 is a moderate strain with a definite loss in strength.
Grade 3 is a complete tear of the hamstrings.

Hamstring injuries occur most often in sports in which the hamstrings can be stretched in an unusual fashion at high speed. Sprinting, track and field, and other running contact sports such as football see their fair share of hamstring injuries. Recreational sports such as waterskiing, in which the knee is fully extended during injury, are also responsible for a number of hamstring injuries. An Australian study involving 1,614 individuals with hamstring injuries revealed that hamstring injuries compose 54 percent of the injuries in rugby, 10 percent of the injuries in soccer, 14 percent of the injuries in track, and less than 2 percent of the injuries in tennis, squash, ballet, and gymnastics.

In track and field events in which the hamstring is unusually contracted, the risk of hamstring injury can be high. Contact sports such as football can result in contusions, or bruises, of the hamstring muscle. The contusion is superficial when the muscle is contracted on impact and deep when the muscle is relaxed on impact. Waterskiing accidents have an association with proximal bony avulsions, or the tearing of the hamstring away from the bone, because the skier's knee is extended when the hip undergoes a violent, forceful flexion as the skier falls forward.

Causes
There are quite a few factors that predispose a person to hamstring injury. Following are some of the most common:

- The major factors that create vulnerability to hamstring injury are lack of warm-up, poor flex-ibility, fatigue, and a hamstring-to-quadriceps strength ratio of less than 50 percent.
- Poor running style, especially overstriding, predisposes some runners to hamstring injuries. Overstriding stretches the hamstring and places it in a position of active insufficiency.
- Abnormal movement of the hamstring muscles also may be a factor contributing to hamstring injuries.
- Rapid growth seen during adolescence sometimes leads to tight hip flexors, resulting in anterior hip tilt. This can cause a natural predisposition to hamstring injuries for this age group.

Diagnosis
Diagnosing a hamstring injury is usually fairly straightforward since pain, loss of strength, and sometimes swelling often accompany the injury and are located at the hamstrings. Laboratory studies typically are not needed to make the diagnosis of hamstring injury. Most often, a diagnosis can be made with history and physical examination alone. In most cases, imaging studies have no role in the workup of hamstring injuries. Following is a list of symptoms that indicate a hamstring injury:

- Onset of pain or weakness is usually sudden and may occur during an explosive movement such as sprinting.
- Patient may report hearing an audible pop at the time of injury.
- Onset of pain in the back of the thigh often occurs near the beginning or near the end of the sport activity, supporting the belief that fatigue and lack of warm-up often contribute to muscle injury.
- Patient may have a sense of apprehension due to a feeling of inadequate leg control as a result of the injury.
- Patient may report pain with sitting or while walking uphill or climbing stairs.
- Swelling and ecchymosis, which is the release of blood into the tissue surrounding broken blood vessels, may accompany more severe injuries.

Treatment
In the past, treatment options for acute hamstring injuries included intramuscular corticosteroids;

however, given evidence of delayed healing in acute muscle injury as well as muscle atrophy, this practice is discouraged. Recommended treatment varies with the severity of the injury. Minor strains may improve quickly so that athletes are able to perform strengthening exercises in PHYSICAL THERAPY within a matter of a few days. Severe hamstring injuries such as ruptures may require surgery.

For rehabilitation, the focus of physical therapy is to limit pain, inflammation, and swelling. Rest, ice, compression, and elevation (RICE) are recommended. Elastic thigh bandages can be useful for compression. Icing for 20 minutes, four times per day provides pain relief. Most patients may begin active range-of-motion (AROM) exercises within their pain tolerance after one to two days. Individuals with more serious injuries benefit from immobilization in knee extension for one to five days to prevent contracture formation, or static muscle shortening, and further damage. Crutches enable the patient to walk while still resting the injured leg.

After several days, most patients may begin pain-free isometrics, pool therapies, and upper body exercises. Isometric exercises are performed at various knee angles in increments of 20 degrees. Patients hold the contraction for five to 15 seconds and perform three sets at each angle.

Prevention

It is most important that the patient not return to normal activities too soon. This can result in delayed healing or reinjury, and in more serious injuries, compartment syndrome, or decreased circulation adversely affecting the tissue, can result from an extending hematoma. The most common symptom of compartment syndrome is increasing pain. Sports-specific training maximizes recovery and minimizes chances for additional injury as do stretching and strengthening exercises to maintain flexibility and an adequate hamstring-to-quadriceps strength ratio.

hamstring tendonitis The hamstring muscles consist of the biceps femoris, semitendinosus, and semimembranosus. These muscles are used to bend the knee. Inflammation of the tendons that connect these muscles to the bone can result from

a partial rupture of the tendon that has not healed properly or overuse of the muscles, especially in sports that involve lots of accelerating and decelerating.

Diagnosis

An athlete with hamstrings tendonitis will have tenderness and swelling over the area where the tendon inserts into the bone. There will also be pain when the athlete tries to bend the knee against resistance. Stiffness following exercise is another common complaint of the athlete who has hamstrings tendonitis.

Treatment

This is an OVERUSE INJURY and requires that the athlete rest the hamstrings in order to avoid further irritation of the tendons. This means that any activity that causes pain or tenderness in the hamstrings must be avoided. Athletes whose sports requires regular use of the hamstring muscles must switch to a different sport for a while in order to allow the hamstrings the rest they need in order to heal. Icing the injury is also helpful and will alleviate some discomfort.

The doctor will probably prescribe anti-inflammatory medication to assist with the discomfort and help the swelling. Ultrasound and laser treatment are also possibilities. A full rehabilitation program that focuses on pain reduction, stretching, strengthening, and sports massage is also part of the treatment for hamstrings tendonitis.

Prevention

As with other overuse injuries, prevention involves proper stretching before and after activity, as well as adequate rest between workouts. It is important to maintain excellent flexibility and strength in the hamstrings so that they can handle the stress of intense physical activity, especially the abrupt stress of sports that require many quick starts and stops.

heat cramps Heat cramps are the mildest form of heat injury and consist of painful muscle cramps and spasms that occur during or after intense exercise and sweating in high heat. They often occur in the muscles at the back of the calves and can be very painful.

Associated with heat, DEHYDRATION, and poor conditioning more than with lack of salt or other mineral imbalances, they usually improve with rest, drinking water, and a cool environment.

Causes

Exposure to abnormal or prolonged amounts of heat and humidity without relief or adequate fluid intake can cause various types of heat-related illness. Sweat is the body's main system for getting rid of extra heat. When the body sweats, the water evaporates from the skin. The heat that evaporates the sweat comes mainly from the skin. As long as blood is flowing properly to the skin, extra heat from the core of the body is "pumped" to the skin and removed by sweat evaporation. Someone who does not sweat enough, cannot get rid of extra heat well. In addition, if blood is not flowing properly to the skin, the body will also be hindered in its efforts to get rid of excess heat.

Dehydration makes this whole cooling process more difficult. The body does not sweat as much when it is dehydrated, and it tries to keep blood away from the skin in order to ensure that blood pressure remains at the right level in the core of the body. The body also does not sweat as much in humid conditions. Humidity makes it harder for the sweat to evaporate off the skin. When the evaporation process is hindered, the body has a harder time cooling off.

In addition to these conditions, children adjust more slowly than adults to changes in environmental temperature. They sweat less than adults and produce more heat with activity than adults, which puts them at an immediate deficit when it comes to preventing heat illnesses since sweating is the body's primary cooling mechanism. In addition, children often do not think to rest when having fun and may not drink enough fluids when playing, exercising, or participating in sports.

Diagnosis

Heat cramps normally cause the following symptoms:

- painful cramps, especially in the legs
- flushed, moist skin
- mild fever, usually less than 102°F

Treatment

Treatment should consist of the following:

- Move to a cool place and rest.
- Remove excess clothing and place cool cloths on skin; fan skin.
- Give cool sports drinks containing salt and sugar such as Gatorade.
- Stretch cramped muscles slowly.

Prevention

It is possible to prevent heat-related illnesses by exercising caution when exerting oneself in hot, humid weather. It is important to stay well hydrated to make sure that the body can get rid of extra heat. The best fluid to drink when sweating is water, although sports drinks are generally fine. Although there is a little salt in sweat, the body does not really lose that much salt with sweat, except in special circumstances; taking salt tablets may raise the body's sodium level to hazardous levels. It is best to check with a doctor before beginning to take extra salt.

The hotter and more humid it is, the harder it will be for the body to get rid of excess heat. Clothing makes a difference as well. The less clothing one wears, and the lighter that clothing is, the easier it is to cool off. Those who wear heavy clothing during exertion, such as football players, are more susceptible. Football players are notoriously prone to heat illness, since football uniforms cover nearly the whole body, and since football practice usually begins in late summer when the outside temperature is highest. Football players should, therefore, pay extra attention to the fluids they drink and lose, and teams should consider limiting practice and wearing light clothing for practice on very hot days, and athletes should be able to drink all the water they want during practice.

People with chronic health problems, those who are overweight, and those who take certain medicines may be more susceptible to heat-related illnesses.

The following guidelines are helpful in preventing heat illness:

- Drink plenty of fluids during vigorous or outdoor activities (including sunbathing), especially on hot days. Drinks of choice include water and sports drinks; avoid alcohol and fluids with caffeine such as tea, coffee, and cola, as these can lead to dehydration.

- Dress children in light-colored, lightweight, tightly woven, loose-fitting clothing on hot days.
- Schedule vigorous activity and sports for cooler times of the day. Take rest periods in shady or cool areas.
- Protect children from the sun by having them wear a hat and sunglasses and by using an umbrella. Use a sunscreen that is at least SPF (sun protection factor) 15.
- Increase time spent outdoors gradually to get a child's body used to the heat.
- Teach children to take frequent drink breaks and "wet down" or mist themselves with a spray bottle to avoid becoming overheated.
- Spend as much time indoors as possible on very hot and humid days.
- Do not leave children unattended in a hot automobile.
- Teach children to warm up and cool down before and after exercising.
- If a child has a medical condition or is taking medication, consult the child's physician for further advice for preventing heat-related illnesses.

heat exhaustion   More severe than HEAT CRAMPS, heat exhaustion is the result of excessive heat and DEHYDRATION, which renders the body unable to cool itself properly. It usually occurs in conditions of extreme heat, and if left untreated, it can progress to heat stroke.

Causes

Exposure to abnormal or prolonged amounts of heat and humidity without relief or adequate fluid intake can cause various types of heat-related illness. A loss of water and salt in the body—due to extreme sweating and inadequate fluid and salt replacement—is the culprit in heat exhaustion.

Sweat is the body's main system for getting rid of extra heat. When a person sweats, the water evaporates from the skin. The heat that evaporates the sweat comes mainly from the skin. As long as blood is flowing properly to the skin, extra heat from the core of the body is "pumped" to the skin and removed by sweat evaporation. If the body does not sweat enough, it cannot get rid of extra heat well. In addition, if blood is not flowing properly to the skin, the body will also be hindered in its efforts to get rid of excess heat.

Dehydration makes this whole cooling process more difficult. The body does not sweat as much when it is dehydrated, and it tries to keep blood away from the skin in order to ensure that blood pressure remains at the right level in the core of the body. The body also does not sweat so much in humid conditions. Humidity makes it harder for the sweat to evaporate off the skin. When the evaporation process is hindered, the body has a harder time cooling off.

In addition to these conditions, children adjust more slowly than do adults to changes in environmental temperature. They sweat less than adults and produce more heat with activity than adults, which puts them at an immediate deficit when it comes to preventing heat illnesses since sweating is the body's primary cooling mechanism. In addition, children often do not think to rest when having fun and may not drink enough fluids when playing, exercising, or participating in sports.

Diagnosis

The signs of heat exhaustion include paleness, dizziness, nausea, vomiting, fainting, and a moderately increased temperature (101–102°F). This is not technically a fever, but is caused by the heat.

Common signs and symptoms of heat exhaustion include the following:

- muscle cramps
- pale, moist skin
- a fever over 102°F
- nausea
- vomiting
- diarrhea
- headache
- fatigue
- weakness
- anxiety and faint feeling

Treatment

Rest and water, as well as ice packs and a cool environment, may help in mild heat exhaustion. More severely exhausted patients may need to go to the hospital for IV fluids, especially if vomiting keeps them from drinking enough.

- Move to a cool place and rest.
- Remove excess clothing and place cool cloths on skin; fan skin.
- Give cool sports drinks containing salt and sugar such as Gatorade.
- If there is no improvement and the patient remains unable to take fluids, he or she should be taken to a doctor or emergency room immediately. IV (intravenous) fluids may be needed.

Prevention

It is possible to prevent heat-related illnesses by exercising caution when exerting in hot, humid weather. It is important to stay well hydrated to make sure that the body can get rid of extra heat. The best fluid to drink when sweating is water, although sports drinks are generally fine. Although there is a little salt in sweat, the body does not really lose that much salt with sweat, except in special circumstances; taking salt tablets may raise the body's sodium level to hazardous levels. It is best to check with a doctor before beginning to take extra salt.

The hotter and more humid it is, the harder it will be for the body to get rid of excess heat. Clothing makes a difference as well. The less clothing one wears, and the lighter that clothing is, the easier it is to cool off. Those who wear heavy clothing during exertion, such as football players, are also more susceptible. Football players are notoriously prone to heat illness, since football uniforms cover nearly the whole body, and since football practice usually begins in late summer when the outside temperature is highest. Football players should, therefore, pay extra attention to the fluids they drink and lose, and teams should consider limiting practice and wearing light clothing for practice on very hot days, and athletes should be able to drink all the water they want during practice.

People with chronic health problems, those who are overweight, and those who take certain medicines may be more susceptible to heat-related illnesses.

The following guidelines are helpful in preventing heat illness:

- Drink plenty of fluids during vigorous or outdoor activities (including sunbathing), especially on hot days. Drinks of choice include water and sports drinks; avoid alcohol and fluids with caffeine such as tea, coffee, and cola, as these can lead to dehydration.
- Dress children in light-colored, lightweight, tightly woven, loose-fitting clothing on hot days.
- Schedule vigorous activity and sports for cooler times of the day. Take rest periods in shady or cool areas.
- Protect children from the sun by having them wear a hat and sunglasses and by using an umbrella. Use a sunscreen that is at least SPF (sun protection factor) 15.
- Increase time spent outdoors gradually to get a child's body used to the heat.
- Teach children to take frequent drink breaks and "wet down" or mist themselves with a spray bottle to avoid becoming overheated.
- Spend as much time indoors as possible on very hot and humid days.
- Do not leave children unattended in a hot automobile.
- Teach children to warm up and cool down before and after exercising.
- If a child has a medical condition or is taking medication, consult the child's physician for further advice for preventing heat-related illnesses.

heat stroke   Heat stroke, the most severe form of heat illness, occurs when the body's heat-regulating system is overwhelmed by excessive heat. A life-threatening emergency that requires immediate medical attention, heat stroke can occur even in people who are not exercising if the weather is hot enough.

Causes

Exposure to abnormal or prolonged amounts of heat and humidity without relief or adequate fluid intake can cause various types of heat-related illness. Sweat is the body's main system for getting rid of extra heat. When the body sweats, the water evaporates from the skin. The heat that evaporates the sweat comes mainly from the skin. As long as blood is flowing properly to the skin, extra heat from the core of the body is "pumped" to the skin and removed by sweat evaporation. If the body does not sweat enough, it cannot get rid of extra heat well. In addition, if blood is not flowing properly to the skin, the body will also be hindered in its efforts to get rid of excess heat.

DEHYDRATION makes this whole cooling process more difficult. The body does not sweat as much when it is dehydrated, and it tries to keep blood away from the skin in order to ensure that blood pressure remains at the right level in the core of the body. The body also does not sweat as much in humid conditions. Humidity makes it harder for the sweat to evaporate off the skin. When the evaporation process is hindered, the body has a harder time cooling off.

In addition to these conditions, children adjust more slowly than do adults to changes in environmental temperature. They sweat less than adults and produce more heat with activity than adults, which puts them at an immediate deficit when it comes to preventing heat illnesses since sweating is the body's primary cooling mechanism. In addition, children often do not think to rest when having fun and may not drink enough fluids when playing, exercising, or participating in sports.

Diagnosis

The victim of a heat stroke will have warm, flushed skin, but usually a noted absence of sweat. Athletes, however, who are stricken by heat stroke after vigorous exercise in hot weather may still be sweating considerably because of the exercise itself. Whether exercise-related or not, a person with heat stroke usually has a very high temperature (106°F or higher) and may be delirious, unconscious, or having seizures.

The presence of the following symptoms will confirm a diagnosis of heat stroke:

- warm, dry skin
- high fever, usually over 104°F
- rapid heart rate
- loss of appetite
- nausea
- vomiting
- headache
- fatigue
- confusion
- agitation
- lethargy
- stupor
- seizures, coma, and death are possible

Treatment

Heat stroke patients need to have their temperature reduced quickly, often with ice packs, and must also be given IV fluids for rehydration. They must be taken to the hospital as quickly as possible and thus should go in an ambulance. They may have to stay in the hospital for observation since many different body organs can fail in heat stroke.

Treatment should consist of the following while the patient waits for medical attention:

- Move to a cool place and rest.
- Call 911 or local emergency medical service. Heat stroke is a life-threatening medical emergency and needs to be treated by a physician.
- Remove excess clothing and drench skin with cool water; fan skin.
- Place ice bags on the armpits and groin areas.
- Offer cool fluids if the patient is alert and able to drink.

Prevention

It is possible to prevent heat-related illnesses by exercising caution when exerting in hot, humid weather. It is important to stay well hydrated to make sure that the body can get rid of extra heat. The best fluid to drink when sweating is water, although sports drinks are generally fine. Although there is a little salt in sweat, the body does not really lose that much salt with sweat, except in special circumstances; taking salt tablets may raise the body's sodium level to hazardous levels. It is best to check with a doctor before beginning to take extra salt.

The hotter and more humid it is, the harder it will be for the body to get rid of excess heat. Clothing makes a difference as well. The less clothing one has on, and the lighter that clothing is, the easier it is to cool off. Those who wear heavy clothing during exertion, such as football players, are also more susceptible. Football players are notoriously prone to heat illness, since football uniforms cover nearly the whole body, and since football practice usually begins in late summer when the outside temperature is highest. Football players should, therefore, pay extra attention to the fluids they drink and lose, and teams should consider limiting practice and wearing light clothing for practice on very hot days, and athletes should be able to drink all the water they want during practice.

People with chronic health problems, those who are overweight, and those who take certain medicines may be more susceptible to heat-related illnesses.

The following guidelines are helpful in preventing heat illness:

- Drink plenty of fluids during vigorous or outdoor activities (including sunbathing), especially on hot days. Drinks of choice include water and sports drinks; avoid alcohol and fluids with caffeine such as tea, coffee, and cola, as these can lead to dehydration.

- Dress children in light-colored, lightweight, tightly woven, loose-fitting clothing on hot days.

- Schedule vigorous activity and sports for cooler times of the day. Take rest periods in shady or cool areas.

- Protect children from the sun by having them wear a hat and sunglasses and by using an umbrella. Use a sunscreen that is at least SPF (sun protection factor) 15.

- Increase time spent outdoors gradually to get a child's body used to the heat.

- Teach children to take frequent drink breaks and "wet down" or mist themselves with a spray bottle to avoid becoming overheated.

- Spend as much time indoors as possible on very hot and humid days.

- Do not leave children unattended in a hot automobile.

- Teach children to warm up and cool down before and after exercising.

- If a child has a medical condition or is taking medication, consult the child's physician for further advice for preventing heat-related illnesses.

herniated disk (slipped disk) A herniated disk, also called a "slipped" or "ruptured" disk, is a common source of lower back pain. It is a disk that has bulged out from its proper place in the back. Disks are small, circular cushions between the vertebrae, or bones of the spine, that make up the spinal column. In the middle of the spinal column is the spinal canal, a hollow space that contains the spinal cord and other nerve roots. The disks between the vertebrae allow the back to flex or bend. Normally, disks act as shock absorbers to cushion the vertebrae from one another as you move.

The outer edge of the disk is a ring of gristlelike cartilage called the annulus. The center of the disk is a gel-like substance called the nucleus. A disk herniates or ruptures when part of the center nucleus pushes the outer edge of the disk into the spinal canal, and puts pressure on nearby nerves, causing severe pain.

Causes

Disks have a high water content. As people age, the water content decreases, so the disk begins to shrink and the spaces between the vertebrae become narrower. Also, the disk itself becomes less flexible. Aging makes the disk more vulnerable to injury. A disk may be damaged in a number of different ways. These include a fall or accident, repeated straining of the back over time due to bad posture or repeated improper lifting techniques, or sudden strenuous action such as lifting a heavy weight or twisting the back violently. A herniated disk may also happen spontaneously without any specific injury.

When a disk is damaged, the fibrous outer ring may tear and the soft rubbery center of the disk can squeeze out through this weak point in the hard outer layer. Pain results when the disk material pinches and puts pressure on the nerve roots.

Sometimes fragments of the disk enter the spinal canal, where they can damage the nerves that control bowel and urinary functions.

Diagnosis

Low back pain affects four out of five people, so pain alone is not enough to recognize a herniated disk. If the herniated disk is in the neck, the symptoms may begin suddenly or gradually. The patient may wake up and feel a sudden aching, or the patient may have a twisted neck that cannot be straightened without extreme pain. There also may be numbness, tingling, or weakness in one or both arms.

If the herniated disk is below the neck, the symptoms may develop gradually or begin suddenly. Symptoms may include back pain, pain down one or both legs, numbness, tingling, or weakness in one or both legs, and changes in bladder and bowel habits. The most common symptom of a herniated disk is sciatica, a sharp, often shooting pain that extends from the buttocks down the back of one leg. This is caused by pressure on the spinal nerve.

The physician attending the patient with a herniated disk will take a complete history of the patient's medical condition, including the description of exact symptoms. A physical examination will follow, which should include examination of the spine and testing the movement and reflexes of the arms and legs. The doctor may also request that certain tests be done on the patient.

It is most likely that the patient will have either X rays, a COMPUTERIZED AXIAL TOMOGRAPHY (CAT) SCAN, or a MAGNETIC RESONANCE IMAGING (MRI) scan of the spine. In addition, a test called electromyography may be used to test the electrical activity in the muscles. Myelography is another test that involves injection of a dye into the fluid around the spinal cord so that this fluid can be seen on X rays. Finally, discography involves injection of a dye into the disks themselves so that they show up better on the X ray.

Treatment

Most cases of herniated disks can be treated successfully without surgery. In these cases, treatment for a herniated disk in the neck will probably include some or all of the following: use of hot or cold packs on the site of injury, anti-inflammatory drugs, muscle relaxants, prescription pain relievers, a neck collar or neck brace to relieve muscle spasms, neck and shoulder massage, and traction, which is a method of putting bones or muscles under tension with a system of weights and pulleys that is designed to keep the muscles and bones from moving and to relieve all pressure on them.

For a herniated disk in the back, treatment may include several days or more of lying flat on the back on a firm mattress or on an ordinary bed with a stiff board under the mattress, or lying on the belly with a pillow under the chest, whichever is more comfortable. In addition, muscle relaxants, anti-inflammatory drugs, and prescription pain relievers may be indicated. Use of hot or cold packs, traction, back massage and PHYSICAL THERAPY, and steroid injections into the space near the herniated disk may be prescribed to control the pain and inflammation and to relieve the pressure on the muscles and bones surrounding the injury.

As the pain lessens, it is important to begin a physical therapy program to help regain the strength and flexibility in the back muscles and joints. A fairly new development in the treatment of herniated disks is the use of stabilizing exercises in physical therapy. These are designed to teach the patient how to control the movement of the spine in all recreation and work activities so that reinjury does not occur.

Patients with recalcitrant pain may have to have surgery. The traditional surgical treatment is called a laminectomy and involves removing a portion of the vertebral bone. The surgery is performed under general anesthesia with an overnight hospital stay. Newer surgical techniques are minimally invasive and use a local anesthetic. Surgery is performed on an outpatient basis, and the patient is able to return to work within two to six weeks.

Most patients, however, recover well with conservative treatment as described above. Typically, the initial intense pain of a herniated disk does not last longer than a few weeks. In rare cases, it can last up to a few months. However, a patient who has experienced a herniated disk may be prone to lifelong backaches and must learn to avoid movements and activities that compromise the spine.

Practicing correct posture when walking, sitting, standing, lying down, and working is very helpful. Some guidelines follow:

- When lifting heavy objects, it is important to kneel or squat, keeping the back as straight as possible, and use the thigh muscles to do the lifting. Never bend from the waist to pick up something, and avoid twisting when lifting.

- When standing, stand straight up with the shoulders back, the abdomen in, and the small of the back flat.

- It is best to sit with the feet flat on the floor or elevated and to get up every 20 minutes or so to stretch.

- When sleeping, use a firm mattress with a bed board under it. Lie on the side with knees bent or on the back with a small pillow under the head and another one under the knees. Never lie on the stomach.

Patients who have experienced a herniated disk should not return to strenuous activities until fully recovered from the injury. The patient should be able to perform all physical therapy exercises without pain, have full range of motion in the back and neck, and no shooting pain at all in the arms and legs. The patient should be able to run, jump, and twist without any pain.

Prevention

Keeping weight down, eating a good diet, and maintaining excellent fitness to keep the muscles firm will help in preventing a herniated disk. The stronger and more flexible the muscles of the back and stomach are, the more protection they provide to the spine. Strong, flexible muscles can stabilize the spine and protect it from injury. Walking and swimming are two good exercises for strengthening and protecting the spine.

hip dislocation Hip displacements are associated with high-energy impact athletic events, such as American football, rugby, waterskiing, alpine skiing, gymnastics, running, basketball, and race car driving. In fact, American football and rugby are the sports in which hip dislocations have been most widely reported. An estimated 3 percent of all football injuries involve hip fracture or dislocation. Rugby, followed by alpine skiing, is the sport with the second-highest number of hip dislocations. One case of hip dislocation has been documented in the literature in both competitive gymnastics and professional basketball. Anecdotal evidence also exists of hip dislocations and fractures to race car drivers.

Although hip dislocations are relatively uncommon during athletic events, they do sometimes occur, and serious consequences can be associated with hip displacements, making it extremely important for the sports medicine physician to diagnose and treat them carefully and with expedience.

The hip is a ball-and-socket joint, which gives it a great deal of stability and allows it to move freely. The round head of the thighbone (femur) fits inside a cup-shaped socket (acetabulum) in the hipbone (pelvis). It requires substantial force to pop the thighbone out of its socket. But that is just what happens in a hip dislocation.

Dislocation occurs when the ball of the hip joint comes out of the socket. This can happen when a patient's leg is put in various positions that can manually pop the ball from the liner of the socket. Initially, it is very painful. The patient cannot walk, the leg shortens and turns outward, and suddenly the hip, thigh, or knee can give pain. Most patients go directly to the emergency room.

Two general categories of hip dislocations exist, anterior and posterior. Posterior dislocations make up 70 to 80 percent of all hip dislocations and 90 percent of all sports-related hip dislocations. A large force is required to strike the flexed knee with the hip flexed, adducted, and internally rotated in order to cause a posterior dislocation. This injury occurs more commonly during contact sports, such as American football and rugby, when a running player is tackled and falls out of control onto a flexed knee.

Anterior dislocations occur when an athlete's hip is flexed with the leg abducted and externally rotated. These injuries are more common in sports such as basketball and gymnastics, in which players are running at high speeds, jumping, and landing awkwardly with the knees flexed. This force tears ligaments and often fractures the femoral head.

Causes

High-speed, high-impact sports are the setting for most hip dislocations. Unsafe playing surfaces, such as a wet basketball court, are responsible for some of these injuries. There have been reports of basketball players slipping on wet courts and dislocating their hips in the fall. Injuries also occur in alpine skiing when snow conditions are icy, making it more difficult for skiers to control their movements.

Since a large amount of force is required to dislocate a hip, these injuries are usually seen among high-performance athletes who travel at higher speeds and are large enough to produce such force with their bodies. The tackling and body contact of sports such as football and rugby can cause hip dislocations.

Diagnosis

A report of the history of a hip displacement injury will normally describe either a situation in which the athlete strikes the ground, as in tackle, and lands out of control of the body with other players piling on top. In this situation, it is usually that the hip is flexed, adducted, and rotated internally. Another common history is that of the athlete landing in a split, with the hip flexed, abducted, and externally rotated, which more often occurs in sports such as gymnastics and basketball.

In either case, patients will usually describe severe pain in the hip area and upper leg. They may also complain of pain in the knee, lower leg, or back. Patients with a displaced hip will normally be unable to walk or move the leg from the hip joint. They may experience numbness and/or tingling in the legs if there has been neurovascular damage.

The physical examination will reveal deformities in the hip region, depending on the exact impact and type of displacement. The affected leg will normally appear shortened, internally rotated, and adducted.

The doctor will want to do a careful assessment of the neurovascular status of the affected leg. Nerve injury is not uncommon with hip displacements, especially injury to the sciatic nerve. The doctor will palpate for bony deformity and observe for skin color and temperature to gather basic clues

about the possibility of nerve injury. Testing reflexes, strength, and sensation in the affected leg and taking pulses will also help in diagnosing the extent of the injury.

It is not uncommon for athletes who experience a hip displacement to also have other bone injuries. The force required to displace the hip is certainly enough to cause fractures in other parts of the body. Knee injuries, such as fractures, dislocations, and ligament damage, are commonly associated with hip displacements. For this reason, the knee should be given special attention in the physical examination.

If the patient has significant trauma to the hip and injury of blood vessels is suspected, it is a good idea to do a hemoglobin/hematocrit test to evaluate the amount of blood loss that has occurred.

A full range of X rays must be taken in order to evaluate the type of hip dislocation that has occurred, where the bones lie in comparison to one another, and if there are any fractures before a reduction is attempted.

Following reduction of the hip, which may require surgery, a full series of X rays will be taken to assess the results of the reduction. In addition, it is important to examine the hip joint following the reduction for the presence of any loose, bony fragments or fractures. These may not be seen prior to reduction, but their presence may interfere with a successful reduction and cause further damage to the joint. COMPUTERIZED AXIAL TOMOGRAPHY (CAT) SCANS are generally more useful in making this evaluation. They are also called for if there exists a widening in the joint spaces following the reduction. Some physicians routinely use a CAT scan following a closed reduction of a displaced hip to check for tiny fractures and soft tissue damage.

Treatment

Closed reduction, repair of the hip without surgery, should be performed as soon as possible, but at least within 24 hours of the injury in order to minimize long-term damage to the joints. The technique should be performed using conscious sedation in the emergency room or under general or spinal anesthesia in the operating room. There are three different methods that doctors routinely use for closed reduction. These include the Allis maneuver, the Stimson maneuver, and the Bigelow maneuver.

In some cases, it is necessary to perform a surgical reduction of the hip when closed reduction techniques are unsuccessful. An orthopedic surgeon should always be consulted. Surgery is also called for when bone fragments or soft tissue remains in the joint space following a closed reduction, or when the joint remains unstable for some other reason. Sometimes plates are used in the reconstruction of the hip.

Immediately following the reduction, it is most important to rest and ice the injured joint and take anti-inflammatory medications to reduce swelling and inflammation. If the patient does not require surgery, the injured leg is held in traction at least until the joint is pain free, which may be up to two weeks.

Hip joints with associated fractures and/or instability are placed in a short leg cast following reduction with a posterior bar, which keeps the leg slightly externally rotated for optimal healing. Within five to seven days of the injury, patients should perform simple range-of-motion exercises with assistance in order to maintain normal flexibility.

Concerns with this injury include the potential of damage to the sciatic nerve, which sits just behind the hip joint and is injured in about 20 percent of all hip dislocations. Any damage to this nerve requires immediate surgical repair. There is also the risk of recurring hip dislocations during the traction period following reduction. If this occurs, a CAT scan should be performed to assess the problem.

Chronic complications such as AVASCULAR FEMORAL HEAD NECROSIS and OSTEOARTHRITIS may not be avoided even with good follow-up care. X rays should be obtained every few months in the first year after injury and a MAGNETIC RESONANCE IMAGING (MRI) scan should be performed within three to six months post injury to evaluate for avascular necrosis. Unfortunately, even with compliant patients, early diagnosis, early and appropriate treatment, and good follow-up, some patients develop these problems.

Avascular necrosis, or deadening of the bone and osteoarthritis are some of the possible complications of hip dislocations. Delayed reduction of

the hip puts the patient at most risk for these complications. For this reason, treatment should begin as soon as possible following the injury. If there has been some delay in the reduction of the hip, an MRI of the hip should be performed within two to three months after dislocation to assess possibility of avascular necrosis of the femoral head. Arthritis is the most common long-term complication after hip dislocation, affecting up to 50 percent of all patients. Arthritis is thought to occur from damage to the articular cartilage from traumatic injury. Open reduction has been said to decrease the incidence of post dislocation arthritis, although this is not widely accepted. Radiographs are important for diagnosing arthritis, and nonsteroidal anti-inflammatory drugs should be prescribed to decrease pain and inflammation in the arthritic hip joint.

Dislocation of the hip joint is an extremely serious injury. The hip joint is crucial for weight bearing and walking. Proper rehabilitation is crucial in order to retain normal musculoskeletal function. Most experts agree that weight bearing should be postponed until patients are pain-free. This may take one to two weeks, and possibly longer, if associated fractures are involved. Weight bearing with the help of crutches should begin immediately after the patient is pain-free.

Cardiovascular activities and stretching exercises are important early in the rehabilitation process to maintain full range of motion around the hip joint. Examples of these activities include WEIGHT TRAINING and floor exercises such as push-ups. These movements also are important in maintaining the integrity of articular cartilage and preventing adhesions from forming. Over the next four to six weeks, exercises should be performed as tolerated, increasing the level of performance with return of full muscle strength by three months post injury.

PHYSICAL THERAPY once the patient is pain-free should include leg muscle strengthening exercises and walking without crutches. Patients may work on Nautilus equipment to strengthen the hip flexors, hip extensors, and the muscles nearest the hip, including the quadriceps and hamstrings. Over the next few months, it is good to gradually increase the level of cardiovascular training, which should include brisk walking and swimming. Jogging and running should be avoided for at least six to nine months following the injury. The patient should regain full function in high-performance sports activities within 12 months of the injury.

In addition, athletes who participate in high-performance activities need to understand the importance of proper warm-up techniques before competition and maintenance of good overall flexibility and strength. These attributes are especially important during athletic events that involve high speeds that can generate relatively large forces and cause serious injuries to competing athletes.

Prevention

Contact sports that are played under high speeds and great force should not be played in wet and icy conditions if possible. These conditions make for adverse footing and the opportunity for serious joint injuries during falls. Alpine skiing is another high-speed sport popular during inclement weather. Icy and foggy conditions make for treacherous times on the ski slopes. These conditions predispose participants to losing their edge on a patch of ice or running into another skier, causing dangerous falls. Adverse weather conditions during high-speed and contact sports should be avoided in order to prevent serious injuries.

In the first six weeks following surgery, helpful prevention tips include the following:

- Do not sit on chairs that are low.
- Do not pick up anything from the floor without using a gadget called a reacher.
- Do not sleep in any position other than on the back with a pillow between the legs.
- Do not cross the legs at the knees.
- Do not drive a car.

Those who have experienced a displaced hip should always refrain from crossing their legs at the knees, squatting, and bringing the knees up to the chest. Constant repetitive motions such as these can stretch muscles and cause dislocation.

hip flexor injury Hip and pelvis injuries represent 2 to 5 percent of all sports injuries. Among these injuries, groin pain is the most common finding. A hip flexor injury is a pull or strain of the iliopsoas muscle and tendon. The iliopsoas muscle is a large muscle that begins deep within the pelvis and inserts into the top part of the thighbone, or femur. Its main function is to flex or bend the hip joint, which allows a person to lift the knee and bend at the waist. Therefore, an injury to this muscle is known as a hip flexor injury. A strain or pull occurs when there is a stretch or tear of a muscle or tendon, a band of tissue that connects muscle to bone.

A hip flexor injury is considered an OVERUSE INJURY, meaning that it occurs from overuse of the muscles that flex the knee and help to kick the leg up high. This injury commonly occurs in bicyclists, athletes who jump or run with high knee kicks, soccer players and others who do forceful kicking activities, ballet dancers, and people who practice the martial arts.

If a hip flexor injury involves the tendon and becomes chronic, it is known as ILIOPSOAS TENDONITIS.

Causes

The injury typically occurs when there is a hyperextension of the leg at the hip joint, which can occur in almost any sport or activity. Tackling in football and collisions in soccer when a player is attempting to kick a ball are two situations that commonly produce hip flexor injuries.

Diagnosis

Most often, this injury causes sudden sharp pain in the groin area. Bending or flexing the hip, as when the knee is raised to the chest, against resistance increases the pain. There is normally pain in the upper groin region where the thigh meets the pelvis.

Typically, these injuries are diagnosed by taking a complete medical history of the patient and performing a physical examination. If the pain is severe or the patient cannot put weight on the affected leg, an X ray should be ordered to rule out a fracture. In some rare cases, a MAGNETIC RESONANCE IMAGING (MRI) scan is needed to fully evaluate the patient.

Treatment

Conservative treatment involves rest and a progressive rehabilitation program, consisting of three to four days of icing and gentle stretching followed by strengthening. During this time, the patient should take anti-inflammatory medication as prescribed by the doctor. The patient should switch to a sport or activity during the recovery period that does not aggravate the injury. Those who normally bike and run may need to switch to swimming while the hip heals. Return to normal sports activity can often occur safely in four to six weeks, depending upon the severity of the injury. The following guidelines should be helpful in determining when the body is ready for a full return to sports. The patient should have:

- full range of motion in the leg on the injured side compared to the leg on the uninjured side
- full strength of the leg on the injured side compared to the leg on the uninjured side
- ability to jog straight ahead without pain or limping
- ability to sprint straight ahead without pain or limping
- ability to do 45-degree cuts, first at half speed, then at full speed
- ability to do 20-yard figures-of-eight, first at half speed, then at full speed
- ability to do 90-degree cuts, first at half speed, then at full speed
- ability to do 10-yard figures-of-eight, first at half speed, then at full speed

In rare cases, surgery is needed to repair the injury.

Prevention

Maintaining excellent flexibility and strength of the hip and leg muscles may help prevent some hip flexor injuries. Hip flexor strains are best prevented by warming up properly and performing weight-bearing exercises to maintain strength in the hip and leg.

hip pointer A hip pointer is a deep bruise, or contusion, on the top portion of the pelvis, called the iliac crest.

Causes

A hip pointer is caused by a direct blow to the iliac crest. This injury most commonly occurs in a con-

tact sport such as football, when a helmet is driven into the iliac crest.

Diagnosis

The primary symptom with hip pointers is tenderness in the top portion of the hip. A physical examination of the hip and pelvis will locate the exact position of the injury. If the doctor thinks there might be a fracture on the top part of the pelvis, an X ray will likely be ordered to confirm the diagnosis.

Treatment

Initial treatment of a hip pointer includes icing the injury for 20 to 30 minutes every three to four hours for two to three days or until the pain goes away. This will help with any swelling as well. Otherwise, it just takes time for a hip pointer to heal itself. During the healing process, place padding over the area to protect from further injury.

Return to sport or activity will be determined by how soon the hip recovers, not by how many days or weeks it has been since the injury occurred. Athletes may return to sport or activity after a hip pointer when they have no pain when walking or running. There will usually be pain with contact to the hip pointer for several weeks after the injury. If a pad taped over the hip pointer provides enough protection during contact, one may continue participating in a sport or activity.

Prevention

Since hip pointers normally result from accidents, it is not possible to prevent them. However, for those who play contact sports, it is necessary to wear the appropriate protective padding to safeguard this area.

hyponatremia Known as water intoxication, hyponatremia is an electrolyte disorder. The specific problem occurs when there is a low concentration of sodium in the blood. When athletes develop hyponatremia, it usually happens during long or ultra-distance races in the heat, but it may occur anytime. It is estimated that approximately 30 percent of the finishers of the Hawaii Ironman are both hyponatremic and dehydrated. Longer races and workouts predispose the athlete to greater risk of hyponatremia.

Sodium is a required element for normal body functions. It is lost in sweat and urine and is replaced in the diet. The body has a remarkable ability to maintain sodium and water balance throughout a variety of conditions, thus ensuring survival, but ultra-endurance events challenge this survival mechanism.

In hot, humid conditions, a large amount of sweat is lost, which can disturb sodium and water balance. Adequate hydration and sodium intake, either using sports drinks or food, becomes vitally important during long races.

In addition to athletes, hyponatremia is most common in the very young and in the very old. These groups are less able to experience and express thirst and less able to regulate fluid intake autonomously.

Causes

Hyponatremia is caused by improper refueling during long periods of extended physical effort, such as endurance cycling or running events, by a disturbance in thirst or water acquisition or by a disturbance in antidiuretic hormone (ADH), aldosterone, or renal sodium transport.

In athletic events hyponatremia comes about as athletes consume large amounts of water during a workout or race. As they do, their blood plasma increases, diluting the salt content of the blood. At the same time, the body is losing salt through sweat. As a result, the amount of electrolytes available to the body's tissues decreases over time to the point where that loss interferes with normal brain, heart, and muscle functioning. This severely compromises the nervous system.

Longer races carry a greater risk of hyponatremia because of the total amount of sweat lost. During exercise in the heat, more salt is lost in sweat per hour than is usually replaced by food and fluids, including sports drinks. The body can tolerate a degree of imbalance for a short period of time, but it may decompensate if this continues for too long.

In addition, aspirin, ibuprofen, and other non-steroidal anti-inflammatory agents interfere with kidney function and may contribute to the development of hyponatremia in athletes. Other drugs that may contribute to hyponatremia are aceta-minophen (Tylenol), diuretics, narcotics, and certain psychiatric medications.

The rate of development of hyponatremia plays a critical role. When serum sodium falls slowly, over a period of several days or weeks, the brain is capable of compensating by extrusion of solutes and fluid to the space outside of cells. Compensatory extrusion of solutes reduces the flow of free water into the intracellular space, and symptoms are much milder for a given degree of hyponatremia. When serum sodium falls rapidly, over a period of 24 to 48 hours, this compensatory mechanism is overwhelmed and severe cerebral edema may ensue, resulting in brainstem herniation and death.

The following is a list of potential causes of hyponatremia:

- excessive fluid loss due to sweating, vomiting, diarrhea, burns, or pancreatitis
- acute or chronic renal insufficiency
- use of diuretics
- prolonged exercise in a hot environment, especially for patients who hydrate aggressively
- taking in excess free water
- dysfunctional kidneys
- uncorrected hypothyroidism
- consumption of large quantities of beer or the recreational drug ecstasy

Diagnosis

The spectrum of symptoms can range from mild to severe and can include nausea, muscle cramps, disorientation, slurred speech, confusion, headache, and inappropriate behavior. As it progresses, victims may experience seizures or coma, and death can occur. The number and severity of symptoms increase with the degree of hyponatremia and the rapidity with which it develops. Severe hyponatremia is a true medical emergency.

Though the condition is opposite to DEHYDRATION, the symptoms generally mirror those of dehydration, although in the mildest cases of hyponatremia, some individuals show no symptoms at all. This can make it very difficult to diagnose.

A physical examination normally reveals a level of alertness ranging from normal to agitation to coma; variable degrees of cognitive impairment, which might include difficulty with short-term memory, confusion, loss of orientation to place and time, and depression; seizure activity; and in severe cases, signs of brainstem herniation, including coma, dilated pupils, and respiratory arrest. Other possible physical findings include dry mucous membranes, swelling, diminished firmness of the skin, and muscle weakness and cramping.

The proper diagnosis of hyponatremia depends entirely on obtaining a sample of the patient's serum and accurately measuring the concentration of sodium in the serum. There is always the possibility of sampling error, so doctors must be careful if the serum findings are not consistent with the history and physical findings. A second sample should be requested in these situations. In addition, there are several situations in which a person may show low sodium concentrations in the serum but not have hyponatremia.

Determining the exact cause of the hyponatremia may require other tests, such as taking urine sodium levels and testing adrenal function. In certain conditions that cause hyponatremia, X rays may be warranted. A COMPUTERIZED AXIAL TOMOGRAPHY (CAT) SCAN may be indicated in a patient with altered mental status in order to ensure that there is no other underlying cause for the mental state.

Treatment

Minor symptoms, such as nausea and mild muscle cramps, can be treated by eating salty foods and hydrating with a sports drink that contains sodium. More severe symptoms require treatment by qualified medical personnel.

In these cases, treatment first must address acute life-threatening conditions. Supportive care for these conditions should be initiated immediately. The doctor or attending medical personnel will need to establish reliable IV access and give supplemental oxygen to patients with lethargy. These patients should also be evaluated for the possibility of hypoglycemia. If hypoglycemia is present, the patients should receive glucose.

Patients with seizures will need to receive standard anticonvulsant therapy. If there are signs of brainstem herniation, steps must be taken to reduce the intercranial pressure.

The next step in treating the patient, once the life-threatening situations have been addressed, is to determine how long the patient has been in a hyponatremic state and to determine the cause. Exact treatment will vary based on the cause, but may include being admitted to the hospital for further inpatient care.

Prevention

When involved in strenuous activity, an athlete should drink the appropriate sports drinks, such as Gatorade, that make an effort to match the body's natural levels of potassium, citrate, and sodium chloride. Avoid using diuretics and over-the-counter drugs that interfere with kidney functioning and may contribute to the development of hyponatremia in athletes.

hypothermia   Hypothermia occurs when the body's temperature becomes dangerously low, placing many organs in danger of permanent damage.

Causes

Body temperature may gradually drop from increased exposure to cold, or it may drop immediately from falling into cold water.

Diagnosis

The symptoms of hypothermia occur gradually and if left untreated, can result in death. They progress in the following order.

- cold shivering
- difficulty thinking and mental confusion
- unable to shiver
- irregular heartbeat
- coma

Once medical attention is located, a doctor will take the body temperature. A hypothermic individual usually has a body temperature of less than 96°F. The doctor will also do a physical examination to check for the symptoms mentioned above.

Treatment

It is important that a person with hypothermia receive immediate attention. If possible, the patient should be taken to a doctor. Depending on the severity of the hypothermia, the person may be given warm oxygen, warm intravenous fluids, or a warming blanket. If any organs are believed to be injured, these will receive specific treatment as well.

If medical attention is unavailable, the person's clothes should be removed if they are wet, then the person should be placed in warm clothing, blankets, or a sleeping bag. A dry hat on the person's head will help keep the heat from escaping the body. It is best to allow the person to warm up gradually in a warm room.

The hypothermic condition lasts for varying amounts of time, depending upon the severity of any damage done to the organs when the temperature fell below normal.

Prevention

It is important to always be prepared for the worst possible conditions and to dress appropriately. Wearing several layers is a better approach than wearing a single thick layer. In addition, the layers should provide good insulation while also keeping moisture away from the skin. Materials that function in this way include polypropylene, polyesters, and wool. The outer garment should be waterproof, and a hat should always be worn to prevent the body's heat from escaping.

The following guidelines are helpful in preventing hypothermia, which often occurs when you least expect it:

- Be prepared for bad weather by carrying proper clothing in a backpack.
- Start outings early in the day to allow time to reach a destination before nighttime and a possible sudden weather change occurs.
- Remove wet clothing as soon as it gets wet and replace it with warm, dry clothes.
- Drink lots of nonalcoholic fluids. Dehydration is often a factor in hypothermia.

iliopsoas tendonitis Iliopsoas tendonitis and iliopsoas bursitis are common hip injuries athletes experience that are closely interrelated because one problem inevitably causes the other, due to their close proximity. Therefore, these two conditions are essentially identical in terms of presentation and management. On the most basic level, iliopsoas tendonitis is an inflammation of the tendon or area surrounding the tendon caused by either acute trauma or overuse due to repetitive hip flexion. Tendonitis may be acute, subacute, or chronic, depending upon the duration of symptoms. Iliopsoas tendonitis is noted to affect young adults more commonly, with a slight female predominance.

Causes

The two most common causes of iliopsoas tendonitis are acute injury and OVERUSE INJURY. The acute injury often involves eccentric contraction of the iliopsoas muscle or rapid flexion against extension force/resistance but also may result from direct trauma. The overuse phenomenon may occur in any activity resulting in repeated hip flexion or external rotation of the femur.

Activities that may predispose to iliopsoas tendonitis include dancing, ballet, resistance training, rowing, running (particularly uphill), track and field, soccer, and gymnastics.

Another predisposing factor is the adolescent growth spurt. During this time, the hip flexors tend to become relatively inflexible. This inflexibility can lead to problems in younger athletes because stress placed on the iliopsoas muscle and tendon increases and general biomechanics are altered. The subsequent changes can lead to patellar tendon injuries and patellofemoral problems.

Rheumatoid arthritis may be a cause of iliopsoas bursitis.

Diagnosis

A medical history of a patient with iliopsoas tendonitis tends to reveal complaints of an insidious onset of anterior hip or groin pain. Initially, the patient may note that the pain comes with certain aggravating activities and resolves when the activity is done. But eventually this condition progresses so that the pain persists beyond the time of performing the aggravating activity. The average time from initial onset of symptoms to diagnosis ranges from 32 to 41 months.

Patients may note pain with specific sports-related activities, such as jogging, running, or kicking. There may also be pain reported with simple activities, such as putting on socks and shoes, standing from a seated position, walking up stairs, or brisk walking.

The patient may describe the pain as radiating down the thigh toward the knee. There are often reports of an audible snap or click in the hip or groin area, which lends the name "snapping hip syndrome" to this condition. There may also be knee pain that is consistent with patellar tendonitis or patellofemoral pain syndrome.

The physical examination should focus on thorough assessment of the abdomen, hip, and groin. In females, a complete pelvic examination should be considered. The doctor may observe that the hip is held slightly flexed and externally rotated to relieve tension in the iliopsoas tendon. In addition, the patient's gait may demonstrate a shortened stride length on the affected side and increased bending of the knee. Palpating the iliopsoas tendon insertion may reveal tenderness. The doctor will want to perform a number of functional tests to see exactly which types of movement create pain.

Laboratory studies are rarely necessary in diagnosing iliopsoas tendonitis. However, if the diagnosis remains unclear following the examination, the doctor may want to pursue a number of different studies to determine the cause of the groin pain. These include a rheumatoid factor study, antinuclear antibody study, and a urinalysis, among others. X rays of the hip may be helpful but often appear normal in cases of iliopsoas tendonitis. They may, however, demonstrate other bony pathology, which may be contributing to the patient's set of symptoms.

Ultrasound has been used more successfully than X rays in diagnosing muscle-tendon injuries. The usual finding in iliopsoas tendonitis is a thickened tendon. An ultrasound may also demonstrate an excessive amount of fluid in the iliopsoas bursa consistent with iliopsoas bursitis, which may be either a primary or secondary problem.

MAGNETIC RESONANCE IMAGING (MRI), however, is the most effective way to gain images of a muscle-tendon injury site. It is much more specific than other types of imaging studies, and it has the added advantage of revealing bony lesions that may have developed as a result of the muscle-tendon injury. A Lidocaine challenge test may also be performed in cases where diagnosis is elusive. This test works by injecting anesthesia into the tendon. Relief of symptoms following the test confirms the diagnosis.

Treatment

Although patients may present in a less acute or chronic phase of the condition, since there is usually a lapse of many months if not years between onset of symptoms and diagnosis, the focus should be on alleviating pain, spasm, and swelling. A secondary issue, if necessary, is to return the patient to activities of daily living, such as walking, if the symptoms are acute. Treatment consists of a combination of medication, ice, rest, and gentle stretching. A pack of crushed ice in a damp cloth-covered ice bag applied for 20 minutes every one to two hours can provide the patient with relief of pain, spasm, and inflammation.

In addition to avoiding the activities that stress the iliopsoas muscle and tendon, a gentle stretch-ing regimen can assist in reduction of spasm in the iliopsoas complex. Note that stretching must not immediately follow icing, when the sensitivity to pain is lessened, because a potential to overstretch exists.

If a normal gait is not present at the time of diagnosis, the patient should begin walking with crutches, gradually moving to more and more weight bearing and finally walking without assistance. If necessary, the patient can practice walking in front of a full-length mirror to ensure that ambulatory rhythm and techniques are correct.

The purpose of rehabilitation is to return the patient to normal range of motion, strength, endurance, and activity specific to the patient's sport. Normal range of motion can be accomplished by sustaining normal gait mechanics, maintaining a stretching regimen, and practicing good warm-up and cool-down techniques with exercise.

Iliopsoas muscle strengthening exercises involve hip flexion and femoral external rotation, but should begin only once a neutral pelvic position can be maintained without pain. Begin all strengthening exercises at a weight that the patient can comfortably lift or with an elastic band resistive device with which the patient controls the tension. Exercises should be pain free and performed daily in four sets of 10 to 15 repetitions. Patients should increase resistance as the weight becomes easier to lift.

Endurance is gained through movement with low resistance over time. Examples of these exercises are cycling with low resistance, stair climbing on a machine with the setting on the lowest resistance, or walking. The workout should not produce pain but could fatigue the iliopsoas muscle. Use caution so that the musculature has time to recuperate prior to the next bout of endurance training. As the muscle recovers, endurance exercises can be performed daily, and resistance gradually can be increased with time of activity.

In the recovery phase, the patient intends to gradually return to sport-specific activities, leading to full pain-free participation. The goal of the maintenance phase of rehabilitation for iliopsoas injury is to challenge the muscles involved to continue to perform their work. Stretching and strengthening must continue and increase as tolerated. Recreational activities that facilitate the recovered iliopsoas muscle to maintain its strength and function include rollerblading, cycling, dancing, skating, horseback riding (especially English riding), and rowing. Other sports, such as soccer, competitive cycling, running, and gymnastics, all have a high demand of hip flexion combined with trunk flexion, which shortens the iliopsoas and can cause stress when the body demands hip flexion independent of trunk flexion. Maintaining a stretching and strengthening program is crucial, and the patient should consider cross-training for lower extremity sports that allow for a more upright trunk.

Return to normal sports activity is allowed once the patient is free of pain and has demonstrated adequate flexibility and strength of the hip flexors. Performance of pain-free, sports-specific activities should be required.

In rare cases, surgical intervention for iliopsoas tendonitis is necessary for relief of pain. It is considered for those patients who fail conservative management and treatment by injections. Surgery involves either complete release of the iliopsoas tendon or partial release. Each approach has produced generally good results in terms of pain relief, with little documentation of significant residual weakness.

Prevention

As in most cases of muscle-tendon injury, the best prevention is a focused flexibility and strengthening program. Exercises should always include hip flexors, hip extensors, knee flexors, and knee extensors. In addition, an organized training program that incorporates rest days and avoids adding too much distance, speed, or resistance too quickly is important in preventing injuries of the muscles and tendons.

iliotibial band syndrome One of the most common, and often most frustrating, running-related injuries, iliotibial (IT) band syndrome is also easily treated if diagnosed and treated before it becomes chronic. Although development of the condition is linked to improper training, such as an overwhelming increase in running distance or improper running technique, a great number of structural abnormalities may predispose the athlete to this condition as well.

The iliotibial (IT) band is a tough group of fibers that run along the outside of the thigh. It is a thickening of the fascia, or the outer casing of the muscle, that runs up the outside of the thigh. Fascia is like a sausage casing, and the IT band is a thickening of that sausage casing. It originates up by the top of the hip and ends on the outside of the knee. The IT band can be felt when standing. The outside of the thigh becomes very firm and tight while the muscles remain more relaxed because of the presence of the IT band. The IT band holds legs straight when one stands, thereby allowing the bigger thigh muscles a chance to rest.

When a person is running, the IT band acts as a stabilizer as well and can become irritated from overuse. If the IT band becomes irritated or inflamed, runners will usually describe pain on the outside part of the knee or lower thigh, often worsened by going up or down stairs, or getting out of a car.

Causes

Predisposing factors for the development of IT band inflammation include training error and abnormal biomechanics.

The lateral knee pain is caused by the IT band pulling up on its insertion on the outside of the knee. Underneath the IT band near its insertion at the knee is a bursa. Bursae are fluid-filled sacs that lubricate areas where rubbing and friction occur. When that IT band was pulled tight, it put too much pressure on the bursa, and that bursa reacted by becoming inflamed and swollen, giving pain.

The IT band can also be aggravated by running on uneven roads. Some runners make the mistake of running only on one side of the road. Most roads are higher in the center and slope off on either side. The foot that is on the outside part of the road is therefore lower than the other. This causes the pelvis to tilt to one side and stresses the IT band. Tight indoor tracks can cause IT band problems for the same reason.

Running in poor running shoes or running with biomechanical problems can also bring on IT band syndrome. If a runner pronates excessively, which means that the arch collapses during running, this may cause problems because when there is a minor abnormality in the foot anatomy, the force of the foot strike is passed to the knee area. In addition, leg length discrepancy, lateral pelvic tilt, and "bowed" legs might also cause stress to the IT band. Tight gluteal or quadriceps muscles may also contribute.

Although IT band syndrome is considered a runner's injury, it can happen to other athletes as well. Increasingly, IT band syndrome is being seen in cyclists whose bikes do not fit properly.

Diagnosis

Athletes will often present with one or more of the following symptoms:

- Lateral (outside) knee pain—very few conditions, other than a ligament sprain, will present as lateral knee pain therefore this alone is often diagnostic.
- Pain is often worse after running, especially after climbing hills and often aggravated by climbing stairs.
- Pain may not be present until midway through a run, often not until climbing a hill.
- Pain can literally bring a runner to his or her knees.
- Sometimes the pain is associated with a "snapping hip," in which the muscles that cross the outside of the hip can be felt to snap or click during walking or running.
- Pain may also present as lateral thigh pain more so than knee pain but is rarely focused primarily in the hip or gluteal muscles.
- The pain can often be attributed to some form of over-training—doubling one's mileage, sudden increase in hill repeats, and so forth.

Once the doctor has taken a medical history of the patient, it is important to do a physical exam. The doctor will want to check where the pain occurs and test the patient's pain with both weight-bearing and nonweight-bearing exercises.

In addition, three different special tests can be performed to confirm a diagnosis of IT band syndrome: Ober's test, Renne's test, and Noble's test,

all of which concentrate an identifying the exact location of the pain and any associated loss of strength.

Treatment

The grade of severity of the present inflammation must first be determined before a treatment approach is adopted. With the inflammation properly assessed and the diagnosis taken into consideration, the athlete may be placed into one of the three phases of IT band care.

In the acute phase, the goal is to control pain and inflammation and correct any poor training habits or structural abnormalities. To do this, the athlete must reduce or stop running and begin taking anti-inflammatory medications. Other appropriate treatments may include ice, heat, ultrasound, stretching, and electrical stimulation.

If the pain does not resolve within about 10 days of the onset, the doctor may consider steroid injections in addition to continuing the previous treatment. It may be advisable to restrict activity further as well. Athletes can maintain fitness levels by running in water, cycling, rollerblading, or doing an activity that does not stress the injured IT band.

Once pain and inflammation have been resolved, the athlete may begin a gradual return to training.

General treatment should continue if there is any flare-up of symptoms. It is important that patients stop running until the pain disappears. General treatment should always include relative rest, ice massage, addressing any biomechanical or training errors, and gentle stretching. When stretching the IT band, the "pulling" sensation is usually felt along the mid to upper thigh. Don't worry if this doesn't seem to exactly hit the site where the pain occurs. The IT band is a long structure, and the goal is to get it to loosen and lengthen. Along the same lines, gentle stretching of the gluteal muscles will also help. Hot tubs and the use of Epsom salts are both valuable in loosening the muscles before stretching.

If the source of the problem is faulty pelvic mechanics, it is difficult to get rid of IT band pain without help from a doctor. Stretching probably will not do it alone. Those who treat IT band pain for more than two weeks with just stretching, ice, exercises, and so forth but without much improvement, should have a chiropractor check the pelvic mechanics. Also, be sure to address any problems in foot mechanics. Orthotics may be helpful for those who tend to pronate excessively.

Surgical release of the IT band is also a treatment option, but is indicated only after extensive nonoperative measures have failed to relieve symptoms. Surgery is usually necessary only for those athletes who are unwilling to modify their sports participation.

Prevention

Prevention of IT band syndrome is achieved by running on a level surface or alternating directions on the road, a balanced approach to training that allows for rest and recovery, and preventive stretching. In some patients, strengthening the external hip rotators will help. This is achieved by doing sets of one-leg squats in front of a mirror. Watch pelvic alignment to ensure that one side does not drop. Finally, orthotics can be quite useful if there is a tendency to develop IT band inflammation.

infraspinatus syndrome Shoulder pain is a common complaint among athletes who participate in overhead sports. Sports such as baseball, volleyball, tennis, and weight lifting demand skills that place substantial load upon the athlete's shoulder when his or her arm is in an overhead or abducted position. The highest incidence of this injury occurs in volleyball players, lending credence to the term *volleyball shoulder*, which is sometimes used to describe this injury. Athletes who participate in these sports are consequently at higher risk for OVERUSE INJURIES of the arms in general and overuse injuries of the shoulder in particular, including ROTATOR CUFF TENDONITIS. One often overlooked cause of shoulder pain in such athletes is infraspinatus syndrome.

A result of compression of the suprascapular nerve, infraspinatus syndrome is a condition in which the infraspinatus muscle in the shoulder atrophies. The syndrome typically causes symptoms that mimic those of rotator cuff tendonitis, and the diagnosis is often overlooked until the con-dition fails to respond to a traditional rotator cuff treatment program.

Causes

Sports that place a substantial load on the athlete's shoulder when it is in an overhead or abducted position cause this condition. The infraspinatus can also be damaged as a result of direct trauma to the shoulder.

The shoulder joint is the most mobile joint in the human body, but this mobility comes at the cost of stability because the bony components in the joint provide little stability. Ligaments do some of the work of providing support, but the supraspinatus and infraspinatus muscles, which are part of the rotator cuff, are essential in stabilizing the shoulder joint. Therefore, any injury to these muscles puts the entire shoulder joint at risk.

Diagnosis

Typically, patients with this injury are young athletes who complain of vague shoulder pain. A history reveals pain typically on just one side of the body, usually the dominant side. The pain is often described as deep, dull, and aching. Activities that involve overhead throwing usually exacerbate the symptoms, causing weakness and hindering the athlete's endurance. Occasionally the injury occurs in such a way that it produces little pain or functional disability.

The physical examination reveals atrophy of the supraspinatus and/or infraspinatus muscles. Manual tests may be performed to determine the exact location of any weakness in the shoulder muscles as well as the exact location of pain. Palpation of the muscles may elicit pain, but muscle reflexes may be unaffected.

X rays usually reveal nothing in the case of simple infraspinatus syndrome, unless there is a bone injury, such as a fractured clavicle, to blame for the shoulder pain.

A MAGNETIC RESONANCE IMAGING (MRI) scan of the shoulder may be useful in revealing muscle swelling in acute cases and muscle atrophy with fatty replacement in more chronic cases. It may also reveal a cyst or other mass that could be responsible for nerve compression. If such a mass is suspected, it is less expensive to screen for this with ultrasound.

Electrodiagnostic testing may be used to help confirm the diagnosis. The physical examination and electrodiagnostic test results should enable the clinician to rule out other possible underlying nerve damage and to specifically locate the site of nerve impairment.

Treatment

The treatment for infraspinatus syndrome depends on the cause, severity, and duration of the symptoms; degree of functional disability; and patient preference. If there are no compressive lesions present, conservative treatment is recommended. For athletes without symptoms, this involves a simple program of exercises for scapular stabilization and rotator cuff strengthening. Such a program should prevent not only progression of the condition but also secondary impingement of the rotator cuff. Athletes with symptoms can follow a similar program but limit their activity in the acute phase so that they minimize the symptoms. The athlete then can follow an exercise program designed to restore flexibility, balance, range of motion, strength, and endurance, resulting ultimately in a full return to sports activity.

Another nonsurgical treatment is injection of a nerve block to help manage the pain. Blocks may provide symptomatic relief, thereby permitting the patient to more fully participate in a rehabilitation program. This type of treatment does not, however, address the underlying cause of the injury. It is designed only to alleviate the symptoms.

If conservative care fails, surgery may be necessary to repair the nerve injury. In general, surgical outcomes are good. Patients in whom the condition is diagnosed promptly and treated with early surgical decompression seem to have a better likelihood of regaining full muscular strength and bulk. The patient should participate in a postoperative program of rehabilitation and/or functional restoration to ensure the return of balanced strength and flexibility.

The goal of the recovery phase of a rehabilitation program is to maintain active range of motion in the shoulder while helping the athlete progress through a strengthening program designed to further stabilize and strengthen the rotator cuff. Ideally, the rehabilitation program should extend beyond the mere resolution of symptoms to include an analysis of the athlete's technique to determine if any flaws or biomechanical issues need to be corrected to minimize the risk of recurrent injury.

Most patients treated nonsurgically recover fully in six to eight months and are able to resume their prior level of function, including high-level sports participation. Studies do show, however, that muscle atrophy is generally not reversible, although the symptoms of pain improve over time.

The athlete may return to play when he or she is able to perform appropriate skills without provoking symptoms. Those who do not show symptoms but still have the injury may return to their sport while continuing to participate in a rehabilitation program. However, to minimize the progression of the condition, athletes should minimize the extent to which they perform overhead skills during training.

Athletes who undergo surgical decompression should participate in an appropriate postoperative rehabilitation program to restore strength, flexibility, and endurance before returning to play.

Prevention

Although some researchers have suggested that the floater serve in volleyball may be responsible for the high incidence of infraspinatus syndrome in volleyball players, no definitive studies have been done. Consequently, it is difficult to make recommendations concerning the appropriate techniques and skills to use to help prevent development of this condition.

injury prevention Injuries are a part of athletics and fitness. Fortunately the body has a remarkable ability to heal itself. Still, the best thing is to avoid injuries in the first place with some of the tips and practices outlined here.

General Tips

Warm up and cool down The most important times for preventing fitness injuries occur while athletes are not even engaged in activity. The periods before and after exercise are critical times for preventing unnecessary pain and injury. By "warming up" for five minutes prior to exercise with gentle activities like running in place, the athlete can increase blood flow to inactive muscles and gradually raise the heart rate to its target zone. Similarly, the heart rate can be gradually lowered to its resting rate by simply walking for five minutes or so after exercise.

Stretch Gentle static stretching is actually a part of the warm-up/cool-down process. Stretching before exercise limbers tight muscles and improves joint flexibility thereby reducing the risk of sprains and tears. Concentrate on stretching those muscle groups used in a particular activity. For example, runners will want to concentrate on stretching out the legs, while swimmers will want to pay extra attention to upper body muscles. Static stretching for a few minutes after exercise is also recommended to prevent muscle soreness.

Use the right equipment Improper equipment—worn exercise shoes, an ill-fitting bicycle, and so forth—can cause more harm than is generally realized. Always check equipment before and after activity and be sure to make replacements or repairs promptly. Worn-out running shoes may bring "good luck," but they can also bring an ankle or leg injury if they fail to support the foot properly. Even though cycling places less stress on bones and joints than other high-impact sports, an ill-fitting bicycle can lead to back and knee pain and/or injury. For any activity, be sure that equipment is in good condition before risking health and safety.

Use safety devices Helmets, goggles, gloves, mitts, braces, guards, pads, even sunscreen, are just a few of the numerous safety "devices" available for today's active person. Each activity carries its own risks, and which devices are used will depend on a particular activity. The point, however, is to use them. While some safety gear may feel awkward or "look funny," keep in mind that these minor inconveniences are far outweighed by risk reduction.

Use common sense The most important factor in fitness injury prevention is common sense. Make sure muscles are conditioned before engaging in vigorous activities, and use the right equipment and available safety devices. Fitness should be fun. The best way to enjoy any activity and prevent unnecessary injuries is to use common sense.

Listen to your body As the body ages, it becomes less flexible and cannot tolerate the same types of activities that it did years before. While no one is happy about getting older, aging athletes can prevent injury by modifying their activity to accommodate the body's needs.

Increase your activity level gradually When increasing activity level, do so in small increments. Athletes who normally walk two miles a day and want to increase their fitness level, should not try to suddenly walk four miles. Slowly build up to more miles each week, until the higher goal is reached. This is true in WEIGHT TRAINING as well when increasing the amount of weight being lifted.

Develop a balanced fitness program A fitness program should incorporate cardiovascular exercise, strength training, and flexibility. In addition to providing a total body workout, a balanced program will stave off boredom and lessen the chance of injury.

Add activity and new exercises cautiously Beginner and veteran athletes alike should not try to take on too many activities at one time. It is best to add no more than one or two new activities per workout.

Be careful with old injuries Those who have had sports or orthopedic injuries or problems such as tendonitis, arthritis, STRESS FRACTURES, or low back pain in the past, should consult an orthopedic surgeon who can help design a fitness routine to promote wellness and minimize the chance of injury.

Injury Prevention for Specific Parts of the Body

Knee Knee injury prevention focuses on ample stretching and warm-up prior to practice or competition. Stretching exercises should concentrate on the quadriceps, hamstrings, and calf muscles. Warm-up should involve jogging, then sprinting and sport-specific functional movements. Examples of sport-specific movements include side-to-side shuffles for tennis players and jumping exercises for basketball players.

There are many different commercially available knee braces that athletes may find helpful. Although they do not cause any harm, knee braces have never been scientifically shown to help prevent knee injuries.

Shoulder   Shoulder injury prevention involves many of the same principles as injury prevention in other parts of the body. Adequate warm-up and stretching are important. For athletes who throw, off-season throwing is important. Many throwing-related shoulder injuries occur because athletes begin throwing hard at the start of a new season despite not having thrown for months.

Pregame warm-up for the throwing athlete should begin with stretching followed by short tosses. Distance and velocity for the throws should be increased gradually. Shoulder warm-up for the nonthrowing athlete is also important and should include multiple different stretches as well as push-up or pull-up exercises to ready the shoulder for activity.

Pain experienced in the shoulder should be addressed by the athlete with rest and ice after competition. Consultation with an athletic trainer or physical therapist can get the athlete evaluated and treated with exercises to help strengthen specific muscles.

Ankle   Ankle injury prevention uses the same principles as the rest of the body. Stretching and warm-up are essential prior to practice and competition. Slow jogging followed by sprinting and more complex cutting and pivoting motions are important prior to competition.

Taping the ankle and wearing an ankle brace are common forms of supporting the ankle, but literature can be found both to support and to refute the use of these aids. The healthy athlete without a history of ankle injuries probably does not require these aids. The most important factor in injury prevention is adequate stretching and warm-up. Shoes that fit properly are also important. This includes selecting the proper type of cleat for the surface. Some terrains are better suited for shorter versus longer cleats, and some are suited for neither.

iron deficiency anemia   Sports medicine experts have observed for years that endurance athletes, particularly females, frequently develop iron deficiencies. Research at Purdue University suggests that even moderate exercise may lead to iron depletion in women. Iron deficiency affects one in four adolescent girls and one in five women ages 18 to 45. It is even more prevalent among active women,

affecting up to 80 percent of female endurance athletes. Women who menstruate, eat little red meat, and/or restrict their caloric intake are at a heightened risk of developing iron deficiency.

The average woman takes in only two-thirds of the recommended daily allowance for iron. Exercise may be all it takes to tip some women over the edge into a serious deficiency. For this reason, sports medicine physicians are becoming more aggressive in their screening of athletes for iron deficiency anemia.

Iron deficiency is a condition in which the blood contains less hemoglobin than usual. The mineral iron is needed to make hemoglobin, which is the protein in blood cells that carries oxygen to the body's tissues. If one is anemic, the body is unable to transport oxygen efficiently and adequately, which results in a feeling of fatigue.

Causes

Iron deficiency may result from a number of situations. The most common are a diet that is lacking in iron, blood loss, or body changes during pregnancy.

Exercise can result in iron loss through a variety of mechanisms. Some iron is lost in sweat, and for unknown reasons, intense endurance exercise is sometimes associated with gastrointestinal bleeding. Athletes in high-impact sports such as running also may lose iron through repetitive trauma to capillaries of the feet, a phenomenon known as "foot-strike hemolysis."

Diagnosis

Patients with low iron stores may show no symptoms at all. Once the iron deficiency is sufficient to affect the production of hemoglobin, the symptoms include fatigue and poor performance. Once the deficiency has reached the level of iron deficiency anemia, the patient will often feel weak, tired, breathless, and the ability to perform activities, especially exercise, will be severely impaired.

Diagnosis of iron deficiency anemia can be done by tracking iron levels through hemoglobin, hematocrit, and ferritin tests. The best of these is the serum ferritin test, which is highly sensitive and specific for iron deficiency anemia. Some athletes can have mild iron deficiency without actually having anemia, or loss of hemoglobin. The ferritin test is most effective in separating out these cases.

Some sports medicine physicians routinely order complete blood counts and ferritin levels for most female athletes and male endurance athletes. Screening is recommended every year before the season begins. Athletes with low iron status should have follow-up tests done monthly to ensure that iron supplementation has sufficiently restored iron stores in the bone marrow.

Treatment

Treatment involves taking iron supplements and increasing the amount of iron in the diet. It is, however, possible to take too much iron, so patients should be careful to follow the prescription of their doctor.

Prevention

While active, reproductive-age women are most likely to have low iron stores, men who are physically active and vegetarian are also quite susceptible. (An estimated 15 percent of male distance runners have low iron stores.) Many experts advise people in these groups to have a yearly blood test to check ferratin levels.

Those with low iron levels should talk with a physician to see if the deficiency should be made up with diet or supplements. In general, it is better to solve the problem by adding more iron-rich foods to the diet, since supplements can cause nausea and carry a risk of toxicity. The best food sources of iron, and the only sources of heme iron (the most readily absorbed by the body), are meat, poultry, and fish. Good, nonheme sources of iron include dried apricots, prunes, dates, raisins, beans, tofu, and some vegetables such as spinach.

It is also helpful to select breads and cereal that indicate they are "iron-enriched" or "fortified" on the label. Eating these foods with a source of vitamin C, such as orange juice or tomato juice, to enhance iron absorption is a helpful strategy. Cooking in an iron skillet is also recommended, since some of the iron actually enters the food.

![J]

jammed finger (PIP joint injuries)   The layman's term *jammed finger* often refers to injuries that are incurred around the proximal interphalangeal joint, otherwise known as the PIP joint, of the fingers. While imprecise in its diagnostic accuracy, *jammed finger* aptly describes a group of injuries that result from excess pressure on this joint.

Injury to the PIP joint is common in athletics, especially ball-handling sports, but it is often minimized by players and coaches. The anatomy of the PIP joint is complex, and several types of injuries can result in permanent disability if they are left undiagnosed or mistreated. The sports medicine practitioner must develop a working knowledge of these common injury patterns, so that timely and appropriate treatment can be provided.

Causes

A common cause of a jammed finger is a basketball hitting the tip of the finger or running into someone with the tip of a finger while the finger is hyperextended and rigid.

One of the joints holding the finger bone may not be totally dislocated, but the bone may have snapped partway out of joint and then snapped back in. This injures the cartilage on the end of the bone, as well as the capsule around the joint, and stretches the ligaments that hold the joint together. The result is a swollen, painful finger that may appear normal on an X ray since the bone snapped back into the joint.

Diagnosis

The athlete with a jammed finger will typically present a history of some type of blow to the finger combined with hyperextension of the finger. The physician should pay close attention to the mechanism of injury in order to help pinpoint the exact type of injury that has occurred, which might include dislocated bones, ligament injury, nerve damage, and other problems. The most common diagnoses involving a jammed finger are volar plate disruption, dorsal dislocation, collateral ligament injury, and boutonniere deformity. Volar plate disruption, dorsal dislocation, and boutonniere deformity involve injury to the slips or bands of the exterior tendon at the level of the PIP joint. A collateral ligament injury may be a partial or complete rupture of the collateral ligament. This injury commonly occurs in conjunction with a volar plate rupture, resulting in lateral dislocation.

The physical examination will include observation and palpation of the point of tenderness and swelling. The doctor will need to assess tendon functioning and range of motion with particular attention to active extension of the finger. The doctor will want to document the integrity of the nerves and assess joint stability. If the finger is too painful to manipulate adequately, the doctor may want to use anesthesia.

X rays may be called for in order to rule out the possibility of fractures or dislocations. Lab studies are not necessary in the diagnosis of PIP joint injuries.

Treatment

A jammed finger typically heals very slowly. It should be immobilized for seven to 10 days and then taped to the finger next to it. It can take six months or more for the joint to return to normal size, and it may never return to completely normal function. The jammed finger will always be somewhat larger than the joint on the opposite hand, and it will have less flexibility than it did prior to injury, though it should not be enough to interfere with dexterity.

Any dislocation that cannot easily be reduced by conservative means may need to be treated surgically by an orthopedic surgeon. Fracture dislocations that are unstable will likely need to be repaired in surgery. Grossly unstable collateral ligament injuries may be considered for surgical repair as well, and surgical reconstruction is always the treatment of choice for chronic boutonniere deformity.

The time frame for an athlete's return to play is dependent on the severity of the injury. A mild sprain without ligament damage may be taped on the sidelines, allowing the player to return to play immediately. More severe sprains or dislocations and fractures require rest from the sport for several weeks. When the athlete does return to play, protective splinting or buddy taping should be used until the finger is completely pain free.

Possible complications following a PIP joint injury include persistent pain and swelling, stiffness, weakness, instability, and chronic boutonniere deformity. In general, however, the prognosis is excellent for a full recovery.

Prevention

In athletics, most cases of jammed finger injuries are not preventable.

jumper's knee (patellar tendonitis) Jumper's knee is inflammation or a rupture in the patellar tendon, which is the band of tissue that connects the kneecap to the shinbone. Under extreme stress, such as that involved in repeated jumping or running, the patella tendon can become inflamed and the surrounding tissue can degenerate.

Causes

The most common activity causing patellar tendonitis is too much jumping. Other repeated activities such as running, walking, and bicycling may lead to patellar tendonitis as well. All of these activities put repeated stress on the patellar tendon, causing it to be inflamed.

Patellar tendonitis can also happen to people who have problems with the way their hips, legs, knees, or feet are aligned. This alignment problem can result from having wide hips, being knock-kneed, or having feet with arches that collapse in walking or running, a condition called overpronation.

The patellar tendon may sometimes tear completely, or rupture, during strenuous activity.

Diagnosis

Symptoms of patellar tendonitis that may be revealed in the medical history of the patient include:

- pain and tenderness around the patellar tendon
- swelling in the knee joint or swelling where the patellar tendon attaches to the shinbone
- pain with jumping, running, or walking, especially downhill or downstairs
- pain with bending or straightening the leg
- tenderness behind the kneecap

If the patellar tendon is ruptured, usually there will be sudden severe pain, and the patient will be unable to straighten the leg or walk.

In a physical examination, the doctor will examine the knee to see if there is tenderness at the patellar tendon. The patient will usually be asked to run, jump, or squat to see if this causes pain. The doctor will also examine the feet to see if overpronation may be playing a role in the patellar tendonitis.

X rays or a MAGNETIC RESONANCE IMAGING (MRI) scan may be necessary in cases of a partial or complete rupture.

Treatment

Treatment may include the following:

- applying ice to the knee for 20 to 30 minutes every three to four hours for two to three days or until the pain and swelling go away
- taking anti-inflammatory medication or a pain medication prescribed by the doctor
- wearing a band across the patellar tendon, called an infrapatellar strap, or a special knee brace to support the patellar tendon, preventing it from becoming overused or more painful
- wearing custom-made arch supports called orthotics if overpronation is a contributing factor

In cases of a rupture of the patellar tendon, the patient will need surgery right away to repair it.

Rehabilitation from this injury involves a program of PHYSICAL THERAPY and changing sports to an activity that does not aggravate the injury. A basket ballplayer, for example, may need to switch to swimming until the patellar tendon is recovered.

The patient's return to his or her sport will be determined by how soon the knee recovers, not by how many days or weeks it has been since the injury occurred. In general, athletes will be ready to return to their sport when the following conditions have been met:

- The injured knee can be fully straightened and bent without pain.
- The knee and leg have regained normal strength compared to the uninjured knee and leg.
- The knee is not swollen.
- The athlete is able to jog straight ahead without limping.
- The athlete is able to sprint straight ahead without limping.
- The athlete is able to jump on both legs without pain and on the injured leg alone without pain.

Prevention

Patellar tendonitis is usually caused by overuse during activities such as jumping, running, or biking uphill. It can best be prevented by having strong thigh muscles.

It is also helpful to avoid activities that put extra stress on the knee. These include the following:

- squatting
- deep knee bends
- excessive bending
- sitting "Indian" style
- sitting back on the heels
- kneeling directly on knee caps
- excessive stair or hill climbing
- wearing high-heel shoes
- riding a bike with the seat too low
- breaststroke in swimming

knee bursitis (pes anserine bursitis, breaststroker's knee) Knee bursitis is an irritation or inflammation of a bursa in the knee. A bursa is a fluid-filled sac that acts as a cushion between tendons, bones, and skin. The pes anserine bursa is located on the inner side of the knee just below the knee joint. Tendons of three muscles attach to the shinbone over this bursa. These muscles act to bend the knee, bring the knees together, and cross the legs. Pes anserine bursitis is common in swimmers who do the breaststroke and is sometimes called breaststroker's knee.

Bursae are small tissue-lined structures that help different tissues glide over one another, such as a tendon sliding over another tendon or bone. Bursae may become painful when irritated, damaged, or infected.

Knee bursitis is a common finding in athletes who complain of anterior knee pain. This condition usually is found in patients who have tight hamstrings, although it also can be caused by a direct blow to the knee. In most patients, it is a self-limiting condition that responds to a program of hamstring stretching and quadriceps strengthening.

Causes

Knee bursitis can result from the following:

- overuse, as in breaststroke kicking or kicking a ball repeatedly
- repeated pivoting from a deep knee bend
- a direct blow to the area

The main cause of knee bursitis is underlying tight hamstrings. The tight hamstrings are believed to place extra pressure on the bursa, causing bursal irritation. In addition, some patients may have bursal irritation due to a direct blow and experi-

ence a contusion to this area, a common finding in patients who have OSGOOD-SCHLATTER DISEASE or other causes of joint irritation, such as arthritis, which may make the hamstrings spasm.

When a patient has tight hamstrings or experiences a blow to the area of the bursa, the synovial cells in the lining of the bursa may secrete more fluid and the bursa becomes inflamed and painful.

Diagnosis

Patients with knee bursitis often complain of pain on the inner side of the knee, just below the joint. There may be pain when bending or straightening the leg. This is the most common symptom described in a medical history of a patient with knee bursitis. While patients sometimes point to an area directly over the pes anserine bursa, they often may point to a rather general area of the knee.

The physical examination usually reveals pain in the area of the bursa and general tightness of the hamstrings. Intense pain is not consistent with knee bursitis and usually indicates a stress fracture in the shin bone.

Patients with signs of infection around the bursa should have a standard work-up for infection. In addition, an X ray or a MAGNETIC RESONANCE IMAGING (MRI) scan may be useful in ruling out a stress fracture and in helping to diagnose other concurrent problems, such as arthritis or OSTEOCHONDRITIS DISSECANS, which could contribute to tight hamstrings and the development of knee bursitis.

Treatment of knee bursitis usually includes the following:

- using ice packs on the knee for 20 to 30 minutes every three to four hours for two or three days or until the pain goes away

- wrapping an elastic bandage around the knee to reduce any swelling or to prevent swelling from occurring
- taking anti-inflammatory medication
- removal by the doctor of some of the fluid within the bursa if it is very swollen
- injection of a medication such as cortisone into the swollen bursa
- stretching exercises to loosen up the hamstrings

Patients with knee bursitis need to work on both a hamstring stretching program and a quadriceps-strengthening program. It is important for patients to stretch their hamstrings frequently during the day, sometimes hourly, to gain the maximum benefit from this program. This usually results in alleviation of the pain from knee bursitis in approximately six to eight weeks. Addition of a nonsteroidal anti-inflammatory medication may help to alleviate some of the pain at this time. Cutting back or eliminating the offending activities also is important. Ice massage may help to reduce inflammation.

Surgical intervention is very rare in cases of knee bursitis. However, patients with weakened immune systems and a localized infection of the bursa that will not resolve with standard antibiotic treatment may be considered for surgical decompression of the bursa.

Patients will need to modify their activity during the recovery period to allow the joint to quiet down and allow the hamstring tightness to resolve.

In most patients, this modification involves minimizing the use of stairs, climbing, and other activities that cause irritation of the joint. Patients can begin to gradually resume their activities once the symptoms improve. In athletes who play contact sports, the use of a protective pad over the area may prove useful. Patients may return to full activity when the following conditions have been met:

- The injured knee can be fully straightened and bent without pain.
- The knee and leg have regained normal strength compared to the uninjured knee and leg.
- The knee bursa is not swollen or tender to touch.
- The patient is able to jog straight ahead without limping.
- The patient is able to sprint straight ahead without limping.
- The patient is able to jump on both legs without pain and jump on the injured leg without pain.
- A swimmer needs to be able to do the breast-stroke kick without pain.

Prevention

Knee bursitis is best prevented by a proper warm-up that includes stretching of the hamstring muscles, the inner thigh muscles, and the top thigh muscles. In addition, athletes should be sure to gradually increase their activity levels, being careful not to add too much additional challenge all at once.

lateral collateral knee ligament injury   Lateral collateral knee ligament injuries are sprains that cause either a stretch or tear in the ligament, which is a strong band of tissue located on the outer side of the knee. The collateral ligaments are located at the inner side and outer side of the knee joint. The lateral collateral ligament (LCL) attaches the thighbone (femur) to the outside bone in the lower leg (fibula). Sprains vary from minor tears in a few fibers of ligament to complete tears of entire ligaments. Complete tears make the joint very loose and unstable.

Causes

The lateral collateral ligament can be injured by a twisting motion of the knee or from a blow to the inner side of the knee. This often occurs in contact sports and in skiing when ski bindings fail to release during a fall.

Diagnosis

A patient with a stretched or torn lateral collateral knee ligament will normally present pain on the outside of the knee. The knee is usually swollen and tender and feels like it will give way any moment. A history of the condition often reveals a pop or snap heard at the time of injury.

During the medical history, the doctor will want to know as many specifics as possible about how the knee was injured. The physical examination will include palpating the knee for tenderness outside and gently moving the knee to see if the joint is stable and if the ligament is stretched or torn. X rays or MAGNETIC RESONANCE IMAGING scans of the knee may be ordered.

Treatment

Remember the acronym RICE with all ligament injuries—rest, ice, compression, and elevation. Rest the knee to give the ligament time to heal. Apply ice two or three times a day for 15 to 20 minutes each time to alleviate inflammation. Compress the injury to limit swelling. A bandage or brace may be worn for a while to achieve this compression. Finally, keep the knee elevated whenever possible.

In addition to following the RICE guidelines, taking anti-inflammatory medication or other drugs prescribed by a health care provider will help in managing the pain. The patient may also need to use crutches until he or she can walk without pain.

While recovering from the injury, the patient will need to change to a sport or activity that does not aggravate the condition. For example, a runner may need to swim until he or she becomes free of the symptoms of the injury.

If the collateral ligament is completely torn or torn in such a way that ligament fibers cannot heal, the patient may need surgery. Repair may bring good results, with a return to good knee stability. After satisfactory rehabilitation, many people resume their previous levels of activity.

A rehabilitation plan is needed in the case of collateral ligament injury. Most rehabilitation plans include range-of-motion exercises designed to restore flexibility, braces to help control movement of the joint, exercises to strengthen the quadriceps in the front of the thigh, and additional exercises as tolerated.

The patient's return to sport will be determined by how soon the knee recovers, not by how many days or weeks it has been since the injury occurred. If the patient feels at any time that the knee is giving way or if the patient develops pain or swelling in the knee, he or she should see the doctor immediately. Guidelines for returning to full activity include the following:

- The health care provider has cleared the patient to advance his or her activities.

- The injured knee can be fully straightened and bent without pain.
- The knee and leg have regained normal strength compared to the uninjured knee and leg.
- The knee is not swollen.
- The patient is able to jog straight ahead without limping.
- The patient is able to sprint straight ahead without limping.
- The patient is able to jump on both legs without pain and jump on the injured leg without pain.

Prevention

Unfortunately, most injuries to the lateral collateral ligament occur during accidents that are not preventable. However, keeping the quadriceps and hamstrings strong and flexible will help in preventing this type of injury. Regular stretching before and after exercise will also help. Skiers should be certain that their bindings are correctly set by a trained professional so that the skis will release during a fall. The lateral collateral knee ligament injury occurs readily when ski bindings fail to release.

Lisfranc fracture-dislocation (tarso-metatarsal fracture-dislocation)

Named for a French field surgeon in Napoleon's army, the Lisfranc fracture-dislocation describes a range of traumatic injuries to the midfoot, specifically to the boundary between the midfoot and the more supple forefoot. A cluster of small bones forms an arch on top of the foot between the ankle and the toes. The five long bones of the foot called metatarsals extend from this cluster to the toes. The second metatarsal meets a row of small bones and acts as a stabilizer for the foot. These small bones are held in place by ligaments, but the first and second metatarsal are not connected by any ligaments, and this is where a problem may occur. Lisfranc fractures or dislocations can be the result of a twist of the foot or fall that dislocates the normal anatomy of this part of the foot. A Lisfranc injury can be anything from a sprain of the midfoot to a complete disruption of the anatomy, including breaks in the bones.

Causes

Generally speaking, the injury results when some type of acute trauma causes the midfoot to fold over the forefoot. Common accidents such as a dropping a heavy box on the foot or stepping in a hole and twisting the foot can produce a Lisfranc dislocation or fracture. The injury is also observed in people involved in industrial and car accidents, as well as in parachute jumpers.

Diagnosis

The patient may complain of pain whenever weight is placed on the foot. In severe injuries, the patient will be unable to bear any weight. The doctor may observe swelling on the top of the foot and sometimes bruising as well.

Lisfranc injuries are often mistaken for sprains. Often the doctor will hold the heel and move the foot around in a circle. In patients with a sprain, this produces minimal pain, but a Lisfranc injury will cause severe pain with this movement. X rays should be taken and sometimes a weight-bearing X ray is helpful. In some cases, a COMPUTERIZED AXIAL TOMOGRAPHY (CAT) scan or MAGNETIC RESONANCE IMAGING (MRI) scan is necessary to confirm the diagnosis.

It is crucial that a Lisfranc injury be properly diagnosed from the beginning. Serious complications can arise from an untreated Lisfranc injury, such as joint degeneration and compartment syndrome, which is an accumulation of pressure within muscles that can damage nerve cells and blood vessels. If the doctor diagnoses a sprain, and rest, ice, and elevation do not relieve the symptoms within a day or two, an orthopedic specialist should be consulted.

Treatment

Treatment for a Lisfranc injury depends on the severity of the injury. If the bones have not been forced out of position, the patient will probably have to wear a cast and refrain from putting weight on the foot for about six to 12 weeks. Surgery is sometimes required to stabilize the bones with pins, wires, or screws until healing can occur. When the cast is removed, the patient may have to wear a rigid arch support for up to one year. Rehabilitation will include foot exercises to build strength and help restore full range of motion. In some cases, if arthritis develops in these joints, the bones may have to be fused together.

Prevention

The injury is most often the result of an accident, but it is possible to avoid reinjuring the area after an initial injury has occurred. It is crucial that patients with a Lisfranc injury allow themselves adequate time to heal before returning to weight-bearing activities because it is very easy to reinjure the same part of the foot, which can result in damage to the blood vessels, the development of painful arthritis, and an even longer period of recovery.

little league elbow (medial apophysitis) Millions of children participate in organized sports every year, sometimes starting at a very young age. This increase in participation has been accompanied by an increase in the incidence of sports-related injuries in children. An emphasis on organized training and competition has led to the development of many injuries that fall into the general category of OVERUSE INJURIES, and one of the most common and widely discussed overuse injuries in children is little league elbow. Caused by repetitive throwing, little league elbow affects an estimated 4.8 million children between the ages of five and 14 each year.

Causes

Little league elbow is caused by too much throwing, which puts stress on the muscles that bend the wrist where they attach to the inner side of the elbow. The elbow joint consists of the bone in the upper arm, known as the humerus, and one of the bones in the lower arm, the ulna. The bony bumps at the end of the humerus are called epicondyles. The bump closest to the body is called the medial epicondyle, and the bump on the outer side of the elbow is called the lateral epicondyle. The muscles that work to bend the wrist attach at the medial epicondyle, and the muscles that work to straighten the wrist attach at the lateral epicondyle. Too much bending of the wrist will irritate the muscles that attach to the medial epicondyle.

In a child, the bones of the body grow from areas called growth plates. There is a growth plate at the medial epicondyle called the medial apophysis. In little league elbow, this growth plate is irritated or inflamed as a result of too much stress being placed on the muscles that attach to the growth plate. In severe cases of little league elbow, the growth plate may actually break away from the upper arm.

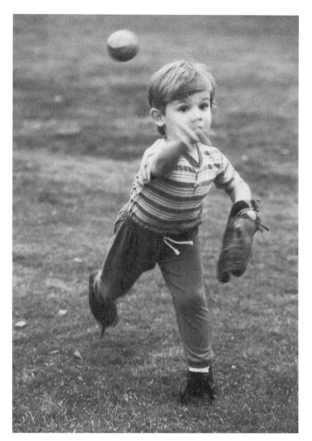

Little league elbow is a common overuse injury among children and is estimated to affect 4.8 million children between the ages of five and 14 each year. *(Fogstock, LLC)*

The following list includes some of the most common causes of little league elbow:

- training errors, such as abrupt changes in intensity, duration, or frequency of throwing activity
- imbalance of strength, flexibility, or bulk of muscles and tendons versus their elasticity
- anatomic malalignment of the lower extremities
- improper footwear or playing surface, which results in an insecure platform for stability in throwing activities
- associated disease state or preexistent injury

- growth
  - The growth cartilage around the growth plate is less resistant to repetitive trauma than fused adult bone.
  - Rapid growth or growth spurts can cause increased muscle and tendon tightness around a joint, resulting in loss of flexibility.

Diagnosis

Patients with little league elbow will usually describe pain at the inner side of the elbow. Swelling and tenderness may also be present.

The doctor will take a complete medical history and perform a thorough physical examination. The history will concentrate on the patient's history of sports and other physical activity, including position played and duration of the pain, which indicates whether the injury is chronic or acute. The patient's position on the sports team will also tell a lot about the magnitude of stress the elbow has endured. Pitchers on baseball teams and quarterbacks on football teams experience the highest incidence of this injury. Infielders, catchers, and outfielders may also experience the injury in decreasing order of prevalence. The patient's age will play a determining factor in regard to diagnosing this injury, which occurs primarily in patients whose medial epicondyle is not yet fused, rendering the growth plate vulnerable to injury.

The physical examination will focus on the arm and elbow. There will be tenderness along the inner elbow and pain when the patient throws a ball. During the initial examination, the doctor will evaluate the patient for loss of motion, muscle atrophy, muscle hypertrophy, bony deformity, elbow asymmetry, and flexion contracture.

The doctor will palpate all areas of the elbow and nerves in the elbow to locate the exact source of the tenderness. Various stress tests will help the doctor determine the damage to the ligaments. The neck, shoulders, wrist, and hand should also be examined thoroughly. Finally, the doctor will request an X ray, which may show irritation or a break in the growth plate.

Treatment

The most important treatment for little league elbow is to not throw if the growth plate is inflamed. Ice packs should be placed on the elbow for 20 to 30 minutes every three to four hours for two to three days or until the pain goes away. An elastic elbow wrap may be placed on the inflamed elbow to give it more support. An anti-inflammatory medication may be prescribed, as well as rehabilitation exercises.

Surgery may be necessary in severe cases of little league elbow where there is an actual break in the bone.

PHYSICAL THERAPY should involve strength and flexibility exercises for the muscles of the forearm, shoulder, and wrist. The patient must limit movement in the affected arm for a period of two to six weeks until the tenderness and swelling disappear. Once the patient is free of pain, physical therapy can progress to active range-of-motion exercises of the elbow. An elbow sleeve may also help provide comfort and support for the elbow during this time.

Initiating physical therapy too early or progressing too rapidly may prolong the healing process. In addition, injuries may be made worse, increasing the possibility of long-term complications. The patient may begin throwing when there is no swelling around the injured elbow, and it has regained its normal strength compared to the uninjured elbow. The patient must have full range of motion of the elbow, and throwing should be gradually increased but stopped if the elbow becomes painful. In most cases, the distance, number of throws, duration of throwing, and velocity should gradually be increased over a period of three weeks before attempts at near maximal effort occur. Any recurrence of symptoms during the return to activity necessitates halting the throwing recovery program and reassessment of the child. This return to throwing activities must be carefully monitored by the patient and his or her family in conjunction with an educated trainer, the coach, and a sports medicine or orthopedic specialist.

In the short term, most cases of little league elbow heal with rest and conservative management, but OSTEOARTHRITIS is a potential long-term complication. In the worst cases, functional disability and permanent deformity can result from proper or improper management of this injury.

Prevention

The best way to prevent little league elbow is to limit the child's amount of throwing. Since this problem occurs the most in pitchers, there are guidelines for how many pitches or innings a child can throw in a week. In general, a child ages nine through 12 years old should pitch a maximum of six innings per week (and no more than 250 pitches). A teenager between the ages of 13 and 15 should pitch a maximum of nine innings per week (and no more than 350 pitches). Since this rule applies only to game play, the number of pitches thrown during practices also should be monitored and limited.

Prevention can be accomplished by educating parents, players, and coaches about the symptoms and progression of little league elbow. Full recovery of strength and range of motion, along with pain-free throwing, should be accomplished before return to competition. Proper warm-up and strength and flexibility exercises should be maintained during the off-season or initiated at least six weeks before the first practice. Emphasis should be placed on proper throwing technique during practices. The prescreening physical allows an excellent opportunity for the doctor to provide this information to parents and coaches.

low back pain Low back pain is one of the most common problems treated by orthopedic surgeons. Four out of five adults will experience significant low back pain sometime during their life. This is especially true of athletes, who sometimes stress the low back in ways that nonathletes do not.

The lower spine is a complex structure that connects the upper body, including the chest and arms, to the lower body. It is the part of the spine that provides mobility and strength, allowing movements such as turning and twisting and bending, and providing strength that allows standing, walking, and lifting. Proper functioning of the lower back is essential in everyday activities and, of course, required in sports endeavors. Pain in the lower back can make it impossible to function properly in life and in sports.

Causes

Low back pain can have numerous causes, including both acute/traumatic injuries and OVERUSE INJURIES, aging, fractures, and osteoporosis, among other factors. Since the muscles of the low back provide power and strength for most basic activities, such as standing, walking, and lifting, these

muscles can be strained when they are poorly conditioned for the work they are asked to perform or when they are overworked and given inadequate rest and time for recovery. A sprain of the ligaments in the low back can occur when a sudden, forceful movement injures a ligament that has become stiff or weak through poor conditioning or overuse. Football, basketball, hockey, golfing, rowing, and many other sports may make an athlete vulnerable to low back injury.

In addition to poor conditioning and overuse, age, obesity, smoking, the presence of osteoporosis, and fractures in the spine can all contribute to low back pain.

Diagnosis

Most cases of low back pain are not serious and respond to simple treatments. They will be diagnosed on the basis of a medical history and a physical examination. In cases of severe pain or pain that does not respond to conservative treatment, the doctor may request an X ray to check for signs of arthritis or bone disease. If there is damage suspected in the soft tissues, such as the disks or nerves of the low back, a COMPUTERIZED AXIAL TOMOGRAPHY (CAT) SCAN or MAGNETIC RESONANCE IMAGING (MRI) will be used for further investigation. Sometimes bone scans are used to assess bone activity, and electrical tests, such as the EMG (electromyography) can be used to diagnose nerve or muscle damage.

Treatment

Most low back pain can be safely and effectively treated with a conservative approach that involves activity modification and some medication to relieve pain and help reduce the inflammation. Although rest may be useful initially, it is not usually recommended for the long term. Light activity has been shown to promote speedy recovery of many causes of low back pain.

Once the initial pain has gone away or lessened considerably, the athlete may begin a rehabilitation program to increase muscle strength in the low back and abdominal muscles and to increase flexibility. This program may include a weight loss component for patients who are significantly overweight. The long-term treatment plan is focused on maintaining physical fitness and observing proper lifting and postural activities to prevent further injuries.

In some cases, conservative treatment is not enough, and surgery may be required. The most common reason for surgery on the lower back is to remove the pressure caused by a "slipped disk." This condition can cause considerable nerve and leg pain that sometimes does not respond to other treatments. Some arthritic conditions of the spine can also cause recalcitrant pain that may only be improved with surgical treatment.

Prevention

The normal effects of aging that result in decreased bone mass, and decreased strength and elasticity of muscles and ligaments, cannot be avoided. However, the effects of aging on the low back can be slowed by regular exercise that maintains strength and flexibility in the muscles of the low back. Proper posture and lifting techniques will also help with preventing low back injuries, as will maintaining an appropriate body weight and avoiding smoking.

lumbosacral disk injuries   Injuries to the intervertebral disks of the lumbosacral spine are responsible for low back pain in many people. There are numerous ways in which a disk can be injured and generate back pain, which is second only to upper respiratory infection as a cause of time lost from work. At any one time, nearly 2.5 million Americans are disabled by lower back pain, with half of these patients experiencing chronic pain.

Athletes may injure a disk in number of ways, but the central aspect of any injury to the lumbosacral disks is the natural aging process and degeneration of these disks. The degenerative process occurs in three stages, with the greatest incidence of injury occurring during the first two phases.

The first phase is known as the dysfunctional phase. During this period of degeneration, tiny tears and fissures develop in the disks. There are also may be a disruption of blood supply, and thus nutrition, to the disk as a result of physical changes that occur in this phase. These changes are thought to occur from repetitive microtrauma to the disks.

During phase two, the unstable phase, multiple tears, internal disk disruption, and loss of disk space height occurs.

Phase three is known as the stabilization phase. During this time, the disks get closer together and further degeneration occurs to the disks themselves.

Causes

For athletes, injury to the spine can happen in numerous ways, including normal participation in contact sports or a fall or twisting motion while running. Repeated small traumatic injuries may accumulate over time, eventually causing serious disk injury. The most important thing that predisposes the athlete to disk injury, however, is disk degeneration.

Disk degeneration that creates anatomic changes is the primary cause of lower back pain. Nerve compression, inflammation, and internal disk disruption are the other primary causes of lumbosacral disk injury.

Diagnosis

By definition, pain is the primary presenting symptom in patients with low back pain. However, a variety of conditions may be signaled by the appearance of pain in the lumbosacral area, so it is extremely important to elicit a detailed description of the pain. The medical history should specify descriptions of the pain, noting the character, intensity, duration, and location, including any radiation to the extremities, groin, or abdomen, or associated pain at any other location. A subjective rating of the intensity of pain by the patient can be helpful in following the patient's progress if used at each visit to assess the patient's perception of pain intensity and progress of treatments. The physician should also try to determine the extent to which the pain is constant or intermittent, and whether there have been any changes in pattern. It may also be beneficial to have the patient complete a pain diagram, which provides a visual representation of the pattern of pain.

The history should also include a list of factors related to changes in pain. These commonly include coughing, sneezing, bending forward, lifting, carrying, sitting, straining at stool, ascending and descending stairs, walking, standing, lying down, and stretching. The patient should be asked specifically about each factor, as he or she may not be able to recall certain information without prompting, and the record should note explicitly whether each of these factors aggravates or alleviates the pain. In addition, the patient should be asked whether the pain is associated with a particular time of day.

In addition to these descriptions of the pain, the history should include information about any previous diagnoses of back problems, including specifics about the therapy prescribed for each problem and the patient's response to the therapy. A review of all previous diagnostic tests, as well as spinal taps, spinal anesthesia, hospitalizations, and surgery should be noted in the record.

Any history of the following diagnoses should also be included: arthritis; other musculoskeletal diseases; congenital abnormalities related to the spine; cancer, including the removal of moles; diabetes mellitus; major cardio- or cerebrovascular disease; peripheral vascular disease; renal and urinary tract disease; gynecologic/obstetric problems, including a notation regarding early menopause (age 35 or younger) and whether the menopause was due to surgical or biological causes; seizure disorders; psychiatric diagnoses and/or emotional problems; chronic pain syndromes; and chronic obesity.

Previous cancer, even 10 years in the past, is extremely important to an investigation of back pain, since the pain may be the first indication of metastatic cancer. A positive history of diabetes has significance both for interpreting any neurologic signs, which may indicate a neuropathy due to diabetes rather than to the back disorder, and for estimating the patient's prognosis. A history of early menopause may suggest the presence of osteoporosis as a cause of spinal deterioration and resulting pain. Endometriosis may also be associated with back pain.

A history of seizures may suggest previous spinal injuries resulting in compression fractures that may be producing pain.

In addition to pain, a description of any associated symptoms, such as numbness, fatigue, depression, muscle weakness, gait disturbances, changes in voiding patterns, and sexual dysfunction should be noted.

Patients who report numbness should be asked what they mean, as this term is synonymous with

pain to some patients. The record should contain a specific notation regarding the distribution, degree (severity), location, and intermittency of the numbness. A functional assessment should be made if the patient reports muscle weakness, with explicit questions regarding any experience of toe scuffing; difficulties in ascending and descending stairs; weakness of ankles, hips, and knees; and whether the muscle weakness occurs on one side or on both sides of the body.

The patient should be carefully questioned regarding his or her regular occupational and sports activities during the year prior to the onset of symptoms, including a notation regarding any recent changes. Stress levels should also be noted.

An assessment should be made of the patient's use of alcohol and tobacco products, with an explicit notation regarding chronic excessive consumption. Excessive alcohol consumption may be related to dietary abnormalities, which can lead to nerve problems. In addition, chronic excessive consumption or binge drinking should also be investigated as a possible cause of back trauma and consequent pain. Some patients may black out after drinking and sustain injuries that they do not remember afterward. Increased consumption of alcohol or cigarettes is also associated with osteoporosis.

Recent changes in the patient's weight should be noted in the record, with a comment as to whether the changes were voluntary. Sudden involuntary weight loss, particularly in a patient with a previous history of cancer, may suggest back pain due to metastatic cancer. Dietary abnormalities should also be included in the record, particularly those which suggest severe vitamin deficiency or excessive caloric intake. Vitamin deficiency, as previously mentioned, may be a clue to a possible neuropathy. Excessive caloric intake may be associated with back pain resulting from obesity and chronic poor posture.

The most common physical finding with injury to a lumbosacral disk is a protrusion or extrusion that results in nerve damage. Physical examination of the lumbar spine should focus on a mechanical and neurologic examination. The mechanical examination should evaluate for posture, range and quality of motion in the spine, and gait changes.

Typical posture problems include a rotation and listing to one side and an inability to stand erect. Examination of the vertebrae in the spine will focus on whether the vertebrae move normally and whether the patient experiences any pain with particular segments of motion in the spine.

The neurologic examination incorporates various tests to evaluate for signs of nerve root inflammation and neural deficit.

Discography is the only way to get an exact image of the location of pain and is necessary prior to most types of treatment. Discography provides information about the structure and sensitivity of disks that may not be learned from other sources. Discographic pain provocation is a very important part of the evaluation. Currently, discography is the only method of directly relating a radiographic image to a patient's pain. Discography is called for in many situations, including the correlation of an abnormal disk with clinical symptoms and persistent severe symptoms without clearly identifying the disk as the pain source. It is also called for in the assessment of failed surgery patients and in the assessment of disks prior to fusion or minimally invasive interventions.

Treatment

Conservative treatment for acute radiculopathy includes prescription for analgesics for management of pain and PHYSICAL THERAPY that includes stretching activities and massage. Once the vertebrae have begun to move more normally and the pain has lessened, the patient may begin a walking program and a program of exercises to help in stabilizing and conditioning the spine.

Surgical intervention may be required, depending upon the pain severity, degree of functional limitation, and status of the nerves. Although certain situations may be considered surgical emergencies, most situations will require a minimum of six to 12 weeks of adequate nonsurgical care prior to considering surgery. Treatment is directed toward alleviating pain.

Other treatments that may be considered in cases of structural abnormalities such as disk herniation and spinal stenosis include epidural steroid injection. In addition, intradiskal electrothermy (IDET) is one of the newest and least invasive treatments for chronic lower back pain. This targeted heat therapy has proven quite successful and has become an important alternative to major spinal surgery.

Athletes must follow a rehabilitation program designed specifically for their sport. Once the athlete demonstrates full pain-free range of motion and proper neutral spine posture with sport-specific activities, he or she can return to full activities.

Prevention

Injury prevention is best accomplished through good coaching, proper techniques during sport-specific activities, adequate preparticipation training, and appropriate safety measures, including proper protective equipment and adherence to the rules of the game. In addition, it is extremely important that athletes maintain strength in the spine and the associated muscle groups to help prevent injury in the future.

lumbosacral facet syndrome   Athletes involved in any type of sport are susceptible to facet joint injury. From the lineman on a football team, who may sustain repetitive and compressive forces to an extended spine, to the baseball player or golfer, who performs constant spinal rotational maneuvers, this syndrome can affect athletes in most sports. In addition, the lumbosacral facet joint is reported to be the source of pain in 15 to 40 percent of patients with chronic LOW BACK PAIN.

Doctors have concluded that, in most cases, facet joints are not the single or primary cause of lower back pain. In many cases, facet pain often can be mistaken for discogenic pain. Thus, many doctors find that it is a challenge to correlate historical or physical examination findings with pain emanating from the facet.

Diagnosis

By definition, pain is the primary presenting symptom in patients with low back pain. However, a variety of conditions may be signaled by the appearance of pain in the lumbosacral area, so it is extremely important to elicit a detailed description of the pain.

However, a variety of conditions may be signaled by the appearance of pain in the lumbosacral area, so it is extremely important to elicit a detailed description of the pain. The medical history should note the character, intensity, duration, and location of the pain, including any radiation to the extremities, groin, or abdomen, or associated pain at any other location. A subjective rating of the intensity of pain by the patient can be helpful in following the patient's progress if used at each visit to assess the patient's perception of pain intensity and progress of treatments. The physician should also determine the extent to which the pain is constant or intermittent, and whether there have been any changes in pattern. It may also be beneficial to have the patient complete a pain diagram, which provides a visual representation of the pattern of pain.

The history should also include a list of factors related to changes in pain. These commonly include coughing, sneezing, bending forward, lifting, carrying, sitting, straining at stool, ascending and descending stairs, walking, standing, lying down, and stretching. The patient should be asked specifically about each factor, as he or she may not be able to recall certain information without prompting, and the record should note explicitly whether each of these factors aggravates or alleviates the pain. In addition, the patient should be asked whether the pain is associated with a particular time of day.

In addition to these descriptions of the pain, the history should include information about any previous diagnoses of back problems, including specifics about the therapy prescribed for each problem and the patient's response to the therapy. A review of all previous diagnostic tests, as well as spinal taps, spinal anesthesia, hospitalizations, and surgery should be noted in the record.

Any history of the following diagnoses should also be included: arthritis; other musculoskeletal diseases; congenital abnormalities related to the spine; cancer, including the removal of moles; diabetes mellitus; major cardio- or cerebrovascular disease; peripheral vascular disease; renal and urinary tract disease; gynecologic/obstetric problems, including a notation regarding early menopause (age 35 or younger) and whether the menopause was due to surgical or biological causes; seizure disorders; psychiatric diagnoses and/or emotional problems; chronic pain syndromes; and chronic obesity.

Previous cancer, even 10 years in the past, is extremely important to an investigation of back pain, since the pain may be the first indication of metastatic cancer. A positive history of diabetes has significance both for interpreting any neurologic signs, which may indicate a neuropathy due to diabetes rather than to the back disorder, and for estimating the patient's prognosis. A history of early menopause may suggest the presence of osteoporosis as a cause of spinal deterioration and resulting pain. Endometriosis may also be associated with back pain.

A history of seizures may suggest previous spinal injuries resulting in compression fractures which may be producing pain.

In addition to pain, a description of any associated symptoms, such as numbness, fatigue, depression, muscle weakness, gait disturbances, changes in voiding patterns, and sexual dysfunction should be noted.

The patient should be carefully questioned regarding his or her regular occupational and sports activities during the year prior to the onset of symptoms, including a notation regarding any recent changes. Stress levels should also be noted.

An assessment should be made of the patient's use of alcohol and tobacco products, with an explicit notation regarding chronic excessive consumption. Excessive alcohol consumption may be related to dietary abnormalities that can lead to nerve problems. In addition, chronic excessive consumption or binge drinking should also be investigated as a possible cause of back trauma and consequent pain. Some patients may black out after drinking and sustain injuries that they do not remember afterward. Increased consumption of alcohol or cigarettes is also associated with osteoporosis.

Recent changes in the patient's weight should be noted in the record, with a comment as to whether the changes were voluntary. Sudden involuntary weight loss, particularly in a patient with a previous history of cancer, may suggest back pain due to metastatic cancer. Dietary abnormalities should also be included in the record, particularly those which suggest severe vitamin deficiency or excessive caloric intake. Vitamin deficiency, as previously mentioned, may be a clue to a possible neuropathy. Excessive caloric intake may be associated with back pain resulting from obesity and chronic poor posture.

Establishing a diagnosis of facet syndrome is difficult due to nonspecific findings and poor correlation between the history and physical examination. The basic history should include a temporal account of the symptoms and a complete description of the complaint, as well as the associated activities that cause or alleviate the pain. The patient should describe the location of pain, whether it is isolated or radiating, and its intensity, character, and frequency. Unexplained weight loss, fever, and chills are symptoms that should be taken seriously.

Often a patient with facet joint problems will complain of lower back pain that has a deep and achy quality. This pain may radiate to the buttocks and back of the thigh, but usually not below the knee. The pain is often exacerbated by twisting of the back, stretching, and side-bending. Some patients describe their pain as worse in the morning, aggravated by rest and hyperextension, and relieved by repeated motion. This type of pain often occurs after an acute injury but may be more chronic in nature.

A physical examination should include an in-depth evaluation of the neurological and musculoskeletal systems to help exclude other possible diagnoses. The doctor will want to palpate along the vertebrae in an attempt to locate the exact point of tenderness. Range-of-motion exercises should be assessed to determine which movements cause an increase in pain. In addition, flexibility of the pelvis and hamstrings should be assessed since these sometimes directly affect the mechanics of the lumbosacral spine. Muscle reflexes should be tested and usually appear normal. In addition, manual muscle testing is important to determine whether weakness is present, and whether the distribution of weakness corresponds to specific nerves.

Lab studies generally are not necessary for the diagnosis of lumbosacral facet joint syndrome.

Plain X rays are normally used to assess for fractures in the case of a sports injury. X rays may detect degenerative changes, but, in general, no abnormalities are seen in facet joint pathology.

Bone scans can be helpful when a tumor, infection, or fracture is present, but they usually are normal in the facet syndrome.

A COMPUTERIZED AXIAL TOMOGRAPHY (CAT) scan is useful in ruling our fractures and arthritic changes.

A MAGNETIC RESONANCE IMAGING (MRI) scan may be called for if degenerative changes are suspected within the disks.

Electrodiagnostic studies, such as nerve conduction studies (NCS) and needle electromyography (EMG), are usually not indicated for suspected facet syndrome. These studies, however, should be considered if the history and physical examination suggest that there is entrapment of a nerve root or if the diagnosis remains unclear after all other testing has been done. The electrodiagnostic testing may be helpful in excluding other causes of pain, such as radiculopathy.

Treatment

The initial treatment plan for acute facet joint pain should focus on education, relative rest, pain relief, maintenance of positions that provide comfort, and exercises. PHYSICAL THERAPY should include instruction on proper posture and body mechanics in activities of daily living that protect the injured joints, reduce symptoms, and prevent further injury. Positions that cause pain should be avoided. It is not recommended that patients rest in bed more than two days since this can have a detrimental effect on bone, connective tissue, muscle, and the cardiovascular system. Thus, activity modification, rather than bed rest is strongly recommended.

Use of superficial heat and cryotherapy also may help relax the muscles and reduce pain. In addition, medications such as nonsteroidal anti-inflammatory medications can also be initiated. Several different types of injection may also be used in the treatment program to help with pain, but their use should be conservative.

At this point, spinal manipulation and massage can also be tried in an attempt to reduce pain. An exercise program to strengthen the muscles of the trunk can also help to reduce the pain.

Once the painful symptoms are controlled during the acute phase of treatment, stretching and strengthening exercises of the spine and associated muscles can be initiated. It will help to stretch the hip flexors, hamstrings, hip internal and external rotators, and lumbar extensors, as these muscles may have been inactive secondary to reduced activity by the patient. In addition, treatment should include strengthening of the abdominal and gluteal muscles.

These exercises are eventually incorporated into a more comprehensive rehabilitation program, which includes spine stabilization exercises. The goal with these exercises is to teach the patient how to find and maintain a neutral spine during everyday activities. The neutral spine position is specific to the individual, and is determined by the pelvic and spine posture that places the least stress on the elements of the spine and supporting structures.

The maintenance phase represents the final phase of the rehabilitation process and should focus on sports-specific activities and conditioning. Goals of the comprehensive spine rehabilitation program have been met when pain is controlled, there is near full range of motion of the spine, and trunk control can be maintained in sport or recreational activities.

Prevention

In order to prevent further injuries to the facet joints, the patient should be instructed on proper posture, modification of activities, and the use of proper body mechanics in activities of daily living and sports that protect the injured joints, reduce symptoms, and prevent further injury. Positions that cause pain should be avoided.

magnetic resonance imaging (MRI) Magnetic resonance imaging, also known as MRI and as nuclear magnetic resonance imaging (NMRI), is a noninvasive procedure that uses powerful magnets and radio waves to construct pictures of the body. An MRI can provide additional imaging information for the clinician, based upon its superior tissue contrast resolution. Combined with other imaging methods, a more definitive diagnosis can be given. Sequences performed with intravenous contrast may provide additional data regarding the vascular nature of masses and tumors. An MRA, or magnetic resonance angiogram, is a special type of MRI that creates three-dimensional reconstructions of vessels containing flowing blood and is often utilized when conventional angiography cannot be performed due to renal failure or other contraindications.

How It Works

Unlike conventional X rays and COMPUTERIZED AXIAL TOMOGRAPHY (CAT) SCANS, which make use of potentially harmful radiation, MRI imaging is based on the magnetic properties of atoms. A powerful magnet generates a magnetic field roughly 10,000 times stronger than the natural background magnetism from the Earth. A very small percentage of hydrogen atoms within a human body will align with this field.

When focused radio wave pulses are broadcast toward the aligned hydrogen atoms in tissues of interest, they will return a signal. The subtle differences in that signal from various body tissues enable MRI to differentiate organs, and potentially contrast benign and malignant tissue.

Any imaging plane, or "slice" of the body, can be projected, stored in a computer, or printed on film. MRI can easily be performed through clothing and bones. However, certain types of metal in the area of interest can cause significant errors in the reconstructed images.

Because of the strong magnets, certain metallic objects are not allowed into the room.

- Items such as jewelry, watches, credit cards, and hearing aids can be damaged.
- Pins, hairpins, metal zippers, and similar metallic items can distort the images.
- Removable dental work should be taken out just prior to the scan.
- Pens, pocketknives, and eyeglasses can become dangerous projectiles when the magnet is activated and should not accompany the patient into the scanner area.

Because the strong magnetic fields can displace or disrupt the action of implanted metallic objects, people with cardiac pacemakers cannot be scanned and should not enter the MRI area.

MRI also should not be used for people with metallic objects in their bodies, such as:

- inner ear (cochlear) implants
- brain aneurysm clips
- some artificial heart valves
- older vascular stents
- recently placed artificial joints

Sheet metal workers, or persons with similar potential exposure to small metal fragments, will first be screened for metal shards within the eyes with X rays of the skull.

No preparatory tests, diets, or medications are usually needed. An MRI can be performed immediately after other imaging studies. Depending on the area of interest, the patient may be asked to fast for four to six hours prior to the scan. The patient will also be asked to sign a consent form confirming that none of the above issues apply before the study will be performed. A hospital gown may be recommended, or the patient may be allowed to wear "sweats" or similar clothing without metal fasteners.

Since MRI makes use of radio waves very close in frequency to those of ordinary FM radio stations, the scanner must be located within a specially shielded room to avoid outside interference. The patient will be asked to lie on a narrow table that slides into a large tunnel-like tube within the scanner. In addition, small devices may be placed around the head, arm, or leg, or adjacent to other areas to be studied. These are special body coils that send and receive the radio wave pulses. They are designed to improve the quality of the images. If contrast is to be administered, an IV will be inserted in a small vein of the hand or forearm. A technologist will operate the machine and observe the patient during the entire study from an adjacent room.

There is no pain. The magnetic field and radio waves are not felt. The primary possible discomfort is the claustrophobic feeling that some experience from being inside the scanner. The table may be hard or cold, but the patient can request a blanket or pillow. The machine produces loud thumping and humming noises during normal operation. Earplugs are usually given to the patient to reduce the noise.

A technologist observes the patient during the entire procedure and may be spoken to through an intercom in the scanner. Some MRI scanners are equipped with televisions and special headphones to help the examination time pass.

Several sets of images are usually required, each taking from two to 15 minutes. A complete scan, depending on the organs studied, sequences performed, and need for contrast enhancement may take up to one hour or more. Newer scanners with more powerful magnets utilizing updated software and advanced sequences may complete the process in less time.

Excessive movement can blur MRI images. If the patient has difficulty lying still or is very anxious, an oral or intravenous sedative may be given. There is no recovery time, unless sedation was nec-essary. After an MRI scan, normal diet, activity, and medications can be resumed.

Risks

There is no ionizing radiation involved in MRI, and there have been no documented significant side effects of the magnetic fields and radio waves used on the human body to date. The most common intravenous contrast agent, gadolinium, is very safe, and although there have been documented allergic reactions to it, this is extremely rare. If sedation is used, there are associated risks of oversedation. The technologist monitors the patient's vital signs, including heart rate and respiration as needed.

Despite the low risk associated with MRI, pregnant women are usually advised to avoid MRI scans because the effects of strong magnetic fields on a fetus have not yet been well documented.

MRI is usually not recommended in acute trauma situations since traction and life-support equipment cannot safely enter the scanner area, and scan times are relatively lengthy.

Finally, there have been instances when people have been harmed in MRI machines because they failed to remove metal objects from their clothes or metal objects were left in the room by others.

History of the Procedure

Magnetic resonance imaging (MRI) is based on a physics phenomenon discovered in the 1930s and 1940s, called nuclear magnetic resonance, in which magnetic fields and radio waves cause atoms to give off tiny radio signals. In 1970 Raymond Damadian, a medical doctor and research scientist, discovered the basis for using magnetic resonance imaging as a tool for medical diagnosis. He found that different kinds of animal tissue emit response signals that vary in length, and that cancerous tissue emits response signals that last much longer than noncancerous tissue. Less than two years later, he filed his idea for using magnetic resonance imaging as a tool for medical diagnosis with the U.S. Patent Office, entitled "Apparatus and Method for Detecting Cancer in Tissue." His patent was granted in 1974 and was the world's first patent issued in the field of MRI. The first whole-body MRI scanner was completed by 1977 by Dr. Damadian. Since that time, MRI has become the primary diagnostic technique for disease processes throughout the body, often replacing CAT scans as the preferred imaging procedure. The special advantages of the MRI include the fact that it is noninvasive and does not use radiation. It also offers extremely high-resolution images and specificity in taking all images of all parts of the body.

medial collateral knee ligament (MCL) injury

Medial collateral ligament (MCL) injuries of the knee are very common sports-related injuries. The MCL is the most commonly injured knee ligament. Injuries to the MCL occur in almost all sports and in all age groups. Knee ligament injuries are sprains that cause either a stretch or tear in the ligament, which is a strong band of tissue located on the outer side of the knee. The collateral ligaments are located at the inner side and outer side of the knee joint. Sprains vary from minor tears in a few fibers of ligament to complete tears of entire ligaments. Complete tears make the joint very loose and unstable.

Causes

Contact, noncontact, and overuse mechanisms are involved in causing MCL injuries. Contact injuries involve a direct load to the outside of the knee. This is the usual mechanism in a complete tear. Noncontact, or indirect injuries, are seen with deceleration, cutting, and pivoting motions. These mechanisms tend to cause partial tears. OVERUSE INJURIES of the MCL have been described in swimmers. The whip-kick technique of the breaststroke has been implicated since it involves repetitive heavy stress across the knee.

Diagnosis

A patient with a stretched or torn medial collateral ligament will normally present pain on the inside of the knee. The knee is usually swollen and tender and feels as though it will give way any moment. A history of the condition often reveals a pop or snap heard at the time of injury.

During the medical history, the doctor will want to know as many specifics as possible about how the knee was injured. The physical examination will include palpating the knee for tenderness on the outside and gently moving the knee to see if the joint is stable and if the ligament is stretched or torn. X rays or MRIs of the knee may be ordered to rule out fractures. Recent studies have suggested that ultrasound may be useful when evaluating a MCL injury.

Treatment

Remember the acronym RICE with all ligament injuries—rest, ice, compression, and elevation. Rest the knee to give the ligament time to heal. Apply ice two or three times a day for 15 to 20 minutes each time to alleviate inflammation. Compress the injury to limit swelling. The patient may have to wear a bandage or brace for a while to achieve this compression. Finally, keep the knee elevated whenever possible.

In addition to following the RICE guidelines, taking anti-inflammatory medication or other drugs prescribed by the health care provider will help in managing the pain. The patient may also need to use crutches until he or she can walk without pain.

While recovering from the injury, the patient will need to change to a sport or activity that does not aggravate the condition. For example, a runner may need to swim until he or she becomes free of the symptoms of the injury.

If the collateral ligament is completely torn or torn in such a way that ligament fibers cannot heal, the patient may need surgery, although this is quite rare. Persistent instability may also indicate surgery. Repair often brings good results, with a return to good knee stability. After satisfactory rehabilitation, many people resume their previous levels of activity.

A rehabilitation plan is needed in the case of collateral ligament injury. Most rehabilitation plans include range-of-motion exercises designed to restore flexibility, braces to help control movement of the joint, exercises to strengthen the quadriceps in the front of the thigh, and additional exercises as tolerated.

The patient's return to sport will be determined by how soon the knee recovers, not by how many days or weeks it has been since the injury occurred. If the patient feels at any time that the knee is giving way or if pain or swelling in the knee develops, see the doctor immediately. Guidelines for returning to full activity include the following:

• The health care provider has cleared the patient to advance his or her activities.

- The injured knee can be fully straightened and bent without pain.
- The knee and leg have regained normal strength compared to the uninjured knee and leg.
- The knee is not swollen.
- The patient is able to jog straight ahead without limping.
- The patient is able to sprint straight ahead without limping.
- The patient is able to jump on both legs without pain and jump on the injured leg without pain.

Prevention

Unfortunately, most injuries to the medial collateral ligament occur during accidents that are not preventable. However, keeping the quadriceps and hamstrings strong and flexible will help in preventing this type of injury. Regular stretching before and after exercise will also help. Skiers should be certain that their bindings are correctly set by a trained professional so that the skis will release during a fall. The medial collateral knee ligament injury occurs readily when ski bindings fail to release.

medial condylar fracture of the elbow Medial condylar fractures are rare in adults but fairly common in adolescents between the age of 10 and 14, especially boys. The injury involves a fracture line that extends through and separates the medial metaphysis and epicondyle from the rest of the humerous bone. Since trauma to the elbow has a high potential for complication and residual functional disability, it is extremely important that these injuries are diagnosed properly and treated effectively.

Causes

Medial condylar fractures generally occur as a result of either a fall onto an outstretched upper extremity or a fall onto a flexed elbow. The mechanism of injury appears to be the same in both children and adults.

Diagnosis

When evaluating a patient with an acute elbow injury, obtain a detailed event history including the injury mechanism and the quality, intensity, duration, and location of symptoms.

Patients will often report falling on an outstretched arm, with the elbow in extension and the wrist in dorsiflexion. This type of injury can cause the medial condyle of the elbow to fracture.

Another mechanism responsible for medial condylar fracture is falling onto the point of a flexed elbow. In this case, it is important for the doctor to elicit and document hand dominance, occupation, and preexisting extremity injury.

The medical history should also include a history of any weakness, numbness, coolness, or other indication of neurovascular damage.

The physical examination includes a visual inspection of the injured elbow and an evaluation beginning at the shoulder and upper arm, and then proceeding to the forearm, wrist, and hand. The elbow should be examined last, as tenderness elicited may interfere with a proper examination of the injured extremity. The doctor should assess vascular status of the extremity. It is important to look for signs of compartment syndrome, including pain out of proportion to the injury, severe forearm pain with passive extension of the fingers, and paralysis.

The doctor should perform tests to assess the functioning of the nerves. Finally, range-of-motion tests should be minimized, especially in children, since they usually are quite painful. Lab studies generally are not indicated for diagnosing condylar fractures of the elbow.

The decision to obtain elbow radiographs is based on the history of the injury and the physical examination of the patient. Standard elbow X rays are often sufficient to diagnose a fracture in the acutely injured elbow. They are often performed on patients who exhibit joint swelling and tenderness of the bony landmarks or a restricted and painful range of motion of the elbow following trauma. X rays will help the doctor to classify the exact type of fracture and thus the specific treatment approach that is needed.

Treatment

Neurovascular complications can occur as a result of medial condylar fractures. One of the most feared is the development of a compartment syndrome. As a result of bleeding and swelling in a closed space, compartment pressures rise, circulation is compromised, and tissue damage occurs.

Failure to make the proper diagnosis during the initial evaluation can complicate the management of these injuries. In young children, the proper diagnosis of a medial condyle fracture may be challenging, but is especially important to ensure proper functioning in the future.

Closed reduction of the fracture is the conservative treatment. It often involves splinting of the arm following reduction to relieve the tension on the forearm. Normally, the arm will remain immobilized for four to six weeks, after which time the patient will perform range-of-motion exercises.

Surgical intervention is recommended sometimes to restore displaced fractures or to repair nerve damage.

Barring any other traumatic injury, patients should try to maintain general fitness levels during rehabilitation. After the initial period of immobilization, patients should begin range-of-motion exercises and implement progressive resistance training with the goal of reaching preinjury strength and flexibility.

The medications used in the management of elbow fractures include analgesics. Conscious sedation may be required for the initial closed reduction of a fracture. Intravenous sedative and narcotic agents are commonly used to perform conscious sedation.

Prior to returning to athletic competition, the participant should regain normal or near-normal strength in the affected arm, and range of motion should be similar to the preinjury status. Some athletes may be able to return to competitive sports prior to reaching these goals. This depends on the type of sport and whether the injury affected the athlete's dominant or nondominant arm. Athletes returning to sports such as gymnastics that require "elbow-loading" maneuvers usually require more extensive rehabilitation prior to returning to competition.

In general, nondisplaced fractures that are managed conservatively with a long arm cast have excellent results. In displaced fractures requiring open reduction and internal fixation, a good outcome can be expected barring complications.

Prevention

Since medial condylar fractures occur as a result of accidental falls, in addition to high-risk sports, it is difficult to prevent them from happening. Proper education and adequate protective gear, such as elbow pads, during sports activities should decrease the frequency of these injuries.

meniscus injuries The meniscus is a cartilage inside the knee joint, whose main purpose is to distribute the forces around the knee joint. It actually bears about 40 percent of the total load transmitted through the knee joint, primarily that transferred from the thigh above the knee to the lower leg. Shaped like a half-moon, the meniscus deepens the relatively flat surface of the upper end of the shinbone and acts like a gasket between the femur and the tibia. By serving this purpose, the meniscus protects the articular cartilage in the knee from excessive wear. If the meniscus is absent or worn, the concentration of force into one small area of the articular cartilage can damage the surface of the joint and lead to OSTEOARTHRITIS.

The meniscus also helps with stability of the knee joint by transforming the surface of the tibia into a shallow socket, making it more stable for the round femur bone.

Meniscus injuries involve some type of tearing of the meniscus. The entire rim of the inner meniscus can be torn in what is called a bucket handle tear. The meniscus can also have a flap torn from the inner rim, or it can have a degenerative type of tear, in which part of the meniscus is frayed and gets torn in multiple directions.

Causes

In younger people the meniscus is fairly tough and rubbery. In order for the meniscus to tear, it usually requires a fairly forceful twisting injury, which often occurs during some type of sports activity.

In older people, the meniscus is normally weaker and can be torn much more easily. Meniscus tears can result from a fairly minor injury or even from the simple up and down motion of squatting. If osteoarthritis develops in the knee joint, meniscus tears can occur as part of the overall condition in the knee without any precipitating injury.

Diagnosis

Patients with a torn meniscus usually describe pain that is fairly significant. It may be felt along the joint line where the meniscus is located, or it may be more vague and involve the whole knee. If the torn portion of the meniscus is large enough, locking of the knee may occur. This inability to completely straighten out the knee happens when a piece of the torn meniscus gets caught in the hinge of the knee and does not allow the leg to straighten completely.

If a torn meniscus goes untreated, there are long-term effects as well. The torn piece of the meniscus may rub the articular cartilage, causing wear and tear on the surface that will lead to degeneration of the joint. When the knee becomes inflamed, fluid will sometimes collect inside the knee joint, causing the knee to swell and become stiff and tight.

The doctor will take a complete medical history of the patient and conduct a thorough physical examination in order to make a diagnosis. The history may reveal a "popping" sound noted at the time of injury. Other common symptoms include joint tenderness, pain that gets worse when gentle pressure is applied, recurrent catching of the knee, and locking of the knee. The physical examination will focus on determining where the pain is located, whether or not locking has occurred, and if there are any clicks or pops as the knee is moved.

X rays will not show a torn meniscus, but a MAGNETIC RESONANCE IMAGING (MRI) scan is very effective at revealing this injury. If there is an uncertainty in the diagnosis following the history and physical examination, or if other injuries in addition to the meniscal tear are suspected, the MRI scan may be suggested.

If the tests suggest a torn meniscus, then ARTHROSCOPY may be used to confirm the diagnosis and treat the problem at the same time. The arthroscope allows the doctor to actually look into the knee joint and see the condition of the articular cartilage, the ligaments, and the menisci.

Treatment

Initial treatment for a torn meniscus usually is directed toward reducing the pain and swelling in the knee. It is important not to force weight bearing on the injured knee if pain is experienced. The physician may recommend crutches for resting the knee for several days and suggest ice to reduce the pain and swelling. If the knee is locked and cannot be straightened out, surgery may be recommended as soon as reasonably possible to remove the torn portion that is caught in the knee joint. Once a meniscus is torn, it will most likely not heal on its own.

If the symptoms continue, surgery will be required to either remove the torn portion of the meniscus or to repair the tear. Most meniscus surgery today is done using the arthroscope. In some cases, the meniscus tear can be repaired with sutures, but repair is not possible in all cases. Young people with relatively recent meniscal tears are the most likely candidates for repair. Degenerative type tears in older people are not usually repairable.

Prevention

It is important to use proper technique when exercising or playing sports and to warm up and stretch before all strenuous physical activity. This helps in the prevention of many injuries, but there are many cases of meniscus tears, especially those that occur in conjunction with osteoarthritis, that still may not be preventable.

metacarpophalangeal joint dislocations (MCP joint dislocations)   Sprains and dislocations of the metacarpophalangeal (MCP) joint of the finger are relatively rare due to the protected position of this joint in the hand. Injuries to the MCP of the thumb and index finger are more common. Prompt recognition of this injury is important to ensure the best possible outcome. In particular, it is important to determine whether a dislocation is simple or complex, because simple dislocations can be treated with closed reduction, whereas complex dislocations usually require surgery. Further, closed reduction must be done properly to avoid converting a simple injury into a complex one.

Cause

MCP dislocations typically occur in football and basketball. The mechanism of injury is usually forced hyperextension of a finger in a fall on an outstretched hand.

Diagnosis

The clinical signs of simple and complex disloca-tions are distinctly different. In a simple disloca-tion, the finger is hyperextended about 60 degrees above the horizontal.

In a complex dislocation, the digit is hyperex-tended about 15 degrees above the horizontal. In addition, the displaced bone usually forms a prominence in the palm of the hand, and the adja-cent skin is puckered.

Reduction refers to the procedure, either man-ual or surgical, in which the dislocated joint is returned to its proper position. This type of com-plex dislocation should not be reduced on the side-lines of a game. The hand needs to be thoroughly examined, including a neurologic exam, before the decision about a closed reduction or a surgical reduction is made.

The patient will often present a sprained or rup-tured ligament as well. The sudden mechanism of injury after a direct fall on to the thumb or palm often causes these to occur.

Physical signs of an MCP injury include various abnormal positions of the finger and tenderness over the joint. The bone may be sticking up and palpable in the palm of the hand and the sur-rounding skin may be puckered, depending on the exact site of injury. There may be swelling and decreased pinch strength even with mild ligament injury.

Lab studies generally are not indicated in the diagnosis of MCP injuries.

Prereduction and postreduction X rays are nec-essary to demonstrate associated fractures and joint congruency. Stress X rays may also be useful but should not be taken until after static X rays have been done in case the stress causes dislocation of the bone.

Treatment

With fractures, closed reduction with local anes-thesia and subsequent splinting is recommended whenever possible.

Sprains should not be overtreated. They may require a brief period of protection, usually con-sisting of buddy taping (taping to the adjacent fin-ger) for two to three weeks, and immobilization in more severe cases.

Certain types of injuries to the metacarpopha-langeal joint will require surgery for repair. When there is gross instability or a significantly displaced or rotated avulsion fracture, surgery is needed.

Recovery following treatment involves progres-sive hand therapy following the initial mobiliza-tion. In most cases, noncontact activities are permitted once the acute injury has healed, usually within six weeks. The injured finger should be buddy taped during this period. Usually, it is safe to return to contact sports after three months. A pro-gressive range of motion program is essential in order for the joint to regain full range of motion and flexibility.

Prevention

Prevention is difficult since this injury normally occurs during an accidental fall. Reinjury may be prevented with appropriate buddy taping of the injured finger to an uninjured digit during forceful activities, especially contact sports.

metatarsalgia Metatarsalgia is a general term used to denote a painful foot condition in the metatarsal region of the foot, which is the area just before the toes, more commonly referred to as the ball of the foot. A common foot disorder that can affect the bones and joints at the ball of the foot, metatarsalgia is often located under the second, third, and fourth metatarsal heads, or more iso-lated at the first metatarsal head, which is near the big toe.

Cause

With this common foot condition, one or more of the metatarsal heads become painful and/or inflamed, usually due to excessive pressure over a long period of time. It is common to experience acute, recurrent, or chronic pain with metatarsal-gia. Ball-of-foot pain is often caused from improper fitting footwear, most frequently by women's dress shoes and other restrictive footwear. Footwear with a narrow toe box forces the ball-of-foot area to be forced into a minimal amount of space. This can inhibit the walking process and lead to extreme discomfort in the forefoot.

Other factors can cause excessive pressure in the ball-of-foot area that can result in metatarsalgia.

These include shoes with heels that are too high or participating in high-impact activities without proper footwear and/or orthotics. Also as people get older, the fat pad in the foot tends to thin out, making them much more susceptible to pain in the ball of the foot.

Diagnosis

A patient with metatarsalgia often reports that one or more of the toe joints becomes inflamed, painful, and stiff. Swelling may be present, and if there is metatarsalgia, the patient will often experience a burning sensation in the joint area. Generally, the swelling and pain become progressively worse with continued activity, especially if the patient's shoes are fairly old or the patient has relatively poor foot and ankle strength. In full-blown metatarsalgia, the pain can be so intense that putting weight on the foot becomes nearly impossible.

In order for the doctor to diagnose metatarsalgia, a complete medical history and a physical examination is taken. The doctor will want to pay particular attention to a history of recent weight gain and a family history of diabetes or gout. Diabetes causes poor blood circulation to the feet, which can lead to pain similar to the discomfort of metatarsalgia. Gout produces profound joint irritations, which can mimic metatarsalgia, too. If there is indeed a family history of either of those conditions, urine and blood samples will often be taken. An X ray and possibly a MAGNETIC RESONANCE IMAGING (MRI) scan may be requested in order to inspect the troubled joint closely, especially if the doctor suspects a stress fracture. In cases that are extremely difficult to diagnose, nerve function in the foot may need to be tested.

The doctor will also want to know about the duration of the symptoms and should ask whether the pain is related to a single event. A description of what activities provoke discomfort and the exact location of the pain is important to define. It is also important to determine if the patient has recently changed a workout schedule, athletic shoes, or the running surface.

Treatment

The first step in treating metatarsalgia is to determine the cause of the pain. If improper fitting footwear is the cause of the pain, the footwear must be changed. Footwear designed with a high, wide toe box (toe area) and a rocker sole is ideal for treating metatarsalgia. The high, wide toe box allows the foot to spread out while the rocker sole reduces stress on the ball of the foot.

Unloading pressure to the ball of the foot can be accomplished with a variety of foot care products. Orthotics designed to relieve pain in the ball of the foot usually feature a metatarsal pad. The orthotic is constructed with the pad placed behind the ball of the foot to relieve pressure and redistribute weight from the painful area to more tolerant areas. Other products often recommended include gel metatarsal cushions and metatarsal bandages. When these products are used with proper footwear, the patient should experience significant relief.

Naturally, it may be necessary to limit training until the symptoms go away. Workouts may be made less lengthy and intense (in severe cases of metatarsalgia, training will have to cease until symptoms subside), and ice and elevation should be used after training sessions are over. The best policy appears to be to rub the painful area with ice for about 12 minutes at a time while the foot is elevated, taking 20-minute recovery periods between icings. Weight loss may be helpful to the overweight athlete suffering from forefoot pain, and nonsteroidal anti-inflammatory medications are often taken to provide pain control.

If a stress fracture is discovered, symptoms may hang around for four to eight weeks, and if obesity, diabetes, gout, or arthritis are present, it is very difficult to predict how long the pain will last. Although athletes will be sorely tempted to train through the metatarsalgia, they need to realize that activity will increase the stresses on the point of injury and slow down the recovery process. Return to normal training and competition should be delayed until underlying causes of forefoot pain have been resolved and until major symptoms have disappeared.

It is generally believed that increasing the range of motion of the ankle, maintaining elasticity of the Achilles tendon, strengthening the muscles and connective tissues of the foot, and enhancing the flexibility of the metatarsal joints help to spur recovery and reduce the possibility of recurrence.

This is important in the recovery from injury as well as in the prevention of future injuries.

Prevention

Athletes in a variety of sports have noticed that when they increase their total training load or engage in an unusually long workout or competition, their feet are likely to pay the price. More specifically, they often begin to experience some discomfort on the bottom of one of their feet or both feet. Careful training programs that do not add too much stress at one time are helpful in preventing this condition.

In addition, metatarsalgia experts indicate that high arches, deformities of the toes, stiff ankles, irritated nerves in the forefeet, bunions, poor circulation to the feet (due to diabetes), gout, arthritis, weight gain, and shoes with too-high heels are also predisposing factors.

The most important preventive strategies include the following:

- Wear athletic shoes that fit properly and are appropriate to the activity.
- Make sure that the insoles and midsoles of athletic shoes have not broken down and that they do retain a healthy measure of support. This loss of resiliency may put extra pressure on the foot and metatarsal joints.
- Increase the intensity and duration of training very slowly and cautiously. Whenever forefoot pain appears, take a day off and then train lightly for a few days to keep inflammation at bay. Resume normal training, using STRETCHING and exercises to ward off future problems.
- Be particularly careful whenever initiating new training methods. For example, a basketball player who begins to work on vertical jumping ability by practicing repeated jumps against extra resistance will find that the increased number of high-impact landings and additional forces placed on the feet will significantly increase the risk of metatarsalgia.
- Athletes prone to metatarsalgia should use shoes with relatively boxy toes and try to avoid shoes that seem to have increased heel height. The latter can pitch the feet forward, putting extra pressure on the metatarsal joints.

- Maintain a healthy weight.
- Athletes with a family history of diabetes, arthritis, or gout should pay particular attention to signs of this condition as they are more vulnerable to developing foot problems.

Morton's neuroma   A neuroma is a noncancerous tumor of nerve tissue. A Morton's neuroma is located in the nerves between either the second and third toes or the third and fourth toes.

Causes

These painful tumors can occur on their own or be caused by excessive running and walking. Running or walking on hard surfaces and wearing shoes that are too tight both exacerbate the pain. The repetitive damage that occurs to the nerve fibers due to either of these conditions may eventually increase the nerve diameter and cause a neuroma.

Diagnosis

A history of the pain in the foot and a thorough physical examination by a doctor will lead to a diagnosis. Morton's neuroma normally causes pain over the ball of the foot, and the patient will normally complain of numbness, tingling, and a burning sensation, all of which ease with the removal of the shoe and rubbing the ball of the foot. Usually, the patient's history will reveal wearing of tight-fitting, high-heeled, or pointed-heel shoes. In addition, jumpers, sprinters, and those who work out on a treadmill or stair climber, using a repetitive step-off motion in their sport, are vulnerable to developing this injury.

Treatment

Treatment is usually conservative and designed to relieve pain while permitting the athlete to continue activity. This often involves a podiatric consultation to ensure that shoes fit properly, as well as rest, icing the injury, and taking anti-inflammatories. Sometimes an injection of a corticosteroid will be effective in reducing the size of the tumor. These injections typically provide relief within a few days to a few weeks.

If none of these approaches works, surgery may be required to remove the neuroma, which provides quick relief from pain and inflammation. Recovery following surgery typically takes up to a month or longer.

Rehabilitation will include range-of-motion and strengthening exercises for the foot. Return to normal activity may occur when the patient has full range of motion and strength in the injured foot and can run and jump without pain.

Prevention

Avoiding repetitive stressful motions will help to prevent the development of a Morton's neuroma, as will walking and running on soft surfaces and wearing shoes that provide adequate room for the toes.

mountain biking   During the past 20 years, mountain biking has grown from a little-known sport made popular in the hillsides of California into a worldwide sport that has spawned a multi-billion-dollar industry. More than half of all bicycles owned in the United States are mountain bikes.

While this phenomenon has fueled the bicycle industry, created a new event in the Olympics, and given rise to the new sport of amateur mountain bike racing, it has also meant an huge increase in the number of bicycle-related injuries that occur each year. Although there are similarities between road biking and mountain biking with some injuries showing up frequently in both, there are injury patterns that are unique to mountain biking.

The differences in equipment, terrain, and competition account for most of these differences. The mountain bike has evolved into a very different machine from the standard road bike. It may be constructed of exotic synthetic and natural materials and shaped in geometries that barely resemble the road bike. It has wide knobby tires, shock absorption systems, and advanced braking systems that allow cyclists to go off road. In competition and in recreational riding, mountain bikers travel on tough terrain and are subject to steep inclines and descents, jumps, and falls from significant heights. All these things make the mountain biker susceptible to serious injury, as well as to many OVERUSE INJURIES.

Traumatic Injuries

Unfortunately, crashes appear to be inherent in off-road bicycling. More than 80 percent of 650 mountain bikers who participated in surveys were injured in off-road crashes during a one-year period. However, many of those injuries were minor and self-treated.

Traumatic injuries range from minor ABRASIONS and contusions to wrist fractures, shoulder injuries, and CONCUSSIONS. Helmet use is important in preventing serious head trauma. Fortunately, most off-road cyclists use helmets. One study found that mountain bikers were more than four times as likely as other cyclists to wear helmets, which probably accounts for the low rate of head injuries in the sport.

Most crashes result in only minor injuries such as abrasions, contusions, and lacerations. Fractures and concussions are less common but have been consistently reported. The majority of fractures occur to the upper extremity and commonly involve the fingers, metacarpals, wrist, and radial head.

The shoulder is particularly vulnerable to injury in mountain biking crashes. Clavicle fractures and acromioclavicular separations commonly occur when a cyclist falls and lands on the shoulder. Shoulder dislocations can occur if the cyclist's arm is raised during a forward fall. Other serious injuries that have been consistently reported include pelvic fractures, intra-abdominal injuries, facial fractures, and severe brain injuries.

A number of factors contribute to acute injuries. A retrospective survey of recreational mountain bikers found that off-road crashes were commonly associated with excessive speed, unfamiliar terrain, inattentiveness, and riding beyond one's ability. A similar survey of recreational and competitive off-road cyclists identified loss of control, high-speed descent, and competition as factors related to acute injuries. Studies have found that those racing in competitions are four times more likely than non-competitors to be acutely injured.

Studies also indicate that the majority of injuries take place on downhill rides. Flat tires and other mechanical problems are more commonly associated with accidents that occur during downhill than during cross-country races. Other causes of accidents include hitting a bump or rock during a high-speed descent, losing traction while turning, or losing control of the bike while riding too fast.

Whatever the cause, injuries tend to be more severe when a rider is thrown forward over the handlebars than when he or she falls off the bike to the side. Some studies have shown that female riders are more likely to go over their handlebars than are their male counterparts.

Injuries commonly associated with mountain biking include ABRASION, ACROMIOCLAVICULAR JOINT INJURY, ANKLE FRACTURE, CONCUSSION, SHOULDER DISLOCATION, and SHOULDER SEPARATION.

Acute Injury Prevention

To prevent acute injuries, the importance of bicycle maintenance, bike-handling skills, and common sense cannot be overemphasized. Helmet use is clearly effective in decreasing head injuries and should remain a key preventive measure. However, most bicycle helmets provide little protection to the lower face. Some newer helmets have been redesigned to offer improved facial protection, and these are especially popular among downhillers.

Other protective gear, such as chest, shoulder, and extremity padding, is also used by many downhill cyclists. These devices probably help decrease superficial injuries to the bicyclist, but their ability to prevent serious injury has not been demonstrated.

Overuse Injuries

Many overuse injuries stem from improper bike fit, anatomic misalignments, and training errors. Treatment includes adjustments to the bike and modification of training habits. Overuse injuries of the knee are common, as are injuries to the spine, upper extremity, and saddle region. Knee pain, low-back pain, and numbness and pain in the wrist and hand are all commonly reported by those who mountain bike.

Overuse injuries in off-road cyclists are related to interactions between the cyclist's body, the bicycle, and the terrain on which they ride. The effects of anatomic variations and small errors in bike fit are magnified by long hours spent riding and by the highly repetitive nature of the leg movements. A combination of these factors is usually responsible for overuse injuries of the lower extremity. In contrast, upper-body overuse syndromes are more often related to weight bearing on the handlebars and the vibrations transmitted from rough riding surfaces to the cyclist via the bicycle.

Training errors also contribute to overuse injuries. The abundance of hills available for off-road riding can easily tempt a rider to push beyond his or her established level of conditioning, especially early in the season. Common training errors include inadequate preseason conditioning, riding in too high a gear by relying too much on the large chain ring, and suddenly increasing mileage, hill climbing, or riding intensity.

Treatment of Injuries

The office evaluation of a cycling overuse injury should include a training history to detect common training errors. Riders should be encouraged to establish a basic level of conditioning at the beginning of the season before increasing their mileage, hill climbing, or intensity. Injured cyclists may require temporary modifications of their riding habits until symptoms decrease. Rather than taking a complete break from cycling, the injured off-road cyclist can often benefit from relative rest. This may mean temporarily decreasing mileage and hill climbing and emphasizing low-resistance easy pedaling with avoidance of the large chain ring. As symptoms subside, the cyclist can gradually increase the amount and level of riding.

The physical examination should include a search for anatomic variations that could negatively interact with the mechanical restraints of the bicycle. When present, these misalignments can usually be compensated for with adjustments to the bicycle. The cyclist's position on the bicycle should be checked whenever possible. Sometimes an overuse injury can be treated simply by putting the cyclist in a neutral riding position. If this treatment does not resolve the symptoms or if a cyclist with an overuse injury already rides in a neutral position, specific adjustments to the bicycle may be indicated. The seat may need to be raised or lowered, for example, or the position of the cyclist's cleats may need to be rotated slightly.

For lower-extremity problems such as tendonitis and patellofemoral pain, the key to successful treatment is usually obtained in detecting anatomic misalignments or errors in bike fit and correcting the rider's position on the bicycle with adjustments to the saddle and pedals. Upper body syndromes, such as ulnar nerve compression and neck soreness, often respond to unloading of the upper extremities by raising the handlebars and/or decreasing the cyclist's reach. Adding or adjusting a front suspension system and allowing the elbows to flex during rough riding may also be helpful in relieving upper-body symptoms. Low-back pain is often related to inflexibility and inadequate conditioning and tends to decrease as the season progresses. Raising the handlebars early in the season and gradually lowering them to the desired position as flexibility and conditioning improve may be helpful to some cyclists with low-back pain.

Other treatment options for overuse injuries in off-road cyclists include all of the same approaches used with other athletes, such as PHYSICAL THERAPY, ice, and anti-inflammatory medication. The biggest difference is that sports medicine professionals must pay attention to the bicycle as well as the bicyclist in order to thoroughly diagnose and treat overuse injuries in cyclists.

Common overuse injuries include ACHILLES TENDONITIS, BICYCLE SEAT NEUROPATHY, HAMSTRING TENDONITIS, ILIOTIBIAL BAND SYNDROME, KNEE BURSITIS, medial synovial plica irritation, patellar tendonitis, patellofemoral pain syndrome, and quadriceps tendonitis.

muscle cramps (charley horse)   A cramp is an involuntary, forcibly contracted muscle that does not relax. Cramps can affect any muscle that is under voluntary control, but muscles in the lower leg, back of the thigh, front of the thigh, feet, hands, arms, abdomen, and along the rib cage are the most commonly affected. In these areas, a muscle cramp may affect all or just part of a muscle. It may even affect several muscles in a muscle group. Muscles that span two joints are more prone to cramping than those that do not.

Causes

Although there are numerous conditions and situations associated with cramped muscles, the exact cause is unknown. Some researchers believe that muscle cramps occur when the muscles are inadequately stretched and experiencing fatigue, which may lead to improper functioning of the mecha-

nisms that control muscle contraction. Muscles are bundles of fibers that contract and expand to create movement. Regular stretching lengthens muscle fibers so that they can contract and tighten more vigorously during exercise. A poorly conditioned body is more likely to experience muscle fatigue, which can lead to a build-up of waste products in the muscle and muscle spasms.

DEHYDRATION can also be a contributing factor. When the body is exercised in hot weather, it sweats, which drains its fluids, including its stores of salts and minerals. Loss of these essential nutrients, such as potassium and magnesium, may lead to a muscle spasm as well. Stress can contribute to muscle cramps, especially in the neck, where many people tend to hold tension. General overuse or an injury can also cause a muscle to cramp. Finally, night cramps are a common form of muscle cramp affecting the muscles in the calf of the leg. They can be extremely painful and often recur.

Certain people are more likely than others to experience muscle cramps. These include people over the age of 65, whose normal muscle loss means that they cannot work as hard as they used to. Infants and young children, and those who overexert during exercise or work, take certain drugs, are overweight, or ill are also quite vulnerable, especially to heat-induced muscle cramps. Athletes are more likely to experience cramps in the preseason when the body is not yet conditioned and at the end of a training session or the night following a hard exertion. Endurance athletes especially are vulnerable to muscle cramps since they tend to have more problems with overuse and fatigue.

Diagnosis

A person experiencing muscle cramps may feel them as a slight, annoying twitch or as an agonizing, gripping pain. It may feel like tightness or like a knot in the muscle. If the cramp is mild, it may hurt to use the muscle. If the cramp is severe, the patient may be completely unable to use the muscle. A cramp during exercise may be extremely painful, and leg cramps that wake one up at night are often debilitating, leaving the muscle feeling bruised and sore.

The cramps may last just a few seconds or up to half an hour or more. They may occur just once or recur several times before finally going away.

A doctor will diagnose muscle cramps by examining the muscles and assessing them for tightness and tenderness to the touch.

Treatment

Cramps usually go away on their own, but those that do not require medical attention.

Self-care tips for treating muscle cramps are usually adequate. A muscle cramp caused by injury should be treated with ice every 20 to 30 minutes, every three to four hours, for the first two or three days following the injury. For immediate relief of a muscle that is cramping, the patient should try to stretch the muscle. This can be done by straightening the lower leg and pulling the foot toward the head, if the cramp is in the calf. Standing on the leg that is cramping may also help. Massaging the affected muscles helps to relieve the tightness. Occasionally, doctors will prescribe medication for the people who experience severe leg cramps when sleeping.

Prevention

To prevent cramps, one should keep the body well conditioned and adequately hydrated. Children especially often do not drink enough liquids to replenish fluid lost during exercise. Some tips to prevent cramps:

• Drink plenty of fluids to maintain adequate hydration.

• Drink water at regular intervals, before getting thirsty.

• Drink more than thirst requires.

• Drink a sports beverage if working in heat or sweating for more than an hour.

• Stretch muscles regularly.

• Loosen the covers at the foot of the bed to help prevent night cramps.

• Practice good posture to help prevent cramps that result from sitting too long in awkward positions.

nasal fractures A nasal fracture is also called a broken nose. Nasal fractures seen in participants of athletic activities occur as a result of direct blows in contact sports and as a result of falls. The nasal bones are the most commonly fractured bony structures of the face. The protruding position of the nasal bone coupled with its relative lack of support predisposes it to fracture. Prompt, appropriate treatment prevents functional and cosmetic changes. The likelihood of other injuries is high when a nasal fracture occurs, so the doctor should carefully search for other facial injuries as well.

Causes

Any force directed to the mid face, either frontally or laterally, could disrupt the nasal anatomy, causing injury to the bones or cartilage. Frontally directed forces must be greater to cause bony injury because the upper and lower lateral cartilages absorb a great deal of impact.

Children are more likely to sustain injury to the cartilage, mainly because children have a greater proportion of cartilage to bone and the cartilage provides increased protection from fracture. Children's bones are more elastic than adults' bones.

Diagnosis

Common symptoms of a nasal fracture include pain, swelling, bruising, and bleeding in the nose. If the break pushed the bones out of place, the nose may appear misshapen.

Sports-related nasal injuries are usually isolated and rarely constitute an emergency, but some situations do require a referral. These include high-speed impact, such as in baseball or bicycling, loss of consciousness, vision problems, associated facial injuries, and nerve damage.

The medical history will normally reveal a fall or force directed to the mid face. The doctor should obtain details of the injury, including the mechanism and location of injury as well as the direction of force. These details will help in estimating the severity of the injury.

The physical exam includes careful inspection and palpation of surrounding structures as well as an intranasal exam.

In cases of nasal fracture, there is evidence of trauma to the mid face. Often, deformity of the nose provides the greatest clue. Other signs include swelling, skin laceration, bruising, bleeding, and cerebrospinal fluid (CSF) discharge.

The intranasal exam is sometimes difficult for physicians without detailed training. In addition, examination within hours of the injury may be compounded by persistent bleeding and/or swelling. Topical decongestants, appropriate lighting, a nasal speculum, and a Frazier suction tip for blood removal are necessary for a thorough exam. However, these aren't usually needed to rule out a septal hematoma, a collection of blood in the septum, if one is comfortable with the variations in normal nasal anatomy. A septal hematoma should be suspected if the septum is bulging into the nasal cavity.

X rays of the nasal bones are not helpful and should be obtained only if needed for potential legal issues and documentation. Plain film nasal X rays are likely to miss nearly 50 percent of nasal fractures, and there is a high incidence of false-positives in these X rays. X rays may be necessary, however, if there is suspicion of other facial injuries.

A COMPUTERIZED AXIAL TOMOGRAPHY (CAT) SCAN provides the best information regarding the extent of bony injury in nasal and facial fractures. Again, cartilaginous injury is likely to be missed.

In cases with a significant amount of bleeding or where a patient may require operative intervention, several blood tests should be obtained, including a complete blood count (CBC), coagulation studies, and blood typing and cross-matching in case transfusion is needed.

Treatment

When the history and exam are benign, it is almost never wrong to treat the patient with ice, elevation, and topical decongestants and to repeat the examination in one or two days. Applying topical decongestants every 10 to 30 minutes is acceptable early treatment for bleeding and preferred over packing in the initial stage.

Closed fracture reductions have a high rate of success and are the treatment of choice for acute, uncomplicated, displaced fractures of the nasal bone. However, certain situations will still require surgical repair. These include persistent functional or cosmetic problems. Surgery allows for more direct manipulation of displaced nasal bones and the septum. In cases where reduction has been delayed beyond several weeks, surgical repair is necessary, even in simple fractures.

In the acute phase, the patient should apply ice to the nose and elevate the head to aid in reduction of any swelling present. Nasal decongestants are prescribed to help reduce swelling and mucosal congestion.

Uncomplicated nondisplaced fractures should not prevent a patient participating in noncontact sports within about two weeks. Athletes involved in contact sports should have adequate head and face protection for several weeks when returning to play.

Another situation that requires surgery is a simple nasal fracture that has subsequently healed in a displaced location. Whereas displacements often require cosmetic surgery to repair the deformity, most nondisplaced nasal fractures heal without cosmetic or functional deformity.

Prevention

Nasal fractures in sports can best be prevented with the use of helmets that have adequate face protection.

neck strain   Often called a muscle pull, a strain is a tear of a muscle or tendon. The neck is sur-

rounded by numerous small muscles that run close to the vertebrae and larger muscles that make up the visible muscles of the neck. When one of these smaller or larger muscles becomes stretched or torn, either in the muscle or in the tendons of the muscle, the result is called a neck strain.

Causes

Neck strains most often occur when the head and neck are forcibly moved, such as in a whiplash injury or from contact in sports. Athletes in sports such as football, hockey, and golf see a fair number of neck sprains.

Diagnosis

The athlete with a neck sprain will experience pain in the neck. When the neck muscles go into spasm, they feel hard and tight and become very tender to the touch. There is pain with movement of the head to either side or when trying to move the head up or down. The spasming muscles can also cause headaches.

A doctor will take a medical history to see what may be causing the neck strain. A physical examination will also be done and will focus on all the muscles of the neck to see exactly which muscles are strained. The doctor will palpate the muscles to check for tenderness and tightness, as well as pain that may occur over the bones in the neck. If there is any suspicion of bones being injured, the doctor will order an X ray to see if any of the vertebrae are injured.

Treatment

Treatment immediately following the injury should focus on icing the neck muscles for 20 to 30 minutes every three or four hours for two to three days or until the pain goes away. In addition, the doctor may prescribe an anti-inflammatory medication and a neck collar to support the neck during recovery and prevent further injury.

If neck pain persists several days after the injury and after using ice, the doctor may recommend using moist heat, either a heat pad or towels soaked in hot water. Alternating the hot treatment with the cold treatment sometimes provides the most relief. Most people recover from neck strains in a few days to a few weeks, but some people take longer to get better.

Athletes who participate in contact sports must be certain the neck is healed before returning to their usual activities. There should be full range of motion in the neck and normal strength. There should be no pain in any position of the neck. If any positions cause pain, burning, or spasming of the neck muscles, the athlete should refrain from activity. Neck injuries can be quite serious, and a sprained neck may lead to a more serious injury of the neck if the athlete returns to activity too soon.

Prevention

Neck strain is best prevented by maintaining strong and supple neck muscles. Athletes who must keep their neck in one position for long periods of time, perhaps while on the job, must be sure to take breaks and relax the muscles so that they do not become too tight. Athletes who play contact sports should always wear protective equipment that fits properly, which will help prevent neck injuries. In many cases, however, neck sprains are caused by accidents that cannot be prevented.

nose injury   Nose injuries are quite common in sports and come in many different forms. They include nosebleeds, bruised noses, broken noses, and damage to the nasal septum, which is the tissue that separates the nasal passages.

Causes

Nose injuries are almost always caused by a direct blow to the nose, which can occur upon impact from another player, or a stick in sports such as hockey or lacrosse, or upon impact with the ground in sports such as football or basketball.

Diagnosis

Patients with an injury to the nose usually have significant pain. Other common symptoms include bleeding, swelling, sometimes deformity or crookedness, difficulty breathing through the nose, and a grating or grinding noise with movement of broken nose bones.

The doctor will take a medical history and perform a physical examination of the nose. He or she will want to know the cause of the injury and will be looking for swelling, tenderness, bleeding, and movement of bones. The doctor will also check inside the nostrils to see if the septum is swollen or bent to the side, which is called a deviated septum.

Depending upon what the doctor sees in the exam, an X ray may be ordered to see if the nose is actually broken. A COMPUTERIZED AXIAL TOMOGRAPHY (CAT) SCAN may also be called for if there is damage to the nasal septum and sinuses.

Treatment

Initial treatment following the injury includes pinching the nostrils firmly together just below the nasal bones for 10 minutes or until the bleeding stops. Icing the nose will help with the swelling and pain, and sitting up and leaning forward will help with breathing during the period of bleeding.

If the bleeding doesn't stop with pressure, the doctor may need to put gauze packing in the nose to stop the bleeding. After the nosebleed stops, it is important to avoid blowing the nose because this may cause the bleeding to start again. The patient should also avoid taking aspirin and other anti-inflammatory medicines because they may make bleeding worse. Acetaminophen is recommended instead.

Although many broken noses heal normally with no special treatment, a broken nose that is crooked may need to be straightened immediately following the injury. This may be done by the doctor who examines the patient initially, or it may be done by a specialist. In some cases, repairing a broken nose requires surgery. Surgery may also be required if the septum has become deviated and the patient is having trouble breathing.

Patients should refrain from all activity when the nose is bleeding. Once the bleeding stops, there may be return to activity if there is no sign of serious damage. If there is significant pain and swelling, the patient will need to wait until the nose has healed before attempting to play sports again. For athletes who play contact sports and have broken their nose, it is especially important to wear a special nose and face shield for four to six weeks after the injury.

Prevention

Nose injuries are usually caused by accidents that cannot be prevented. However, wearing proper protective face gear, including a face shield, in contact sports such as hockey and lacrosse will help athletes avoid injuries to the nose.

orthopedic medicine   Orthopedics is the medical specialty devoted to the diagnosis, treatment, rehabilitation, and prevention of injuries and diseases of the body's musculoskeletal system. This complex system includes bones, joints, ligaments, tendons, muscles, and nerves and allows a person to move, work, and be active.

The discipline was formerly devoted to the care of children with spine and limb deformities but now cares for patients of all ages. Newborns with clubfeet, young athletes requiring arthroscopic surgery, and older people with arthritis are all cared for by orthopedists.

An orthopedist is skilled in the diagnosis, treatment, rehabilitation, and prevention of injuries and disorders to the musculoskeletal system. Most orthopedists practice general orthopedics, but some may specialize in one or more areas. This might include a specialty in a certain part of the body, such as treating the foot, hand, shoulder, spine, hip, or knee. It also might mean specializing in treating certain populations, such as sports medicine, which treats athletes, or pediatrics, which treats children.

Orthopedic Training

Orthopedic surgeons are medical doctors with extensive training in the proper diagnosis and treatment of injuries and diseases of the musculoskeletal system. An orthopedist normally completes up to 14 years of formal education, which includes four years of study in a college or university, four years of study in medical school, five years of study in orthopedic residency at a major medical center, and one optional year of specialized education.

The orthopedic surgeon is required to exhibit mastery of the discipline by passing both oral and written examinations given by the American Board of Orthopedic Surgery. In addition, each year an orthopedist spends many hours studying and attending continuing medical education courses to maintain current orthopedic knowledge and skills.

Sports Medicine Careers for Orthopedists

Among the sports medicine careers an orthopedist may choose are team physician and orthopedic surgeon specializing in sports medicine.

A team physician plays a central role in coordinating the medical care of athletes. Working closely with athletic trainers, physical therapists, nutritionists, and other health care professionals, the team physician is the athlete's advocate in all health matters.

Injury prevention is, of course, the primary goal, but when injuries occur, the team physician evaluates the athlete to determine the proper diagnosis. Often special tests are required and referral to another physician may be necessary. Once the extent of the injury is understood, proper treatment can be initiated.

Team physicians are also responsible for preseason physical examinations and determining playability during the season. One of the great challenges for any team physician is medical coverage of athletic events. In a game setting, injuries are evaluated without benefit of MAGNETIC RESONANCE IMAGING (MRI) and other technologies, and quick decisions must be made regarding the advisability of returning the athlete to the game. The team physician draws upon his or her training and experience to make the right call and also works with other health care practitioners, including cardiologists, ophthalmologists, dentists and oral surgeons, and podiatrists to complete the medical care of athletes on a sports team.

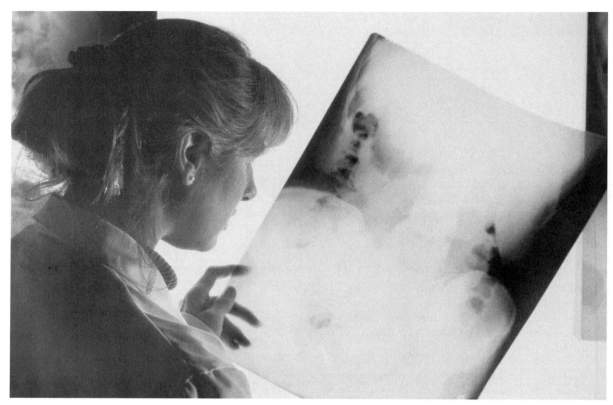

An orthopedic doctor working in a sports medicine clinic examines the X ray of an athlete who may have sustained a whiplash injury while playing football. Orthopedic doctors often work in a health care facility that specializes in sports medicine or for a sports team, where they are responsible for coordinating and overseeing the medical care of all players on the team. *(Fogstock, LLC)*

Orthopedic surgeons are physicians specially trained to diagnose and treat musculoskeletal problems. In spite of the label "surgeon," orthopedists devote much of their efforts to helping athletes recover with nonsurgical measures. After carefully examining the injured athlete, the orthopedist may order and interpret tests such as X rays, bone scans, or MRIs. Treatment may involve medicine, physical therapy, or in some cases, surgery. Major advances in sports medicine over the past two decades have enabled orthopedists to treat many musculoskeletal problems without hospitalization, and postoperative rehabilitation has also been improved through the combined efforts of surgeons, athletic trainers, and physical therapists.

Orthopedic Treatment

Normally a visit to the orthopedist will start with a personal interview and physical examination, which may be followed by diagnostic tests, such as blood tests, X rays, or MRIs. Treatment of orthopedic injuries and disorders may involve a number of different methods including counseling, casts, splints, physical therapy, and surgery. It may also involve various medical professionals, in addition to the orthopedic surgeon. These include physical therapists, rheumatologists, occupational therapists, podiatrists, primary care physicians, and nurses.

Osgood-Schlatter disease   Osgood-Schlatter disease (OSD) is one of the most common causes of knee pain in active adolescents. A temporary condition, Osgood-Schlatter is not really a disease, but rather an overuse syndrome, a set of symptoms that happen at the same time and with excessive activity. Young athletes usually get Osgood-Schlatter during their rapid growth years, between the ages of nine and 13. The condition has been more frequent in boys, although the ratio may be equalizing with girls' increased participation in sports. In addition, girls tend to develop the condition at a slightly younger age than boys.

Osgood-Schlatter is a generally benign disturbance at the junction of the patellar tendon and the tibial tuberosity, which is a bony prominence on the leg bone. In this condition, there is pain and swelling below the knee joint on the tibial tuberosity. There may also be inflammation of the patellar tendon, which stretches over the kneecap and attaches to the top of the shinbone.

Young people who participate in jumping and cutting sports, such as basketball, volleyball, figure skating, gymnastics, and soccer, are most vulnerable to developing Osgood-Schlatter.

Causes

The exact cause of Osgood-Schlatter is unknown, but it probably results from repetitive overuse. In most cases, the condition affects just one knee, but in about 20 percent of cases it occurs on both sides of the body.

Osgood-Schlatter occurs when there is irritation of the bone growth plate in the area of the tibial tuberosity. Bones generally do not grow in the middle but at the ends near the joint at an area called the growth plate. These areas of growth are made of cartilage and not bone. The cartilage is never as strong as the bone, so high levels of stress can cause the growth plate to begin to hurt and swell. In Osgood-Schlatter, the tendon from the kneecap (patella) attaches to the growth plate in the front of the leg bone (tibia). The thigh muscles (quadriceps) attach to the patella, and when they pull on the patella, there is a pull on the patellar tendon. The patellar tendon then pulls on the tibia in the area of the growth plate. Any movements that cause repetitive extension of the leg can result in tenderness at the point where the patellar tendon attaches to the top of the tibia. Activities that put stress on the knee, especially squatting, bending, or running up hills or stairs, cause the tissue around the growth plate to hurt and swell. It also hurts to hit or bump the tender area. Kneeling can be very painful.

Diagnosis

If a young athlete has swelling, tenderness, and aching pain beneath his or her knee joint, it may be Osgood-Schlatter disease. Normally, the pain gets worse when the child is active and better when he or she rests.

Usually Osgood-Schlatter affects only one knee, but in about 20 percent of cases, it affects both sides of the body. Patients will usually point to a slightly swollen, warm and tender bony bump below the kneecap. The bump hurts if pressure is applied. It may hurt at night. It also hurts when the patient kneels, jumps, climbs stairs, runs, squats, lifts weights, or participates in any activity that bends or fully extends the leg.

The pain comes from repeated pulling of the patellar tendon at the kneecap. Repetitive, OVERUSE INJURIES may make the tendon inflamed at the spot where it connects to the shinbone. Fast-growing bone is susceptible where the tendon pulls on it. The tendon may get inflamed or even tear away, sometimes taking a tiny piece of shinbone with it.

This condition is characterized by swelling and tenderness where the patellar tendon attaches. It is typically swollen only in the front, so swelling all over the knee may indicate another condition. There should not be a history of the knees giving way, locking, or catching, and the patient normally has full range of motion with the knee.

Osgood-Schlatter disease is diagnosed by grade. Grade I is the least severe and is characterized by pain after activity that resolves within 24 hours Grade II involves pain during and after activity that does not limit activity and resolves within 24 hours. Grade III, the worst diagnosis, is a condition of constant pain that limits sports and daily activity.

An X ray that shows that the growth plate is wider than usual best confirms the diagnosis of Osgood-Schlatter disease. The X ray may show small bones in the growth plate that have not fused or become solid due to the stress. Sometimes the X ray will appear normal when Osgood-Schlatter is diagnosed, but the imaging studies are useful for ruling out other possible causes of chronic knee pain. These include Sinding-Larsen-Johansson (SLJ) disease, PATELLOFEMORAL PAIN SYNDROME, and OSTEOCHONDRITIS DISSECANS. SLJ disease and patellofemoral syndrome occasionally coexist with OSD in adolescents. Osteochondritis dissecans is the most serious of these conditions and can lead to permanent knee damage, thus is crucial that the physician rule out this possibility when making a diagnosis. X rays are normally required to diagnose osteochondritis dissecans because there are no reliable tests.

It is also important to assess hip range of motion in any adolescent with knee pain. Limitation or pain with internal rotation calls for X rays to rule out the possibility of a slipped capital femoral epiphysis. X rays are also useful in ruling out the possibilities of fractures, tumors, and infections.

Treatment

Treatment for Grades I and II Osgood-Schlatter disease consists of decreasing the activity that makes it worse, icing the painful area, using knee pads for protection, and taking anti-inflammatory medication. Osgood-Schlatter usually goes away with time and rest. Sports activities that require running, jumping, or other deep knee bending should be limited until the tenderness and swelling subside. Kneepads are recommended for athletes who wish to continue participating in sports where the knee might make contact with the playing surface or other players. Ice packs after activity are helpful, and ice can be applied two to three times a day, 20 to 30 minutes at a time, if necessary.

With rest, Osgood-Schlatter usually heals itself within six to 18 months. Resting does not mean doing nothing. Patients can play sports as long as pain is tolerated and resolves within 24 hours. When symptoms flare up, short-term rest from the offending activity typically eliminates pain. Total rest is not recommended as it can lead to deconditioning and increase the chance of recurrence with return to sports.

Shock-absorbent insoles in sports shoes may decrease peak stress on the tendon and tuberosity. Icing the knee for 20 minutes after activity may also be beneficial. Hamstring and quadriceps stretching is recommended as well.

The standard neoprene knee sleeve is generally not beneficial, but other types of knee sleeves that pad the tibial tubercle can help, especially for preventing repeated contusions to the tender tubercle. Wrestling gel pads and basketball kneepads are inexpensive and are sold at sporting goods stores.

Anti-inflammatory medications may be administered as needed after sports activity, but routine usage and routine pretreatment is not recommended. Cortisone injection is not recommended.

Treatment for Grade III Osgood-Schlatter is more intense. Sometimes, a three- to four-week period of immobilization with a cast or brace is necessary when more conservative treatment has failed to produce any results. Forced immobilization is sometimes the only way to achieve the necessary amount of rest in an adolescent. Following this period, the young athletes can begin a rehabilitation program of progressive quadriceps exercises. As soon as the pain stops, they can return to sports with the same precautions mentioned above.

Surgery is almost never required with Osgood-Schlatter because the cartilage growth plate eventually stops its growth and fills in with bone. Once this happens, the bone receives the stress and not the cartilage. The pain and swelling go away because there is no new growth plate to be injured. If one waits until the adolescent is done growing, the pain almost always goes away. Surgery is never performed on a growing athlete since the growth plate can be damaged.

In rare cases where pain persists after the growth of the bones has stopped, surgery may be indicated if there are bone fragments that did not heal.

Prevention

Following an organized training program will help young athletes avoid Osgood-Schlatter disease and other overuse injuries. It is important that athletes not increase the intensity and length of their workouts too much at one time. Progress should occur gradually, in order to give the body time to adjust to the additional stresses of the workout.

osteitis pubis   Osteitis pubis is an inflammation of the pubic symphysis, where the right and left pubic bones meet, and the surrounding muscle insertions. Pubic bones are a part of the pelvis at the lower abdomen and groin. The condition is thought to be about five times more common in males than in females and occurs most often in athletes whose sports involve frequent repetition of the same movements, such as twisting, cutting, pivoting on one leg, excessive side-to-side motion, or multidirectional motions with frequent acceleration and deceleration.

Causes

Osteitis pubis may result from activities that create either acute or continuous shearing forces across the pubic symphysis. In acute situations, this is usually the result of an accident, such as trauma from a fall, being kicked in the hip, or receiving some other direct blow to the hip. Continuous situations result from abnormal pelvis biomechanics. These include muscle imbalance, poor flexibility, and joint dysfunction. When such conditions are present in the pelvis, the patient is susceptible to injury from multiple repetitions of aggravating motions that cause trauma to the pubic symphysis. These multiple traumas result in inflammation and muscle spasm.

Athletes involved in sports that require running, kicking, or quick lateral movements are most susceptible to osteitis pubis. These include soccer players, sprinters, ice hockey players, and football players.

Soccer involves a great deal of running and rapid change of direction. These movements can lead to strained muscles in the buttocks, which can result in stress on the pelvis. In addition, soccer players also do a lot of kicking, which is also problematic. When athletes are not well balanced during the kick, they can place a great amount of strain on the muscles they are using to stabilize themselves. This often translates into abnormal stress on the pelvis.

The multiple repetitions of movements involved in sprinting can create minor traumas to the pelvis. In addition, the rapid acceleration often causes muscle strains, which can also put undue stress on the pelvis. This combination of situations, quite similar to that found in soccer, makes for cumulative stress on the pubic symphysis and increased vulnerability to developing osteitis pubis.

The various risk factors involved in ice hockey include the repetitive strains of the skating motion as well as the often traumatic contact with other players and the dasher boards around the rink. The result of these cumulative stresses can put enough stress on the pelvis to cause the development of this condition.

Many of the skills involved in football make the player vulnerable to pelvis injury. These include the amount of sprinting, the number of violent collisions between players, and the frequent need to run backward, which can lead to muscle strains that put stress on the pubic symphysis.

Diagnosis

The medical history will include detailed description of the symptoms. The patient may describe tenderness at the pubic bone or at the muscles that attach to the pubic bone. The most common symptom is pain directly over the pubic symphysis. The pain may begin gradually and may sometimes move to different places along the groin and pelvis. The patient may have pain in the groin, the testicles, at the muscles that attach to the pelvis, and at the pubic bone. Pain is often described as sharp, stabbing, or even burning and is exacerbated by running, pivoting (especially one-legged), twisting, climbing stairs, kicking, sit-ups, and leg raises. More often than not, the pain is unilateral and has been present for a few days to weeks.

Patients may have difficulty lying in bed at night. If instability is present, patients may describe an audible or palpable clicking sensation with certain activities, such as rising from a seated position or walking on uneven surfaces. Rest usually relieves these symptoms partially.

The doctor will need to inquire about the nature of the patient's activity or sport and the motions required. Any symptoms associated with the pain and any history of a trauma or fall should be noted, but in most cases there is no history of injury. If the patient has received any prior treatment, this should be well documented.

The physical exam usually reveals tenderness on palpation of the area over the pubic symphysis. Hip motion can be restricted. Specific tests can be done to assess weak muscles and the location of pain. In severe cases, patients may have a significant gait disturbance.

When discrepancies of leg length are involved, the athlete may complain of hip pain in the longer limb. This also can be seen in runners who run in the same direction and functionally have one leg shorter due to the slant of the running surface.

X rays of the pelvis are an integral part of the diagnosis. However, it is important to realize that early in the course of the condition X rays are often normal. They tend to show more after a month or more of symptoms.

Bone scans and MAGNETIC RESONANCE IMAGING (MRI) scans can also be valuable for early detection.

Although not very specific, tests such as urinalysis, erythrocyte sedimentation rate (ESR), and a complete blood count (CBC) test can assist in determining if there is any evidence of infection.

It is important to rule out osteomyelitis, a sports-related hernia, and pelvic inflammatory disease in particular.

Treatment

Osteitis pubis requires rest until the symptoms go away. Initially, the athlete will be pulled from all activities. Sometimes it takes two to three months for symptoms to abate. Anti-inflammatory medicines, such as ibuprofen, and use of an ice pack on the area for 20 to 30 minutes three to four times a day will help. Osteitis pubis requires more rest than rehabilitation and most of all requires patience.

PHYSICAL THERAPY may include therapeutic ultrasound and electrogalvanic stimulation. Thermally protective compression shorts have also been advocated.

When pain and inflammation are reduced, patients should begin a physical therapy program that progresses to a graduated exercise program. Exercises for the hip flexors, hip adductors, lumbar stabilizers, and abdominal muscles are started. Hamstring and quadriceps exercises also are necessary, with squatting and leg presses added last due to the increased load used in these exercises. Stretching is performed at least daily, with flexibility as the main focus of therapy. Aquatic conditioning can begin at this time, and many patients can tolerate stair-stepping machines as well. Cycling is usually not possible for a while due to the pressure caused by the seat, though some patients can tolerate a recumbent cycle. Sports-specific activities are added late in this phase, with offending motions added last. In the beginning, pain may increase a bit with the exercise but should eventually subside.

Return to full activities can take up to six months or longer, but the prognosis for full recovery is very good. Residual symptoms may occur but do not usually prohibit the patient from participating in activities.

The patient may safely return to his or her sport when the following criteria have been met:

- There is no pain or tenderness over the pubic bone.
- The patient can jog straight ahead without pain or limping.
- The patient can sprint straight ahead without pain or limping.
- The patient can perform various cutting motions while running without pain.

Prevention

Flexibility in athletes is the most important component of prevention. Proper body mechanics must be stressed in athletes who participate in activities that yield a higher incidence of osteitis pubis. Joint dysfunctions in athletes that can affect the pelvis should be aggressively treated so that the pubic symphysis does not become the victim of poor mechanics in the pelvis. In addition, early recognition of the symptoms of osteitis pubis can prevent chronic and more severe symptoms.

osteoarthritis Arthritis is inflammation of a joint—the point where two or more bones meet. There are many different types of arthritis, but the most common form is osteoarthritis, which affects up to 12 percent of the population. Also called degenerative arthritis, osteoarthritis causes the progressive breakdown of cartilage in the joints and may affect any of the body's 147 joints, although it most commonly occurs in weight-bearing joints, such as the neck, lower back, knees, and hips. It is three times more likely to occur in women than in men, and it normally appears by middle age, although it may be too mild to cause symptoms.

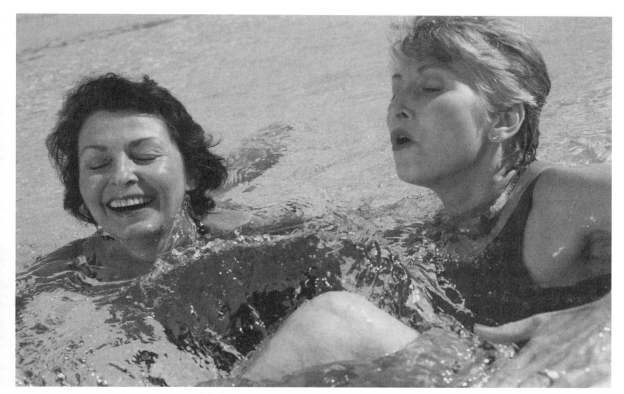

Osteoarthritis is three times more likely to occur in women than in men. Swimming can be an excellent activity for people suffering with arthritis because it allows the joint to continue exercising without having to experience much stress. *(Fogstock, LLC)*

Causes

Osteoarthritis is caused by excessive wear on the joints. For anyone involved in sports activities, injuries are a way of life. It doesn't matter if athletes engage in these activities professionally or for recreation, they are at risk all the time. When arthritis develops as a result of injuries, it is generally referred to as "secondary" osteoarthritis. That means the deterioration of the cartilage was caused by a traumatic injury to begin with. As a general rule, it takes years after the injury to develop.

In addition, any joint that suffers from overuse may be more vulnerable to developing osteoarthritis later in life. Obesity, bad posture, and heredity also appear to play roles in causing osteoarthritis.

Cartilage normally acts as a smooth, cushioning surface between the bones and the joints, but when there is a traumatic injury to a joint or excessive wear on a joint, the cartilage can become rough and flaky, and small pieces begin to break off. Even the bone surface of the joint becomes rough, resulting in pain whenever the joint is moved.

Diagnosis

Osteoarthritis leads to altered activities, increased pain, episodic swelling, altered motion, and occasional mechanical symptoms such as locking, catching, clicking, and giving way of the joint. It may cause destruction of cartilage, overgrowth of the bone, bone spur formation, and impaired function.

The following symptoms are characteristic of osteoarthritis:

- mild to severe pain in a joint, especially after overuse or long periods of inactivity, such as sitting for a long time

- creaking or grating sound in the joint
- swelling, stiffness, limited movement of the joint, especially in the mornings
- weakness in muscles around the sore joint from lack of use
- deformity of the joint

A doctor will take a medical history and do a physical examination in order to make a diagnosis. X rays may be necessary to show the extent of damage in the joint. Blood tests and other lab tests may also be needed. These include the following:

- antinuclear antibody (ANA) test to check levels of antibodies in the blood
- arthrocentesis (joint aspiration) to remove a sample of the synovial fluid to determine if crystals, bacteria, or viruses are present
- complete blood count to determine if white blood cell, red blood cell, and platelet levels are normal
- creatinine to monitor for underlying kidney disease
- erythrocyte sedimentation rate to detect inflammation
- hematocrit to measure the number of red blood cells
- rheumatoid factor test to determine if rheumatoid factor is present in the blood
- urinalysis to determine levels of protein, red blood cells, white blood cells, and casts
- white blood cell count to determine level of white blood cells in the blood

Treatment

The goal of treatment for osteoarthritis, which is chronic, is to keep the joint working by reducing the strain on the joint and be relieving the pain, stiffness, and swelling.

Acetaminophen, aspirin, or an anti-inflammatory are usually prescribed to help with the pain and swelling. In addition, it may be helpful to rub anti-inflammatory or deep-heat creams into the joint. Icing the joint several times a day may help relieve pain as well. If none of these methods pro-

duces relief, the doctor may inject steroids into the painful joint.

Overweight patients will often be advised to restrict their calories and increase their physical activity in order to lose some weight, which helps to relieve stress from the painful joint. Aerobic exercise is also advised because it helps to control the spread of osteoarthritis. Physical and occupational therapy will sometimes be prescribed to help the patient regain normal movement.

With severely damaged joints, especially in the hips and knees, doctors will sometimes advise surgery to replace the joints.

Osteoarthritis is a chronic disease that can worsen over time. It is very important to avoid repeated injuries to the joints and to take all preventive measures to ensure that the joints do not worsen. Once the cartilage is damaged, it cannot repair itself.

Prevention

Although it is not yet known how to prevent osteoarthritis, following these guidelines will help avoid developing symptoms:

- Keep the joints in good working order by staying fit and exercising regularly. Do any exercises recommended by a doctor or physical therapist for posture, muscle strength, and joint mobility. Daily moderate exercise is much better for joints than occasional strenuous exercise. Be sure to wear comfortable, well-cushioned walking shoes. Otherwise, exercise while sitting down or by swimming. The water in a warm swimming pool can help support the body's weight during exercise, and the warmth helps improve joint movement.
- Protect joints by doing warm-up exercises before strenuous activity.
- Use a kneepad to protect knees when kneeling.
- Take the medication a doctor recommends for controlling osteoarthritis.
- Keep the body healthy by eating a healthy, varied, low-fat diet.
- Follow a doctor's recommendations for weight control.

osteochondritis dissecans Osteochondritis disse-cans is an unusual but significant disorder that can lead to breaking down of the cartilage that covers bone. It can affect the talus bone of the ankle or other bones such as the femur in the knee and the capitellum in the elbow. It is not completely under-stood, but it can have a profound effect on joint function if it is severe. Usually a flap of surface car-tilage breaks down because the underlying bone in this disorder does not support it. This usually occurs when there has been something to disrupt the blood supply to the bone. The breaking down of cartilage causes loose pieces of bone and carti-lage to separate from the end of the bone. When this happens, they may stay in place or fall into the joint space, causing the joint to become unstable. This creates pain and can cause the feeling that the joint is catching or giving way. These loose pieces of bone are sometimes called "joint mice." If osteo-chondritis is not treated early, arthritis and signifi-cant pain can occur.

Anyone can get osteochondritis dissecans, but it happens more often in boys and young men 10 to 20 years old, while they are still growing. Osteo-chondritis dissecans is being diagnosed more often in girls as they become more active in sports. It affects athletes, especially gymnasts and baseball players. The adult form occurs in mature bone, and the juvenile form occurs in growing bone.

Causes

It is believed to be caused by either a loss of blood supply to a segment of bone and cartilage or by a traumatic injury.

The condition is often brought on by a traumatic injury, but may be caused by anything that blocks blood supply to bone and cartilage. However, the exact cause is unknown.

Diagnosis

The diagnosis of osteochondritis dissecans of the talus is made by a history of pain around the ankle, knee, or elbow that is sometimes associated with clicking or catching. It can be a dull toothache-like pain or a sharp, stabbing pain. The patient may or may not describe a history of an injury to the area. X rays are used to initially evaluate the bone. Typ-ically, however, a COMPUTERIZED AXIAL TOMOGRAPHY (CAT) SCAN or a MAGNETIC RESONANCE IMAGING

(MRI) scan is needed to confirm the diagnosis and evaluate the extent of the problem.

If a person has a sore joint (especially the knee, elbow, or ankle), it is important to see a doctor. In cases of osteochondritis dissecans, there might be swelling, and the patient might not be able to extend an arm or leg fully. The pain may or may not be related to an injury and may occur during activity, then feel stiff after resting.

The doctor will check the stability of the joint and examine for extra fluid as well. If the doctor rules out the possibility of a fracture or sprain, an X ray will likely be ordered to check for osteo-chondritis dissecans.

If signs of osteochondritis dissecans are seen on X rays of one joint, it will be necessary to X ray the other joints to compare them. An MRI can show whether the loose piece of bone is still in place or whether it has moved into the joint space. If the loose piece is unstable, surgery may be required to remove it or secure it. If the loose piece is stable the patient may not need surgery, but may need other kinds of treatment.

Treatment

Occasionally in very young patients, osteochondri-tis dissecans will heal with immobilization and rest. Most often, however, it requires surgical treat-ment. Initial treatment involves ARTHROSCOPY to remove severely damaged fragments or drilling through the area with no blood supply into adja-cent healthy bone. This drilling allows the blood supply to enter the injured area and encourage healing. In severe cases, when drilling is not effec-tive, a plug of cartilage and bone is taken from a safe area in the joint and implanted into the defec-tive area.

Conservative treatment is indicated for patients who do not have any loose pieces of cartilage or bone in the ankle. This treatment consists of rest from any impact-type activities, casting, and a pro-gressive rehabilitation program. Anti-inflammatory medication and bracing of the ankle during activity may also be required.

If the patient has loose bone or cartilage in the ankle by clinical examination or as seen on a CAT or MRI scan, surgical intervention is required. Options for operative treatment include drilling of the involved area of bone, fixation of the loose bone/cartilage, and removal of the loose pieces of bone/cartilage. Grafting of cartilage and transplantation of cartilage are other possible forms of surgery for this disorder.

If a nonsurgical treatment is recommended, the patient should avoid activities that cause discomfort and refrain from competitive sports for six to eight weeks. Stretching exercises or swimming may be permitted during this time.

Young people have the best chance of returning to their usual activity levels, although they might not be able to keep playing sports with repetitive motions, such as baseball pitching. Adults are more likely to need surgery and are less likely to recover fully. They may later get arthritis in the joint.

In general, return to sports is permitted when the following criteria are met:

- The injured knee can be fully straightened and bent without pain.
- The knee and leg have regained normal strength compared to the uninjured knee and leg.
- The knee is not swollen.
- The patient is able to jog straight ahead without limping.
- The patient is able to sprint straight ahead without limping.
- The patient can perform cutting and twisting motions while running.
- The patient can jump on both legs without pain and jump on the injured leg without pain.

If the knee feels like it is giving way or there is pain or swelling in the knee, the patient should see his or her health care provider.

Prevention

Maintaining excellent balance, coordination, and strength of the foot, ankle, knee, elbow, and arm may help prevent osteochondritis dissecans. Occurrences of this condition that are caused by traumatic injury are unavoidable.

overtraining syndrome Overtraining syndrome occurs when athletes try too hard to improve performance and train beyond their body's ability to recover. Hard training breaks down the body and makes the athlete weaker. Physiologic improvement in sports occurs only during the rest period following hard training. This adaptation occurs in response to maximum loading of the cardiovascular and muscular systems. It is accomplished by improving efficiency of the heart, increasing capillaries in the muscles, and increasing glycogen stores and mitochondrial enzyme systems within the muscle cells. During recovery periods, these systems build to greater levels to compensate for the stress they have experienced during training. The result is that the body is able to perform at higher levels.

If sufficient rest is not included in a training program, then regeneration cannot occur and performance plateaus. If this imbalance between excess training and inadequate rest persists, performance will eventually decline and a state of overtraining will exist.

Overtraining syndrome is the name given to the collection of emotional, behavioral, and physical symptoms that result from overtraining that has persisted for weeks or months. Sometimes called burnout, overtraining syndrome is different from the tiredness that follows a hard workout. It is marked by cumulative exhaustion that persists even after recovery periods.

Diagnosis

The symptoms of overtraining syndrome include feeling exhausted, achy, edgy, and burned out. Although these symptoms can be present during a slump in training or following a particularly difficult workout, when they become chronic they are an indication of overtraining syndrome. The athlete may also complain of the following common warning signs:

- mild leg soreness, general achiness
- pain in muscles and joints
- washed-out feeling, tired, drained, lack of energy
- sudden drop in ability to run "normal" distance or times
- insomnia
- headaches

- inability to relax, twitchy, fidgety
- insatiable thirst, dehydration
- lowered resistance to common illnesses such as colds, sore throat, and so forth
- increased resting heart rate

Since the symptoms of overtraining syndrome are similar to many other medical problems, the doctor will need to take a thorough medical history of the patient and conduct a full examination to rule out other possible causes for the problems. The doctor will want to check for a decrease in normal strength and coordination, a faster heart rate than normal, a loss of appetite, and depression, among other possible conditions.

The most common symptom is fatigue that limits workouts and may even be present during periods of rest. The athlete may also become moody, easily irritated, have altered sleep patterns, become depressed, or lose the competitive desire and enthusiasm for the sport. Some will report decreased appetite and weight loss. Physical symptoms include persistent muscular soreness, increased frequency of viral illnesses, and increased incidence of injuries.

Medically, the overtraining syndrome is classified as a neuro-endocrine disorder. The normal fine balance in the interaction between the autonomic nervous system and the hormonal system is disturbed and athletic "jet lag" results. The body now has a decreased ability to repair itself during rest. Heaping more workouts onto this unbalanced system only worsens the situation. Additional stress in the form of difficulties at work or personal life also contributes.

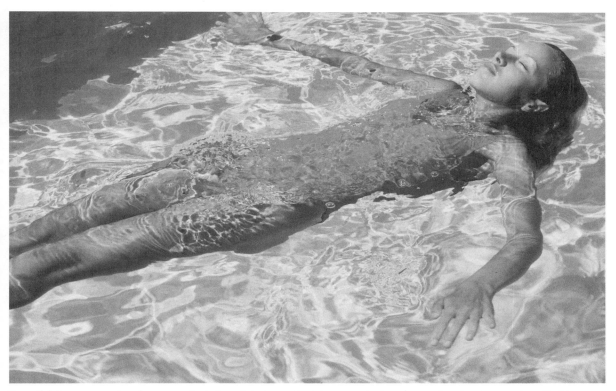

For athletes recovering from overtraining, it is important to cross-train when returning to sports activities. Swimming is an excellent sport for runners, cyclists, and others who want to maintain cardiovascular fitness while giving their joints and muscles a needed break from their regular workouts. *(Fogstock, LLC)*

There is no single test that will confirm the presence of overtraining, but this syndrome should be considered in any athlete who manifests symptoms of prolonged fatigue and performance that has leveled off or decreased. It is important to exclude any underlying illness that may be responsible for the fatigue.

Treatment

Overtraining is a serious condition, and rest is the primary treatment. The period of time the athlete will need to rest corresponds directly to the period of time of overtraining. It is possible that the doctor will allow some light cross-training during the recovery, but the athlete will be encouraged to spend time on something other than sports. It is important to keep well hydrated and to eat a balanced diet when recovering from overtraining. Sleep is also very restorative for the athlete suffering from overtraining.

Depression is one of the biggest problems among overtrained athletes. Training history, discussions with coaches and other athletes, and a family history can help clarify this question. Overtrained athletes should be treated for depression as soon as possible because it can speed up the recovery.

Adequate nutrition will play a big role in helping the overtrained athlete recover. The most common deficiencies, especially in female endurance athletes, are iron, zinc, and magnesium. Calcium deficiencies have also been reported in endurance athletes, especially those who deliberately restrict their diets. In those cases, supplementation is needed.

Sleep will help the athlete to regain strength and to handle any stress that is present. In general, it is probably a good idea to minimize traveling, since it can increase fatigue. However, in some cases, a change of environment may be helpful to an overtrained athlete. Sexual activity can also be restorative since it may help to relax the athlete.

Massage and soaking in a hot tub can also be therapeutic, but the athlete should wait a couple of weeks before beginning these therapies. Massage generally will help speed recovery, but it is also a kind of an exertion for the muscles and may slow the recovery process if initiated too soon. Saunas and hot tubs may also increase the feeling of fatigue and should be initiated only after the athlete has begun to feel better.

After the resting period, the athlete can start light training but should try different sports, refraining from the training modality and intensity that caused the overtraining state. Training should progress very slowly, with the pace determined by carefully listening to the patient's feelings.

Prevention

Prevention is the best line of defense when it comes to overtraining. It is much better to follow an organized and appropriate training schedule than it is to overtrain and then have to recover from the negative effects of this condition. The most important factor in the training schedule is periodization of the workouts. This means that appropriate amounts of training are followed by adequate recovery periods.

A simple strategy athletes can use to prevent overtraining syndrome is to monitor their feelings of fatigue and reduce their training whenever lethargy persists for more than a day or two. The problem with this approach is that it relies upon the athlete's perception of how he or she is feeling, which is not always reliable.

When used in conjunction with a simple heart rate monitoring technique, however, this can be a fairly accurate way of determining when the body is becoming overtrained. To perform the heart rate monitor test, the athlete needs to lie quietly for 10 minutes at the same time every day while monitoring heart rate, which should stay constant during the 10-minute period. It is best to do this test in the morning just after waking up. Then the athlete should stand up and check the heart rate exactly 15 seconds after standing, and then again after about 90 to 120 seconds of standing. It is easiest to use a Polar heart monitor for this, but the athlete can count the heart rate manually as well.

For athletes who are beginning to become overtrained, the heart rate usually shows a rise over a period of about four weeks, which allows ample time to ease up on the training. In addition to these techniques, keeping a training log may help some athletes keep track of progress and watch for signs of overtraining. In addition to keeping track of distance and intensity, the athlete can record the resting morning heart rate, weight, general health, how the workout felt, and levels of muscular soreness and fatigue. The latter two can be scored on a 10-point scale. Significant, progressive changes in any of these parameters may signal overtraining. Avoiding monotonous training and maintaining adequate nutrition are other recommendations for prevention. Vigorous exercise during the incubation period of a viral illness may increase the duration and severity of that illness. Athletes who feel as if they are developing a cold should rest or reduce the training schedule for a few days.

overuse injuries   There are basically two types of sports injuries: acute injuries and overuse injuries. Acute injuries are usually the result of a single, traumatic event. Common examples include wrist fractures, ankle sprains, shoulder dislocations, and hamstring muscle strain.

Overuse injuries are more subtle and usually occur over time. They are the result of repetitive microtrauma to the tendons, bones, and joints. Common examples include ACHILLES TENDONITIS, JUMPER'S KNEE, LITTLE LEAGUE ELBOW, RUNNER'S KNEE, SHIN SPLINTS, SWIMMER'S SHOULDER, and TENNIS ELBOW. In most sports and activities, overuse injuries are the most common and the most challenging to diagnose and treat.

Many of the injuries addressed in this book can be classified as overuse injuries. In-depth information on many of the injuries mentioned above is covered. But overuse injuries can occur to just about any part of the body, and some of them are not covered individually in this book. This entry is intended as a general overview of overuse injuries.

Causes

Overuse injuries occur due to intrinsic and extrinsic factors. Intrinsic factors are those related to the athlete, such as anatomic alignment, growth, muscle-tendon imbalance, and underlying disease. Extrinsic factors include training errors and environmental and equipment factors.

Training errors are the most common cause of overuse injuries. These errors involve a too rapid acceleration of the intensity, duration, or frequency of the activity. A typical example is a runner who has run several miles three times a week without any problem. The runner then begins advanced training for running in a marathon, running a longer distance every day at a faster pace. Injury or breakdown is inevitable. Overuse injuries also happen in people who are returning to a sport or activity after injury and trying to make up for lost time.

These training errors result in a failure of the body to recuperate following a hard workout. The human body has a tremendous capacity to adapt to physical stress. In fact, many positive changes occur as a result of this adaptation. With exercise and activity, bones, muscles, tendons, and ligaments get stronger and more functional. This happens because of an internal process called remodeling. The remodeling process involves both the breakdown and buildup of tissue. There is a fine balance between the two, and if breakdown occurs more rapidly than buildup, injury occurs. This can happen when someone first begins a sport or activity and tries to do too much too soon. If a person begins playing tennis and plays several hours in an attempt to improve rapidly, he or she is apt to develop an overuse injury because the body is not being allowed adequate time to recover from the damage being done in workout. In addition, the poor techniques of most beginners predispose them to common overuse injuries.

Technical, biomechanical, and individual factors can also play a role in developing overuse injuries. Proper technique is critical in avoiding overuse injuries. Slight changes in form may be the culprit. For this reason, coaches, athletic trainers and teachers can play a role in preventing recurrent overuse injuries.

Some people are more prone to overuse injuries simply because of anatomic or biomechanical factors. An imbalance between strength and flexibility around certain joints can predispose a person to injury. Body alignment, such as knock-knees or flat feet, can also present a problem. Old injuries or incompletely rehabilitated injuries may make a person vulnerable to an overuse injury.

Finally, faulty equipment can cause an overuse injury. Inadequate shoes or poor training surfaces can greatly increase the risk of injury.

Diagnosis

The diagnosis of an overuse injury can usually be made after a thorough history and physical examination. This is best done by a sports medicine specialist with specific interest and knowledge of the athlete's sport or activity. The specific requirements of the physical examination vary depending on the injury. In some instances, X rays are needed and occasionally additional tests such as a bone scan or MAGNETIC RESONANCE IMAGING (MRI) scan are needed.

Sports medicine physicians grade overuse injuries based on the symptoms and impact on the athlete's performance. This grading helps guide the treatment and rehabilitation process.

Grade 1: no pain with activity, but some discomfort afterward (either immediately or during the evening or the following days)
Grade 2: some discomfort with activity but does not interfere with performance
Grade 3: discomfort with activity; interferes with performance
Grade 4: discomfort so intense that activity cannot be performed at all

Treatment

Treatment of an overuse injury depends on the specific diagnosis. In general, for minor symptoms, it is sufficient to cut back the intensity, duration, and frequency of the offending activity. The patient will find relief from adopting a modified workout schedule and cross-training with other activities that help maintain overall fitness levels while the injured part of the body recovers. More complex overuse injuries require various treatments that may include surgical repair. Treatment may also include modifying techniques, implementing new warm-up and cool-down activities, taking anti-inflammatory medications, physical therapy, and even surgery in injuries that are resistant to more conservative treatments.

Treatment guidelines for the above grades of injury follow:

Grade 1. Usually, reducing the intensity or duration of the activity by 25 percent is all that is required. Activity can be gradually increased as symptoms allow. A runner, for example, should never increase weekly mileage by more than 10 percent.
Grade 2. Reduce intensity or duration of the activity by 50 percent. In addition to ice and stretching, consider using nonsteroidal anti-inflammatory agents. PHYSICAL THERAPY can be considered but is not absolutely necessary at this point. When pain is gone, the therapist should teach an endurance program, in addition to concentrating on strengthening exercises.
Grade 3. Active rest is recommended. The athlete should stop performing the offending tasks but is allowed to move the affected part for daily activities. Physical therapy is used to speed resolution of the discomfort and to strengthen, increase endurance, and restore coordination in the injured area. In addition to the oral nonsteroidal anti-inflammatory agents, a corticosteroid injection may be considered at this time.
Grade 4. Injuries of this severity require complete rest of the affected part, usually involving the use of a sling or splint, even casting in more severe cases. If the athlete shows no improvement, and the condition recurs despite adequate treatment, then surgical intervention may be required.

Prevention

Most overuse injuries can be prevented with proper training and common sense. It is essential that athletes learn to listen to their bodies. They must allow adequate time for recovery following hard workouts and increase their training programs gradually, keeping increases in volume and intensity below 10 percent per week.

painful plica (synovial plica syndrome)   During embryonic development, the knee is initially divided into three completely separate compartments. Synovial membranes divide the compartments. By the third or fourth month of fetal life, the membranes are reabsorbed, and the knee becomes a single chamber. If the membranes reabsorb incompletely, various degrees of separation may persist. These embryonic remnants are known as synovial plicas. In some individuals, the synovial plica is more prominent and prone to irritation, but most of the time a plica does not cause pain. However, if it becomes inflamed due to overuse or a direct blow to the knee, it can become a significant source of pain. Endurance athletes, especially runners and cyclists, are especially prone to developing painful plicas.

Causes

Trauma to the knee, either in the form of the repetitive microtraumas of overuse or a direct blow to the knee, can cause a plica to become painful. Anatomical abnormalities may also be culprits, as they can cause an overuse injury that creates inflammation around the plica. Other problems in the knee joint, such as arthritis or a meniscal tear, can cause changes around the knee that irritate the plica.

Painful plicas are commonly seen in runners or cyclists who increase the distance of their training dramatically, causing inflammation, or who participate in hard workouts without proper stretching in advance.

Diagnosis

Patients with painful plicas complain of pain in the front or just to the inner side of their knees. They often describe swelling, a clicking sensation, and locking and weakness of the knee. Deep bending of the knee worsens the pain or may cause the band to snap across the knee. Sitting in a car or movie theater, climbing stairs, and prolonged walking may produce discomfort similar to runner's knee. The knee will be tender to the touch, and a thickened cordlike structure can usually be felt. Localized swelling may accompany the tenderness.

Because the symptoms are similar to symptoms of some other knee problems, plica syndrome is often misdiagnosed. Diagnosis usually depends on the exclusion of other conditions that cause similar symptoms. X rays are taken to rule out bony causes of the pain. Occasionally, a MAGNETIC RESONANCE IMAGING (MRI) scan will be employed to either confirm the diagnosis or rule out a meniscus tear on the inner part of the knee.

Treatment

The overwhelming majority of painful plicas can be treated conservatively. The treatment is focused on controlling the pain and inflammation through rest and anti-inflammatory medications, restoring full function to the knee, and returning the athlete to sports. Flexibility of the muscles around the knee and tissues around the kneecap are emphasized. Patients should recognize that a hamstring-stretching program, which is an essential part of the treatment, must be performed several times daily to maximize recovery. Approximately 50 percent of patients notice a significant improvement with an exercise program in the initial six weeks, with a larger percentage of the remaining patients improving with an additional six weeks of rehabilitation.

In patients who have continued pain after a rehabilitation program, a combination of a local anesthetic and corticosteroid injection may help to decrease the inflammation and associated pain.

Patients who undergo this injection need to recognize the importance of continuing physical therapy to address the underlying quadriceps weakness and hamstring tightness. In addition, nonsteroidal anti-inflammatory drugs (NSAIDs) may be used to try to supplement the physical therapy program.

In rare cases, arthroscopic surgery is needed to remove the inflamed and scarred plica to eliminate the pain.

Following recovery, athletes may return to participation in sports based upon their symptoms. It is recommended that patients start out slowly and observe how their knee responds to exercise before advancing further in the workout program. This gradual progression is important to follow because plical irritation appears to involve some tissue inflammation, which may not develop in patients until hours after finishing an activity. In general, if there is no pain or swelling with an activity, it is safe to continue.

Prevention

Maintaining strong and flexible muscles around the knee, especially through strengthening and stretching of the quadriceps and hamstrings, will help prevent the development of a painful plica. In patients who play contact sports, using knee pads to avoid direct blows to the front of the knee will also help.

patellofemoral pain syndrome Patellofemoral pain syndrome is a term used to describe pain originating from the region of the patella (kneecap) and femur (thighbone). It is extremely common among athletes, probably the most common knee complaint that doctors see. Other names for this syndrome include retropatellar pain, anterior knee pain, and chondromalacia patellae. None of these terms accurately describe the cause of this pain, which remains elusive and poorly understood, despite the frequency of its occurrence.

Causes

Several anatomic and congenital factors may lead to a predisposition toward patellofemoral pain and/or instability. Tightness of the quadriceps muscles, hamstrings and iliotibial band, and relative weakness of the quadriceps muscle are probably the most common causes. Other factors that can contribute to this problem include femoral anteversion (excessive rotation of the hips), tibial torsion (excessive rotation of the shin bone), genu valgum (knock knees), genu recurvatum (hyperextended knee), and excessive pronation (flat feet).

In addition to these predisposing factors, other problems, such as prepatellar bursitis, tendonitis in the quadriceps, or meniscal injury may contribute to the development of patellofemoral pain syndrome.

Diagnosis

Patients with patellofemoral pain syndrome describe pain primarily in the front of their knees. It may be on just one side or on both sides. Patients describe pain with stair climbing and especially going down the stairs. They frequently experience pain with prolonged sitting (watching a movie, riding on an airplane) and feel that they have to occasionally straighten their legs out to decrease discomfort. The pain is usually exacerbated by squatting and kneeling. It is generally an aching pain, but can become sharp in nature and even be associated with a burning sensation. On occasion, patients may describe a sense that their knee may give out on them. This occurs particularly when going down the stairs. The onset of symptoms is frequently associated with the start of a new activity or increase in level of intensity of a preexisting activity.

To diagnose patellofemoral pain syndrome, a doctor will take a thorough medical history and conduct a physical examination.

Treatment

Treatment for patellofemoral pain syndrome involves a combination of activity modification, taking anti-inflammatory medication, and participating in a comprehensive stretching and strengthening program. Surgical intervention is rarely necessary and is generally reserved for cases of chronic instability that cannot be corrected or malalignment of the lower leg.

To the extent that patellofemoral symptoms are caused by a change in activity level, or exacerbated by specific activity, activity modification is the mainstay of treatment. Treatment of acute onset of patellofemoral pain syndrome from a specific event, such as running a marathon or initiating a new exercise program, is relatively straightforward. In general, this would involve an initial period of rest, ice, over-the-counter anti-inflammatories and a slow, gradual resumption of activities in a progressive manner.

Chronic patellofemoral pain syndrome is much more difficult to treat. It can be a frustrating problem for physicians and patients alike. The mainstay of treatment for chronic patellofemoral pain syndrome is a combination of quadriceps strengthening exercises in addition to quadriceps, hamstring, and iliotibial band stretching exercises. It is often helpful to refer patients to a physical therapist for one or two sessions of hands-on instruction in the appropriate exercise program. Occasionally, electric stimulation and biofeedback are useful. Prolonged PHYSICAL THERAPY with modalities such as ultrasound is generally not helpful or cost effective. Orthotics and soft braces with patellar cutouts may provide modest symptomatic relief in selected cases.

Prevention

For the most part, this condition is difficult to prevent. However, maintaining strength and flexibility in the hamstrings and knees will help to control the problem somewhat.

peroneal tendonitis The peroneal muscles run along the outer side of the lower leg, and their tendons attach to the foot. These muscles and tendons help move the foot to the outside, but the tendons are relatively weak and poorly anchored, making them vulnerable to strains, when the muscle fibers or tendons are stretched or torn.

Causes

Peroneal tendon strain can result from running on sloped surfaces or running in shoes with excessive wear on the outside of the heel. The tendons may also be stretched or torn during an inversion injury, when the foot and ankle are rolled inward, or in an injury that forces the foot upward toward the shinbone. In addition to these situations, iliotibial band restriction increases force on the peroneal tendons and may contribute to peroneal tendonitis.

Diagnosis

Patients with this type of injury to the foot typically complain of acute pain and swelling centered in the lower leg and ankle. They may recount hearing a pop or snap when the injury occurred. In addition, athletes normally complain of a snapping sensation and sharp pain whenever they change directions or push off with the foot. Swelling is normally visible around the ankle.

In a physical exam, doctors will move the ankle and leg to test the movement in the tendons. X rays may be needed to rule out a break in the ankle or in one of the bones of the foot.

Treatment

Conservative treatment involves the application of icepacks to the ankle for 20 to 30 minutes every three to four hours for two or three days or until the pain goes away. The patient should also keep the injured foot elevated at a level above the heart and wrap the ankle with an elastic bandage, both of which will help reduce swelling. If the doctor prescribes a stirrup splint (often called Aircast or Gelcast), this should be worn instead. Finally, the patient should perform exercises that will strengthen the peroneal muscles and tendons and the ankle joint.

Surgery is reserved for those in whom conservative therapy has failed or for those who are high-level athletes.

While the patient is recovering from the injury, it is important to change to a sport or activity that will not make the condition worse. For example, if the patient is a runner, he or she should try cycling or swimming for a while. Return to the patient's chosen sport should occur when the patient has full range of motion and strength in the leg and ankle and there is no pain or limping when jogging, sprinting, jumping, or running figure-eights. These sprinting and cutting activities should not be resumed for at least six weeks following the injury as they put the most stress on the peroneal tendons. Long-distance running also can aggravate this condition. Returning to normal activities too soon may result in a worse injury and an even longer period of recovery.

Prevention

Avoiding peroneal tendon strains is a matter of keeping the ankles and peroneal muscles strong. High-top shoes or a supportive ankle brace often help by providing extra support for these traditionally weak tendons. It is also important to warm up properly so that these tendons have a chance to get limber before they are put to any strenuous tests. Finally, choosing to run on level, soft surfaces, where there are no rocks or holes, will also help avoid injuring the peroneal tendon.

physical therapy Physical therapy is the health profession that focuses on the neuromuscular, musculoskeletal, and cardiopulmonary systems of the human body, as these systems relate to human motion and function. This direct form of professional patient care can be applied in most disciplines of medicine to provide a hands-on component in partnership with physicians who have medical expertise in neurology, neurosurgery, orthopedics, general surgery, family practice, pediatrics, geriatrics, rheumatology, internal medicine, urology, cardiovascular medicine, cardiopulmonary medicine, psychiatry, and sports medicine. Physical therapists, or PTs, are very important members of the health care team. They evaluate and provide treatment for persons with health problems resulting from injury, disease, or overuse of muscles or tendons. A medical referral is often made for physical therapy postoperatively or following injury or illness.

Training

Physical therapists have an undergraduate degree in physical therapy, and many have a master's degree. In order to practice, all graduates must be licensed by their state and pass a national certification examination.

Careers

There are more than 90,000 physical therapists practicing in the United States today in a variety of settings. Physical therapists who work in the sports or fitness industry are usually employed by sports medicine clinics or consult with professional sports organizations. They may also work in hospitals, rehabilitation centers, home health agencies, schools, sports facilities, community health centers, and in private practice.

Physical therapists who add a credential as a strength coach or athletic trainer are even more marketable to the sports and fitness industry.

Treatment by a Physical Therapist

Physical therapists assess, design, and administer rehabilitative programs that improve mobility, relieve pain, increase strength, and reduce or rehabilitate an injury. They provide comprehensive training that includes, but is not limited to, the following:

- functional mobility
- balance and gait retraining
- soft-tissue mobilization
- body mechanics education
- casting and splinting
- wheelchair safety and management
- neuromuscular re-education
- exercise programming
- family education and training
- assistance with pain relief and management
- instruction in safe ambulation

The objectives of physical therapy are the prevention of disability and pain, the restoration of function and relief from pain, the promotion of healing, and the adaptation to permanent disability.

The physical therapist selects appropriate tests to evaluate and quantitatively measure the patient's problem. Then, in consultation with the referring physician, an appropriate rehabilitation plan is developed.

The physical therapist uses numerous techniques and procedures to expedite healing, and instructs the patient in a home program. There may be follow-up visits for re-evaluation and update of the home exercise program.

piriformis syndrome Piriformis syndrome is a condition in which the piriformis muscle irritates the sciatic nerve, causing pain in the buttocks and referring pain along the course of the sciatic nerve. The piriformis is one of the small muscles deep in the buttocks that rotates the leg outward. It runs from the base of the spine and attaches to the thighbone (femur) roughly where the outside crease in the buttock is located. The sciatic nerve runs very close to this muscle and sometimes even through it. Inflammation of the sciatic nerve, called sciatica, causes pain in the back of the hip that can often travel down into the leg.

Causes

If the piriformis muscle is unusually tight or if it goes into spasm, the sciatic nerve can become inflamed or irritated. Piriformis syndrome may also be related to intense downhill running. A common cause of piriformis syndrome is having tight adductor muscles, which are the muscles located on the inside of the thigh. When the adductors are tight, the abductors on the outside of the thigh cannot work properly, which places more strain on the piriformis.

Diagnosis

Symptoms of piriformis syndrome include pain deep in the buttock that may feel like a burning pain. The pain usually travels down across the lower thigh. The pain may increase with movement of the thigh outward, such as when sitting cross-legged. Climbing stairs and performing squats will usually increase the pain as well.

The doctor will need to take a complete medical history and perform a physical examination to diagnose the problem. A good description of the symptoms and when they began is necessary. Since the sciatic nerve begins in the back, it can be irritated from a back injury, such as a herniated disk. Any history of back or hip injury is especially important to note.

The physical exam will include palpating around the sciatic nerve to check for irritation or tenderness. The doctor will also examine the patient's hips and legs and check to see if movement in them increases the pain.

The piriformis syndrome is diagnosed primarily on the basis of symptoms and on the physical exam. There are no tests that accurately confirm the diagnosis, but X rays, MAGNETIC RESONANCE IMAGING (MRI), and nerve conduction tests may be necessary to exclude other diseases. Some of the other causes of sciatica include disease in the lumbar spine (e.g. disc herniation), chronic HAMSTRING TENDONITIS, and fibrous adhesions of other muscles around the sciatic nerve.

Treatment

Treatment may include:

• placing ice packs on the buttock for 20 to 30 minutes every three to four hours for the first two to three days or until the pain goes away
• rest
• taking prescribed anti-inflammatory medications or muscle relaxants
• performing stretching and exercises for the piriformis muscle
• applying sports massage techniques
• applying ultrasound

If these conservative approaches fail, then injections of a corticosteroid into the piriformis muscle may be tried. Finally, surgical exploration may be undertaken as a last resort.

The goal of rehabilitation is to return the patient to sport or activity as soon as is safely possible. If one returns too soon the injury may worsen, which could lead to permanent damage. Everyone recovers from injury at a different rate. Return to sport or activity will be determined by how soon the nerve recovers, not by how many days or weeks it has been since the injury occurred. In general, the longer symptoms are present before treatment starts, the longer it will take to get better.

Patients may safely return to their sport or activity when, starting from the top of the list and progressing to the end, each of the following is true:

• They have full range of motion in the affected leg compared to the unaffected leg.
• They have full strength of the affected leg compared to the unaffected leg.
• They can jog straight ahead without pain or limping.
• They can sprint straight ahead without pain or limping.
• They can do cuts and figure-eights while running without pain.
• They can jump on both legs without pain and can jump on the affected leg without pain.

Prevention

Piriformis syndrome is best prevented by stretching the muscles that rotate the thigh inward and outward. It is important to have a good warm-up before starting a sport or activity.

plantar fascitis OVERUSE INJURIES, which occur more frequently than traumatic injuries and develop over a long period of time from repetitive stress of mild-to-high intensity exercise, are all too common among the recreational exerciser and athlete. They can be painful, bothersome and frustrating. Often, they can become chronic. One of the most common overuse injuries is plantar fascitis. Those involved in running or any pounding-type activities, such as basketball and tennis, are especially prone to this condition and more than 2 million Americans receive treatment for plantar fascitis every year.

Plantar fascitis is the inflammation of the plantar fascia, which is a tight band of elastic, connective tissue that runs vertically along the bottom of the foot from the five toes to the bottom of the heel. Its primary function is to protect the foot and support the arch. This support allows the foot to be an effective shock and stress absorber. When irritated through overuse, the plantar fascia becomes inflamed and painful, causing muscle tightness and movement limitations that can result in overstretching and tiny tears in the fascia. Treatment for the condition is normally successful, but if left untreated, plantar fascitis can lead to the formation of heel spurs and even surgery in some cases.

Causes

There are numerous causes of plantar fascitis, and those who develop this condition may experience one or any combination of problems that leads to plantar fascitis. The most common causes include use of improper footwear, incorrect exercise techniques, tight calf muscles and/or Achilles tendons, excessive stress on the bottom of the foot, anatomical problems in the foot, and overpronation problems that cause the foot to flatten and become unstable.

Diagnosis

Patients with plantar fascitis will most often complain of pain in the bottom of the foot when exercising, pain that is centered around the front of the heel, stiffness and extreme pain first thing in the morning when getting out of bed, reduced flexibility in the arch of the foot, and decreased strength in the bottom of the foot.

Treatment

A wide range of treatments can help alleviate the symptoms of plantar fascitis. Rest is the very first step, as it is with any overuse injury. Rest allows the plantar fascia time to heal, but it is not necessary to be totally inactive. With plantar fascitis, the most important thing is to refrain from pounding activities that put excessive stress on the bottom of the feet. Activities such as swimming, biking, and using the elliptical trainer at the gym take most the weight off the feet but still allow the athlete to get a good workout. Once the pain and other symptoms cease, the athlete can slowly return to normal activities. Icing the bottom of the foot will also speed the healing process. During an injury, fluid and cells rush to the wounded area, causing inflammation. Ice constricts the blood vessels, limiting the amount of fluid that comes through to the area and therefore decreasing the swelling. Applying a traditional ice pack will produce the desired anti-inflammatory effect, but using a frozen juice can allows the athlete to actually massage the bottom of the foot with the ice. Athletes must be sure to wear shoes with proper arch supports and cushioned heels. Wearing inappropriate shoes can contribute to the development of plantar fascitis and other injuries as well, such as tendonitis and arthritis. Athletes should also engage in proper warm-up and stretching exercises. Stiffness is one of the main symptoms of plantar fascitis, so it is especially important that athletes dealing with this condition incorporate the proper warm-up and stretches into every workout. They should also do some warm-up exercises in the morning before even getting out of bed. It is crucial to make sure that the bottom of the foot is loose and flexible before beginning to exercise on it. Finally, strengthening the plantar fascia muscles on the bottom of the foot will help in prevention of this injury and in recovery for the athlete who has already developed the problem.

If conservative treatment fails to produce good results, bracing or splinting the foot may be advisable. Hot whirlpool therapy may also be recommended. Orthotics to help limit pronation and lift the arch may be considered as well.

Prevention

As with other overuse injuries, prevention is primarily a matter of engaging in a carefully organized training program that builds intensity and duration in workouts gradually. Use of proper shoes and technique is also essential. Engaging in regular stretching and warm-up exercises for the feet before participating in a workout will also help the athlete to avoid plantar fasciitis.

posterior cruciate ligament (PCL) injury   A stretch or tear in the ligament that connects the thighbone (femur) to the shinbone (tibia) is called a posterior cruciate ligament (PCL) injury, or a posterior cruciate ligament sprain. Ligaments are the strong bands of tissue that connect one bone to another bone. The posterior cruciate ligament is one of the major ligaments in the knee. Along with the anterior cruciate ligament (ACL), the posterior cruciate ligament helps keep the knee stable and protects the thighbone from sliding or turning on the shinbone.

Posterior cruciate ligament injuries are much less common than ANTERIOR CRUCIATE LIGAMENT INJURIES and often go unrecognized when they do occur. In part, this is because the PCL is wider and stronger than the ACL.

Causes

The posterior cruciate ligament can be injured by a direct blow to the front of the knee while the knee is bent and the foot is planted. This type of injury usually results in a sprain to the ligament and is most commonly seen in football injuries, running injuries, and in motor vehicle accidents. Injuries to the PCL and ACL also occur during falls while skiing when ski bindings fail to release the foot.

Diagnosis

Patients with a posterior cruciate ligament injury usually recount a history of a direct blow to the knee. Knowledge of the exact mechanism of the injury can be helpful to the doctor in making a diagnosis. Patients often will describe discomfort or pain when walking up or down stairs, starting to run, lifting heavy objects, walking longer distances, as well as swelling, stiffness, and a sensation of instability when walking on uneven ground. In patients who have sustained an injury to the posterior cruciate ligament in the past but have never had reconstructive surgery, there may be the feeling that the knee is about to give way during sporting activities.

The physical examination may reveal swelling with fluid in the knee joint. There may be minimal pain or no pain with various tests performed by the doctor. These include a positive quadriceps active test, a posterior drawer test, among others. There is usually full or functional range of motion in the knee. There may be a contusion present over the front of the shinbone if the patient has indeed had a direct blow to the knee.

An X ray may be taken to see if there are any injuries to the femur or tibia. A MAGNETIC RESONANCE IMAGING (MRI) scan may help diagnose posterior cruciate ligament tears as well and are usually recommended if there is evidence of multiple injured ligaments.

Injuries are graded for severity on a scale:

Grade I sprain involves pain with minimal damage to the ligament.
Grade II sprain involves more ligament damage and mild looseness of the joint.
Grade III injury describes complete tearing of the ligament with a very loose and unstable joint.

Treatment

Conservative treatment for a PCL injury depends on the severity of the injury. The key to nonoperative treatment is to control the swelling, instability, and pain. This is normally quite successful in Grade I and Grade II injuries and is done by using the following techniques:

- applying ice packs to the knee for 20 to 30 minutes every three to four hours for two or three days or until the pain goes away
- elevating the leg with the knee straight, ideally with the ankle above the heart
- wrapping an elastic bandage around the leg to keep the swelling from getting worse
- using crutches

- doing knee rehabilitation exercises
- using electric stimulation or a cold whirlpool

Patients with Grade I and Grade II injuries can bear weight as tolerated immediately, though some may require crutches. The physical therapist should instruct the patient in exercises for quadriceps and hip strengthening.

In cases that do not respond to conservative treatment, surgical reconstruction of the torn PCL may be required. The torn PCL cannot be sewn back together, however, so the ligament must be reconstructed by taking ligaments or tendons from other parts of the leg and connecting them to the tibia and femur.

Rehabilitation following surgery involves controlling the pain and swelling through the use of cold therapy, compression, and elevation, use of crutches initially, exercising the knee and being instructed by the physical therapist to prevent fibrosis during healing and to assist in ensuring full range of motion for the knee.

In general, athletes may safely return to their sport or activity when each of the following is true:

- The injured knee can be fully straightened and bent without pain.
- The knee and leg have regained normal strength compared to the uninjured knee and leg.
- The knee is not swollen.
- The patient is able to jog straight ahead without limping.
- The patient is able to sprint straight ahead without limping.
- The patient is able to do cuts and figure-eights while running without pain.
- The patient is able to jump on both legs without pain and jump on the injured leg without pain.

Prevention

Unfortunately, most injuries to the posterior cruciate ligament occur during accidents that are not preventable. However, athletes who maintain strong thigh and hamstring muscles and participate in a good leg-stretching routine before exercise will have a better chance of avoiding these injuries. Some physicians advocate the use of functional

knee braces for reducing the risk of a recurring PCL injury when returning to activity.

It is also important to be sure that ski bindings are set correctly by a trained professional so that the bindings release during a fall. The failure of bindings to release during falls is a common cause of PCL and ACL injuries.

posterior tibial tendonitis   Posterior tibial tendonitis causes pain along the inner side of the lower leg, ankle, or foot. Tendons are strong bands of connective tissue that attach muscles to bones. The posterior tibial tendon helps point the foot down and in. If this tendon becomes inflamed, stretched, or torn, it causes pain along the inner side of the lower leg, ankle, or foot.

Causes

Commonly found in overpronators, people whose arch flattens out more than normal when they walk and run, posterior tibial tendonitis results from overuse of the tendon. When they overpronate and the arch flattens more than it should, they strain this tendon, whose purpose is to help stabilize the arch.

Posterior tibial tendonitis is also seen in middle-aged women who are unfit as a result of chronic degeneration and in older athletes. Middle-aged women who play stop-and-start or push-off activities, such as soccer, football, and basketball commonly develop this type of tendonitis.

Diagnosis

If the patient complains of pain or tenderness on the inner side of the shin, ankle, or foot, pain with lifting up the foot, and pain when walking or running, posterior tibial tendonitis is a possibility. A physical examination by a doctor will likely reveal tenderness along the tendon, a flattened arch, and pronation of the foot. The patient may be asked to walk or run so that the doctor can observe the degree of pronation that occurs. In some cases, an ultrasound examination may be used to confirm the diagnosis.

Treatment

Initial treatment includes applying ice to the injury every 20 to 30 minutes every three to four hours or until the pain goes away. Once the pain has subsided, it is still advised to ice at least once a day. Ice massages, where the patient applies a block of ice directly to the tendon in a massaging motion, are also beneficial. The injured leg should be elevated above the level of the heart to help reduce swelling, and the foot should be taped to provide extra support to the arch and tendon. In severe cases, a cast may be necessary for a few weeks until the pain and inflammation abate. Crutches are advised for walking to alleviate pressure on the tendon until the pain subsides. Anti-inflammatory medication or other pain medication will help until the tendon has a chance to heal. Finally, patients should begin a program of exercises to help strengthen the tendon and increase flexibility.

A medial arch support is recommended with the heel up for patients with tenosynovitis and partial tears of the tendon. Those with complete tears must undergo surgery to reconstruct the tendon.

PHYSICAL THERAPY is effective in treating inversion injuries and tendonitis of the foot, particularly in athletes who are continuing competition. Rehabilitation involves exercises to build strength and flexibility in the tendon and muscles surrounding the tendon. Recovery will depend upon the severity of the injury and the type of treatment. Patients who have partial or complete tears of the tendon will experience a longer recovery period than those whose tendon is strained and will likely have to participate in more physical therapy when their casts are removed.

Return to normal activities should be gradual, especially in regard to cutting and jumping activities and running for any significant length of time. When full range of motion and strength are restored, one can jog and sprint without pain or limping, and can do 45-degree cuts and figure-eights at slow and fast speeds, the tendon is healed enough to return to sport or activity.

Prevention
Maintaining strong muscles in the lower leg and ankle, warming up regularly before beginning strenuous exercise, and running on even surfaces that are not too hard will help prevent developing posterior tibial tendonitis. In addition, always take care to wear shoes that fit properly and provide adequate cushion. Those who overpronate, should choose shoes, and possibly orthotics, that help compensate for this.

rhomboid muscle injury The rhomboid muscles are located in the upper back, where they connect the inner edges of the shoulder blades to the spine. A rhomboid muscle injury is normally either a strain or a spasm in these muscles. A strain is an injury in which muscle fibers or tendons are stretched or torn. A muscle spasm is an involuntary contraction of the muscle.

Causes

A rhomboid muscle strain or spasm is usually caused by overuse of the shoulder and arm, especially during such overhead activities as serving a volleyball or tennis ball or reaching to put objects on a high shelf. Other activities that often bring about rhomboid injuries include rowing and carrying a backpack with heavy weight resting on the shoulder. Poor posture can also help to cause a rhomboid injury, especially during prolonged use of a computer.

Diagnosis

Patients with a rhomboid strain usually complain of pain in the upper back between the shoulder blades and the spine. Patients with a rhomboid spasm describe discomfort that feels like a knot or tightness in the muscle. There is often pain associated with moving the shoulders and with breathing.

The doctor will take a complete medical history and do a thorough physical examination, focusing on the back and shoulder. Normally, the exam will reveal tightness and some tenderness in the rhomboid muscles.

Treatment

Initial treatment for this injury is icing the shoulder for 20 to 30 minutes every three to four hours for two to three days or until the pain goes away.

Sometimes the best method for applying ice to these muscles is to place a frozen gel pack on the floor, cover it with a towel, and then lie down on top of it. Anti-inflammatory medication may also be prescribed.

Massage is also very helpful. The patient can perform self-massage by placing a tennis ball on the floor, lying down with the rhomboid muscles against the tennis ball, and gently rolling back and forth over the ball, so that the muscles are massaged.

Once the pain has begun to subside, the patient should be given some rehabilitation exercises to help return flexibility and strength to these muscles. During recovery, it is important to refrain from the aggravating activities that caused the injury. Tennis players and rowers may need to switch to running or biking during their recovery, but once the symptoms have resolved, and they can move their arms and shoulders without pain, they can begin a gradual return to their primary sport.

Prevention

Rhomboid strains and spasms are best prevented by warming up properly and doing stretching exercises before activities such as tennis, rowing, or overhead movements.

RICE (rest, ice, compression, and elevation) Few athletes manage to avoid injuries entirely, but not all injuries require a trip to the doctor. Minor sprains and strains can often be effectively treated at home using the RICE method. The RICE approach is designed to help the athlete control pain and swelling and minimize any side effects of the injury. RICE refers to rest, ice, compression, and elevation. It is the front line treatment of choice in many sports injuries during the first 24 to 48 hours following injury.

How It Works

Rest is the first step in treating many injuries. Although the athlete may not need to be totally inactive, it is important to stop the aggravating activity. If an activity is causing pain, it is time to switch to an activity that does not cause pain or to rest entirely for a period of time. Runners who experience pain in the knee may need to try swimming for a while; while swimmers with pain in the shoulder may want to try running or biking. The bottom line is that if the activity hurts, it is important to stop, but maintaining fitness levels can often be accomplished by simply switching to a sport that does not cause pain.

Ice is effective in decreasing the pain from an injury. It deadens the sensation of pain and increases blood circulation to the skin while decreasing circulation in the deeper tissues where the bleeding from an injury may be occurring.

Ice packs can be used directly on an injured body part for up to 20 minutes at a time. Small areas can be treated with an ice massage by using a frozen juice can or a small paper cup filled with frozen water.

The athlete should take care to notice if the skin begins to change color. If it turns white or blue, the icing should be stopped immediately since there is a risk of frostbite. Cold treatments can be repeated every two hours.

Compression of the area that is injured helps prevent swelling, which is fluid accumulating around the injury. An elastic wrap or stocking can be used effectively. It should be tied firmly but not too tight. If the part of the limb that is farthest from the heart begins to throb, the wrap is too tight and should be loosened. Compression wraps should be reapplied every four hours. Compression will help if the swelling is a result of bleeding. It may also help ease pain.

Elevation of the injured body part helps to eliminate the swelling by using gravity to drain fluid away from the injury. It maybe hard to accomplish with some parts of the body, but if at all possible, the athlete should raise an injured arm or leg above the level of the heart whenever resting.

The RICE method will help athletes when they begin to recover from symptoms and are able to return to sports activities. Athletes can use RICE to help control the pain as they begin to gradually return to normal activities. It is important, however, that athletes not forget that full range of motion and strength must be present in order for the injury to be healed. Until it is completely healed, athletes are at greater risk of reinjuring the area.

Many people ask about the use of heat when instructed to use the RICE method. Heat does often feel good and can help alleviate pain, but it promotes swelling, which is something athletes need to avoid following an injury. Heat can also promote blood circulation at the deeper tissue level, which is devastating if bleeding is occurring there.

In the later stages of recovery from an injury, heat may be used to help with stiffness. However, if swelling develops around the injury, it is important to stop using heat and return to ice.

rotator cuff tear   The shoulder is the most mobile joint in the body and therefore is prone to injuries, including injuries to the rotator cuff, which are a group of muscles that plays a major role in the stabilization and movement of the shoulder. They also are important in initiating movement of the arm in various directions.

The rotator cuff is made up of four muscles and their tendons, which insert on the top of the arm bone, or humerus. These muscles function along with the deltoid muscle to elevate and rotate the arm. The four muscles, beginning in the front and moving up over the top to the back are the subscapularis, the supraspinatus, the infraspinatus, and the teres minor. Rotator cuff tears may involve one or all of these four muscles and essentially involve separation of the attachment the muscle makes to the arm bone. Sometimes, the tendons are also involved. The supraspinatus tendon is the one most commonly involved in rotator cuff tears. A partial tear may cause pain when the arm is lifted in a certain arc away from the body, and a complete tear may limit the ability to raise the arm. Rotator cuff tears are seen most commonly in people over the age of 40.

Causes

Rotator cuff tears can be caused by a traumatic injury such as the severe impact of a car crash or by a simple motion such as pulling a child in a wagon. In sports, the most common cause of rotator cuff tears is overuse. The kind of overuse that can cause a rotator cuff tear occurs mostly in throwing sports such as baseball and in sports where the shoulder might have to endure excessive external force, such as football or ice hockey. Complete tears in younger patients are almost always from trauma, such as falling on an outstretched hand, or after a shoulder dislocation caused by trauma such as skiing accidents and football tackles. In individuals over the age of 50, however, tears can occur with only minor trauma, often because scarring from past episodes of tendonitis has weakened the tendons.

Diagnosis

Diagnosis of a rotator cuff injury is often made on the basis of history of trauma or overuse activities in combination with physical findings of pain and weakness as discussed below. Patients with a rotator cuff tear usually describe pain along the outside of the shoulder that becomes worse at night and with attempts to raise the arm. Depending on which of the four muscles is affected, the pain can occur with moving the arm forward, moving the arm straight out from the side, or rotating the arm in and out at the shoulder with the arm held in various positions.

Other symptoms and signs of a rotator cuff tear include muscle weakness, catching of the arm associated with grating and cracking sounds, limited motion, and occurrence in the dominant arm. It can be triggered by a single event, but is often the result of accumulated stress over time.

The physical examination normally reveals weakness in elevating and externally rotating the arm.

X rays can be useful in showing degeneration where the muscle attaches to the arm bone. In cases that are difficult to diagnose based on clinical findings, a MAGNETIC RESONANCE IMAGING (MRI) scan might be useful since it will actually reveal a tear.

Treatment

Treatment is directed toward elimination of pain. Normally, the elimination of pain is achieved repairing the attachment of the rotator cuff to the arm and removing any associated bone spurs.

In most cases, the initial treatment involves rest, use of nonsteroidal anti-inflammatory medications to help control the pain, strengthening and stretching exercises as part of a physical therapy program, corticosteroid injections in some cases, and ultrasound. If the injury fails to respond to conservative treatment, there are several surgical options for the repair of a rotator cuff tear, depending on the size, depth, and location of the tear. These options include open surgery, mini open surgery that utilizes a two-inch incision, and arthroscopic surgery.

Prevention

Rotator cuff tears that result from traumatic injuries are usually caused by accidents and thus are not preventable. But rotator cuff tears caused by overuse may be prevented with careful training that includes adequate rest between workouts and regular stretching and strengthening exercises.

rotator cuff tendonitis (supraspinatus tendonitis, painful arc syndrome) Also called supraspinatus tendonitis or painful arc syndrome, tendonitis in the rotator cuff is the inflammation of the tendon of one of the main muscles that form the rotator cuff—the supraspinatus. This is one of the most common causes of shoulder pain and is usually characterized by pain and weakness on the tip of the shoulder when the arm is moved sideways or upward above the head. Rotator cuff tendonitis is an OVERUSE INJURY and is associated with overhead sports, such as tennis, badminton, volleyball, and baseball, as well as swimming.

Causes

Rotator cuff tendonitis in athletes is caused primarily by repetitive overarm motions or a sudden increase in the frequency, intensity, and/or duration of workouts that brings about inflammation of the supraspinatus tendon and causes it to rub up against the outside tip of the shoulder blade when the arm is raised. This rubbing is what causes the pain. Other risk factors implicated in the development of rotator cuff tendonitis include a spur-shaped shoulder blade, which is a congenital condition; shoulder instability; and a previous history of tendonitis.

Diagnosis

Patients with rotator cuff tendonitis usually describe pain and weakness on the tip of the shoulder when the arm is moved sideways or upward above the head. A medical history reveals that the onset of the condition is gradual. The physical examination will focus on the arm and shoulder and may include tests to assess the patient's range of motion and strength. Swelling and tenderness of the front and upper part of the shoulder may be present.

X rays may be used to rule out certain other problems, but MAGNETIC RESONANCE IMAGING (MRI) scans are the imaging study of choice in shoulder injuries because they are noninvasive, involve no radiation, and they detect partial tears and degeneration within the tendons, as well as inflammation, swelling, hemorrhaging, and scarring.

Treatment

Initial treatment involves icing the shoulder three times a day for 20 to 30 minutes; maintaining activities with modifications to avoid pain; taking anti-inflammatories; ceasing any activity that causes pain; and implementing a conditioning program to stretch and strengthen rotator cuff muscles.

If these conservative measures are not successful in relieving the symptoms, other possible treatments include cortisone injections and surgery. The injections take about 48 hours to relieve the tendonitis symptoms, but the patient must refrain from all aggravating activities for at least two weeks. The tendonitis is normally resolved in three weeks. Surgery is the last resort if rest and cortisone fail to relieve the tendonitis. The goal of the surgery may be to make more room for the tendon in the shoulder, which involves removing ligament, trimming calcium deposits, and cutting out the bursa that is located near the rotator cuff. It may also include stitching together tendons that have been severely torn.

If diagnosed early, supraspinatus tendonitis can be cleared up in one to three weeks with another three weeks needed for recovery in cases that are more severe. Recovery from surgery takes between six and 12 weeks of rest and rehabilitation before returning to physical activities (sports).

The initial goals of rehabilitation include normalizing the range of motion of the shoulder, improving neuromuscular control and strength, and maintaining joint motion.

Prevention

The best prevention for rotator cuff tendonitis is a careful training program that involves strengthening and stretching exercises for the rotator cuff, avoidance of repetitive overarm motions and adequate rest between training that does involve overarm activities, and use of rest, ice, compression, and elevation as a treatment whenever symptoms begin to flare up. Athletes, particularly those involved in throwing and overhead sports, should be instructed in proper warm-up techniques, specific strengthening techniques, and warning signs of early impingement of the rotator cuff tendon.

runner's knee (patellofemoral pain syndrome)

Runner's knee is an OVERUSE INJURY that causes pain behind the kneecap. It has been given many names, including patellofemoral pain syndrome, patellofemoral disorder, patellar malalignment, and chondromalacia. The kneecap (patella) is attached to the large group of muscles in the thigh called the quadriceps. It is also attached to the shinbone by the patellar tendon. The kneecap fits into grooves in the end of the thighbone (femur) called the femoral condyle. With repeated bending and straightening of the knee, the inside surface of the kneecap can become irritated and cause pain.

Causes

Runner's knee occurs most often in runners, as one would suspect from the name. But walkers, cyclists, and those who jump a lot in their sports can also be vulnerable to developing runner's knee.

It is caused by the maltracking of the kneecap in the groove on the lower end of the thighbone. Normally, the kneecap, which is lined by smooth cartilage, tracks directly within this groove. When it runs out of this track, it may cause pain and discomfort in the front of the knee. Factors that may cause this include tight muscular and soft tissue structures, particularly on the outside of the knee, and weak stabilizing muscles of the kneecap, particularly the inner quadriceps of the thigh.

Other conditions that can cause this maltracking of the kneecap include anatomical abnormalities, biomechanical problems in a runner's stride, and the breakdown of articular cartilage under the kneecap. It may result from the way the hips, legs, knees, or feet are aligned. Alignment problems can stem from having wide hips or underdeveloped thigh muscles, being knock-kneed, or having feet with arches that collapse when walking or running, a condition called overpronation.

Occasionally, the pain may begin after a blow to the knee or a minor injury, but usually this disorder arises without a history of significant trauma. The pain may be initiated by overuse, such as a rapid increase in running distance or bicycle riding up hills, or by a twisting injury to the knee.

Diagnosis

The main symptom is pain behind the kneecap. There may also be pain when walking, running, or sitting for a long time. In most athletes, the pain worsens when running or walking downhill or down stairs. The knee may sometimes swell, and there may be a popping or grinding sound in the knee.

On inspection of the knee, an assessment of the alignment of the kneecap is done. The kneecap should fall in the center of the thigh. If it is riding on the outside portion of the knee or appears to tilt with knee bending, the patient is at higher risk for runner's knee. Evaluation of the quadriceps muscle strength is essential. Palpation of the kneecap and finding the area of maximal tenderness is done next. Assessing the kneecap for restricted movement and possible instability are other important components of the physical exam. Checking the knee for fluid should also be done. Finally, it is critical to evaluate the patient's quadriceps flexibility. This can be done by having the patient lie on the stomach and attempt to pull the heel toward the buttock. Comparison to the opposite side will help in this assessment.

Diagnosis can normally be made on the basis of the medical history and physical examination, although sometimes X rays may be ordered to confirm the diagnosis.

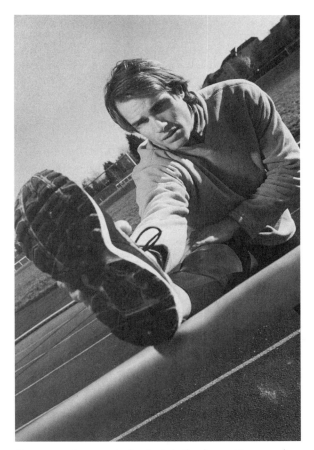

Runners who regularly stretch the hamstrings and quadriceps are less likely to develop overuse injuries that affect the knee. *(Fogstock, LLC)*

Treatment

Treatment for runner's knee is much like treatment for other overuse injuries. Rest is required in order to give the knee a break from all aggravating movements. In addition, the athlete should ice the knee for 20 to 30 minutes every three to four hours for the first two to three days or until the pain goes away. Elevating the knee by placing a pillow underneath the leg when the knee hurts will also help. Anti-inflammatory pain medication, such as ibuprofen, may be useful in managing the pain and swelling.

Depending on the exact source of the problem, it may be helpful to wear orthotics in the running shoes. This is especially true for athletes who overpronate. A patellar knee strap may also be placed beneath the kneecap, over the patellar tendon, to provide extra support. If this does not help, the athlete may want to try a neoprene knee sleeve, which supports the knee and kneecap.

In cases of severe runner's knee, surgery may be required to smooth the articular cartilage or release tight structures around the kneecap.

During recovery from the injury, it is very important to change to a sport or activity that does not make the condition worse. Runners may need to bicycle or swim, or at least try running in water, in order to give the knee the rest it needs.

Once the pain begins to subside, athletes may want to begin exercises to help strengthen the quadriceps. Strong quadriceps help to keep undue stress off the knee and will thus help in preventing recurrences of this injury.

Athletes may safely return to their normal activities when all the pain has subsided and the injured knee can be fully straightened and bent without pain. The knee should have regained normal strength compared to the uninjured knee.

Prevention

Runner's knee is best prevented by strengthening the thigh muscles, both quadriceps and hamstrings, and keeping them as flexible as possible. The muscles on the inside of the thigh are particularly important. Proper shoes with good arch supports are also helpful in preventing runner's knee. Athletes can make prevention easier by avoiding activities that put undue stress on the knees. These include squatting, deep knee bends, excessive bending, sitting "Indian" style, sitting back on the heels, kneeling directly on the kneecaps, excessive climbing of stairs, wearing high-heel shoes, riding a bike with the seat too low, and breaststroke in swimming.

scaphoid fractures A navicular fracture is a break in one of the bones in the wrist. The wrist is made up of eight bones between the forearm and hand. The navicular, or scaphoid, bone is a cashew-shaped bone near the thumb. Fractures to this bone sometimes have trouble healing because the bone has a unique blood supply that can be easily disrupted by a fracture. It is the most frequently injured of the carpal bones and is crucial to the intricate function of the wrist, enduring a myriad of complex forces. Scaphoid injuries are most commonly seen in young men and are often misdiagnosed as sprained wrists. A dull, deep pain in the wrist after a fall on an outstretched hand is the hallmark of a scaphoid fracture.

Scaphoid fractures have a warranted reputation for needing close attention. They can be difficult to treat due to instability and a tenuous blood supply. However, with proper diagnosis and immobilization, the vast majority of scaphoid fractures heal successfully.

Causes

A navicular fracture is caused by a fall onto the wrist or a direct blow to the bone.

Diagnosis

Patients with a scaphoid fracture usually report dull pain, swelling, and tenderness in the wrist, usually just below the thumb.

A doctor will take a medical history that usually involves a fall on an outstretched hand. Patients may not report severe pain and may even continue to use the wrist. Scaphoid fracture pain is usually described as a dull, deep discomfort in the wrist on the thumb side. The swelling and bruising of an isolated scaphoid fracture is usually mild.

Physical examination of the wrist should be done with one fingertip, carefully palpating the major structures of the wrist, including the eight carpal bones. The doctor will want to test for motions that cause pain and compare them in the opposite wrist.

Radiographs are crucial in determining the location, stability, and orientation of the fracture. Sometimes, a fracture may not show up in the first X ray and the provider may recommend a repeat X ray in one to two weeks. In some cases, a COMPUTERIZED AXIAL TOMOGRAPHY (CAT) scan or bone scan may be used to confirm the fracture.

Treatment

The wrist and hand are the most common sites for upper-extremity injuries in sports activities, and the wrist joint can be daunting in its complexity. Until recently, unless a fracture was seen on an X ray, clinicians too often resorted to the vague diagnosis of wrist strain or sprain in active patients. Now, however, a greater understanding of specific injuries has led to greater sophistication in the diagnosis and treatment of wrist injuries. Accurate diagnosis of wrist pain will most often allow a safe and speedy return to sports activity. Treatment ranges from immobilization to corticosteroid injections to surgical repair of a fracture or underlying cause.

In most cases the patient will need to wear an arm cast that includes the thumb. The cast may or may not extend above the elbow and will need to be worn for up to 12 weeks or longer to be sure the bone heals. In some cases, healing does not occur and the pieces of bone do not grow back together. This situation usually requires surgery.

Sometimes the failure of the pieces of bone to grow back together leads to a problem called avascular necrosis. In avascular necrosis, part of the bone dies because it does not get enough blood. If this happens, then an operation is necessary to remove part of the injured bone, insert grafted bone to help heal the fragment, or insert an artificial bone.

Following a scaphoid fracture, the wrist may return to full functioning or there may be some permanent stiffness or loss of range of motion as a result of the injury.

Because of the long immobilization time needed to treat most scaphoid fractures, a rehabilitation program should be instituted after immobilization. A thumb spica splint can be used for protection until range of motion and strength improve. PHYSICAL THERAPY is required for elderly patients because of their increased risk of losing strength and range of motion.

Range-of-motion exercises for the wrist can be started after immobilization, followed by progressive strengthening exercises for the wrist flexors and extensors.

The decision to allow the athlete to return to a sport is based on the location, patient age, sport, and level of competition. At a minimum, the fracture should exhibit healing and be properly immobilized and protected before return is considered.

In general, the patient should have full range of motion in the wrist without pain before returning to full activities. Taping or bracing of the wrist may be advised when the athlete returns to play. It is also important that the injured wrist, hand, and forearm have the same strength as the uninjured side. There should be no pain when swinging a bat or a racket or placing weight on the injured wrist.

Prevention

A navicular fracture usually occurs during an accident that is not preventable. When involved in activities such as skating, it is important to wear wrist guards to protect the wrist from traumatic injury.

sciatica (lumbosacral radiculopathy) One of the major causes of acute and LOW BACK PAIN is sciatica, also known as lumbosacral radiculopathy. Sciatica is nerve root impingement and/or inflammation in the low back. The sciatic nerve is the largest nerve in the body, and sciatica is impingement or inflammation of the roots of this nerve.

Dancers are prone to both acute and chronic back problems, including sciatica, but this condition can be seen in many different sports. It is characterized by pain that radiates into the hip, buttock, and leg. Numbness and weakness may also occur.

Causes

Many different medical conditions of the spine can cause sciatica, including PIRIFORMIS SYNDROME, spinal stenosis, a HERNIATED DISK, and degenerative disk disease. Dancers who place unusual pressures on their spines and runners with chronically tight hamstring muscles are some of the athletes most prone to developing sciatica.

Diagnosis

Doctors will need to take a complete medical history and conduct a thorough physical examination to diagnose sciatica.

Patients normally experience lower back pain that radiates into the hip, back, and leg. Specific notation should be made in the history regarding the character, intensity, duration, and location of this pain, including any radiation to the extremities, groin, or abdomen, or associated pain at any other location. A subjective rating of the intensity of pain by the patient can be helpful in following the patient's progress. The physician should also try to determine the extent to which the pain is constant or intermittent, and whether there have been any changes in pattern. It may also be beneficial to have the patient complete a pain diagram, which provides a visual representation of the pattern of pain.

The record should also include a list of factors related to changes in pain. These commonly include coughing, sneezing, bending forward, lifting, carrying, sitting, straining at stool, ascending and descending stairs, walking, standing, lying down, and stretching. The patient should be asked specifically about each factor, as he or she may not be able to recall certain information without prompting, and the record should note explicitly whether each of these factors aggravates or alleviates the pain. In addition, the patient should be asked whether the pain is associated with a particular time of day.

A specific comment should be made concerning any previous diagnoses of back problems, with a description of the therapy prescribed for each problem and the patient's response to the therapy. A review of all previous diagnostic tests, as well as spinal taps, spinal anesthesia, hospitalizations, and surgery should be noted in the record.

Any history of the following diagnoses should be included: arthritis, other musculoskeletal diseases; congenital abnormalities related to the spine; cancer, including the removal of moles; diabetes; major cardiovascular disease; renal and urinary tract disease; gynecologic/obstetric problems, including a notation regarding early menopause (age 35 or younger) and whether the menopause was surgical or biological; seizure disorders; psychiatric diagnoses and/or emotional problems; chronic pain syndromes; and chronic obesity.

Previous cancer, even in the distant past, is extremely important to an investigation of back pain, since the pain may be the first indication of metastatic cancer. A positive history of diabetes is also significant as it may affect the interpretation of neurological signs. A history of early menopause may suggest the presence of osteoporosis as a cause of spinal deterioration and resulting pain. Endometriosis may also be associated with back pain. A history of seizures may suggest previous spinal injuries resulting in compression fractures, which may be producing pain.

In addition to the medical information, the patient should be carefully questioned regarding his or her occupation during the year prior to the onset of symptoms, including a notation regarding any recent change in occupation. The doctor should get a brief description of the patient's activities at work, including such things as heavy lifting, excessive bending or repetitive back movements, and excessive time standing on hard floors or sitting for prolonged periods. The patient's stress level at work should also be determined. Both the work history and the onset of pain are important for evaluating the patient with regard to the possibility of a work-related injury.

There should be a notation regarding the patient's usual physical activities outside of work, especially regular exercise habits and sports participation. It is especially important to ask about any recent change in type or level of physical activity at work or home, or in exercise habits.

Any significant personal stress should be noted, and an assessment should be made regarding the patient's use of alcohol and other drugs. Recent weight changes and dietary abnormalities should also be reported.

Doctors should also keep in mind that patients under the age of 20 and over the age of 50 are at increased risk for tumors and infections that can cause lower back pain.

The comprehensive physical examination should include an in-depth evaluation of the neurological and musculoskeletal systems. The neurological examination should always include an evaluation of sensation, strength, and reflexes in the lower extremities. The patient should be tested for lower extremity flexibility, muscular balance, and stability of ligaments to help rule out other possible causes of the pain.

X rays are commonly used in making the diagnosis of a patient with lower back pain, but they often reveal nothing. In patients with routine lower back pain, it is advisable to wait a month before taking the first X rays. MAGNETIC RESONANCE IMAGING (MRI) scans do a better job of revealing nerve root impingement but should be reserved for patients who show progressive neurological deficits and patients who have a known history or high risk of cancer or inflammatory disease. They may also be used in patients who are candidates for surgery. Diskography may sometimes be helpful as well but is generally not recommended during the first three months of symptoms. Electrodiagnostic studies may be useful in certain situations as well.

Treatment

Treatment during the acute phase of sciatica focuses on PHYSICAL THERAPY for four to six weeks and refraining from any activity that aggravates the condition. Physical therapy may involve various exercises for the spine, as well as teaching the patient back-protection techniques, such as proper lifting techniques and posture awareness. They also learn various techniques for controlling back pain and exercises to help strengthen the stabilizing muscles of the back. Massage may be incorporated into the treatment approach as well.

In certain situations, surgery is the treatment of choice. These situations include conditions that involve progressive motor deficits and bowel and bladder dysfunction. A number of surgical options are available, depending upon the exact location and type of problem.

Epidural steroid injections are another possible treatment option for acute cases of sciatica that do not respond to more conservative treatments.

In the recovery phase, patients should gradually progress with their physical therapy program to continue to decrease pain and focus on functional stabilization and back safety techniques. By the end of this phase, patients should be independent with an appropriate home exercise program. Once discharged from physical therapy, the patient must continue exercising at home with the understanding that managing sciatica is a long-term process.

In terms of medication, nonsteroidal anti-inflammatory drugs (NSAIDs) are the mainstay of initial treatment. Muscle relaxants may be considered for patients experiencing significant spasms.

Prevention

Patient education regarding proper care and exercise for the back is the most important component in preventing episodes of sciatica. In addition, following an organized training program that includes adequate stretching and strengthening exercises for sports is also quite important.

second-impact head injury syndrome Primary head injury can be catastrophic, but the effects of repetitive head injury also must be considered. Second-impact syndrome (SIS) occurs when an athlete sustains a second head injury before symptoms from the first head injury have resolved. When this happens, the patient's condition gets worse immediately, and coma and death may result. For this reason, identification of initial concussions when they occur is absolutely essential so that precautions can be taken to protect the athlete from another impact before the damage of the first impact has had a chance to heal.

The results of studies of athletes who have incurred multiple concussions have been somewhat conflicting. However, numerous studies have shown a correlation between repeated brain injury and chronic encephalopathy, or swelling of the brain.

Causes

Second-impact head injury syndrome occurs because an athlete endures some sort of impact to the head while still recovering from an initial impact. The factors that predispose an athlete to this happening include the occurrence of a previous head injury and the persistence of symptoms from that injury. These symptoms may include headache; balance disorder; visual, motor, or sensory changes; and mental difficulties that affect thinking processes and memory. The use of alcohol or illegal drugs is also implicated as a risk factor in second-impact head injury syndrome.

Diagnosis

Emergency management is often needed in the case of traumatic injuries. This includes assessment and management of the airway, breathing, and circulation. Once this has been taken care of, the doctor can proceed to the medical history and physical examination of the patient.

A complete medical history is a key element in diagnosing an athlete with suspected head injury. However, the athlete may not be able to provide a good history because of confused thinking and loss of memory. In this case, the doctor should obtain the history from a teammate, coach, or observer.

Patients with head injury normally experience headache, confusion, memory impairment, fatigue, blurred vision, dizziness, nausea, poor hand-eye coordination, irritability, depression, and sensory loss.

A physical examination will usually focus on determining the severity of the head injury and deciding if the athlete needs immediate attention at a hospital or just some time to rest. In the physical examination, the doctor will look for the following:

- altered levels of consciousness
- amnesia
- gait abnormalities
- weakness
- visual abnormalities
- sensory loss
- changes in the pupils
- poor concentration

- apprehension
- increased symptoms with exertion

Head injuries are diagnosed on a scale with Grade I being the most minor and Grade III being the most severe concussion.

Grade I concussion is defined by the experience of transient confusion, no loss of consciousness, and a duration of mental status abnormalities of less than 15 minutes.
Grade II concussion is defined by the experience of transient confusion, no loss of consciousness, and a duration of mental status abnormalities of more than 15 minutes.
Grade III concussion is defined by the experience of loss of consciousness, either brief (seconds) or prolonged (minutes or longer).

There are no lab studies that help in diagnosing repetitive head injury. These cases are diagnosed on the basis of the medical history and physical examination.

In athletes with loss of consciousness, symptoms that do not improve, and significant neurological problems, COMPUTERIZED AXIAL TOMOGRAPHY (CAT) scans or MAGNETIC RESONANCE IMAGING (MRI) scans should be ordered. All patients who have experienced more than one concussion should have an imaging study done.

X rays usually reveal very little when there is mild brain trauma. They may be used to assess neck injuries, however. CAT scans of the head are useful in detecting mild head injuries and are generally preferred over MRIs because they offer better depiction of the bones, cost less, have better sensitivity in detecting skull fractures, and are processed more quickly in the emergency room situation. In addition, CAT scans are better at showing hemorrhages, clots, and swelling of the brain.

MRI is preferable in situations where there is a very small change, such as a small hemorrhage or swelling that may not show up on a CAT scan.

Other neuropsychological tests may be used in diagnosing the patient with head injuries. Patients with multiple concussion often show a reduction in cognitive performance, so it is important to get an accurate assessment of cognitive functioning.

Treatment

In the case of an initial head injury, the patient may need to rest and refrain from sport for a period of time until fully recovered from the injury. If the injury is severe, the patient will need to be taken to the hospital for evaluation and monitoring of symptoms.

Guidelines for removing players from the sport when they have suffered a head injury are as follows:

Grade I concussion.   The athlete should be removed from sports activity, examined immediately and at five-minute intervals, and allowed to return that day to the sports activity only after symptoms resolve completely and the athlete has been medically examined and found to be asymptomatic.
Grade II concussion.   The athlete should be removed from sports activity, examined immediately and frequently to assess the evolution of symptoms. The athlete should return to sports activity only after a full week has elapsed without symptoms. Any athlete who incurs a Grade II concussion subsequent to a Grade I concussion on the same day should be removed from sports activity until asymptomatic for two weeks.
Grade III concussion.   The athlete should be removed from sports activity for one full week without symptoms if the loss of consciousness is brief, or two full weeks without symptoms if the loss of consciousness is prolonged. If abnormal neurological signs are present at the time of initial evaluation, the athlete should be transported by ambulance to the nearest hospital emergency department. An athlete who suffers a second Grade III concussion should be removed from sports activity until asymptomatic for one month. Any athlete with a brain scan that reveals brain swelling, contusion, or other intracranial problems should be removed from sports activities for the season and discouraged from future return to participation in contact sports.

Impairments caused by concussions vary depending on the severity and location of the injury. Although the patient may have experienced only mild injuries, the long-term effects may be profound. Common problems associated with concussion include difficulties with memory, mood, and concentration. Others include significant deficits in organizational and reasoning skills and in learning, cognitive, and executive functions. In

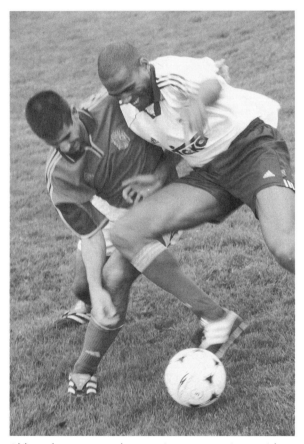

Although most people associate concussions with football, concussions often occur in soccer, when a player hits the ball with his or her head. The problem is serious enough that it has generated a movement among some in the sport to change the rules so that head butting is no longer allowed. *(Fogstock, LLC)*

addition, changes in memory and organizational skills after a brain injury make it difficult to function in complex environments.

Recovery from a concussion may be inconsistent and thus frustrating to both the patient and family members. Sometimes the patient will improve only to experience a setback or a plateau, during which time no progress occurs, but plateaus are quite often followed by more progress.

By definition, repetitive head injury is worse than a single minor concussion; neuropsychological test results are worse in patients with repetitive minor concussions. With a second head injury, it is essential that the patient receive emergency medical support immediately. Neurosurgical specialists may prevent or limit the rapid decline often seen with SIS.

In the recovery and rehabilitation from head injury, much depends on the severity of the injury. The goal of all therapy, however, is to maximize the patient's strength and functional independence. Athletes who have severe head injuries may require rehabilitation for a prolonged period. In most patients, mild brain injuries do not require extensive rehabilitation. Patients with motor deficits following a head injury may benefit from PHYSICAL THERAPY. Range-of-motion (ROM) exercises are helpful in managing many motor problems. In addition, occupational therapy, speech therapy, and recreational therapy may all be useful in dealing with the patient's particular set of problems.

Doctors must be extremely careful in prescribing medications to patients with head injury. Medications that may have sedative effects should not be used since sedation may complicate the monitoring of the patient's symptoms.

Prevention

In preventing second-impact syndrome, the recognition of a concussion is the key factor. Preventing an athlete from returning to play while symptoms from a concussion are still evident and following the guidelines for concussion management may help avert a catastrophic outcome.

In addition, equipment and rule changes have helped to reduce the overall number and severity of head injuries in American football, which has historically been one of the sports with the highest risk for head injuries. This improvement in football has created a debate among those involved in soccer concerning equipment and rule changes in that sport since a significant number of concussions are now known to occur when players hit the ball with their head in soccer.

sesamoiditis Sesamoiditis is a form of tendonitis that affects the sesamoids in the forefoot. The sesamoids are a very small cluster of small bones that unlike most bones are not connected to any other bones. The sesamoids located at the bottom of the forefoot near the big toe (the kneecap is the other sesamoid in the body) are connected only to tendons and found in two places—one sesamoid is on the outside of the foot, and the other is closer to the middle of the foot. These little bones act like pulleys, providing a smooth surface over which the tendons slide, thus assisting the tendons in their effort to transmit muscle forces. They also aid the foot in weight bearing and provide lift to the bones of the big toe.

The sesamoids, like other bones, are vulnerable to fracture, but a more common problem involving the sesamoids is inflammation of the tendons surrounding them, a condition called sesamoiditis that is often seen in ballet dancers, baseball catchers, and runners.

Causes

As with all types of tendonitis, sesamoiditis can be caused by overuse of the tendons that surround the sesamoids. Baseball catchers who squat with their toes bent beneath them apply much pressure to these tendons, keeping them constantly stretched. In addition, cleats or other athletic shoes with little padding in the forefoot can also help to bring on this condition.

Diagnosis

Generally, patients with sesamoiditis will complain of pain under the big toe in the ball of the foot that develops somewhat gradually, worsening with continued play in the aggravating sport. If there is a fracture involved, the pain will be acute and will come on immediately following the break. Swelling and bruising may occur but does not always occur. Some patients find it hard to bend and straighten the big toe.

In a physical exam, the doctor will check for tenderness around the sesamoid bones. Manipulation of the forefoot and toe to see what causes more pain will help the doctor to determine the exact location of the injury. Jumping and pushing off to run are usually painful. X rays should be done to ensure a proper diagnosis. Sometimes, an X ray will fail to detect the problem. If X rays come back normal, the doctor may want to request a bone scan as well.

Treatment

Conservative treatment is usually effective, but occasionally surgery is necessary to remove the sesamoid bones. With sesamoiditis, the patient should cease all activities that cause pain, take anti-inflammatories to help with pain management, and ice the sole of the injured foot for 20 to 30 minutes, two to three times a day until the pain subsides. It is important also to wear low-heeled shoes with soft soles. A felt cushion insert in the shoe may also be helpful.

Patients should return to normal activity gradually, while continuing to use some type of cushioning pad in the shoe. Activities that put weight on the ball of the foot should be avoided until the injury is completely healed. It may help to tape the big toe so that it is pointed down.

If pain persists after four to six weeks, the patient may need to wear a fracture brace on the injured foot to help remove pressure from the foot.

If the sesamoid is fractured, the patient will wear a stiff-soled shoe or fracture brace for four to six weeks or longer. The doctor may take the big toe to limit movement. Cushioning pads and other types of orthotics may be prescribed during the healing process. A fracture of the sesamoid may take several months to completely heal. During this time, the patient may need to take anti-inflammatories or other pain medication to help manage the discomfort.

Prevention

As with all forms of tendonitis, the best way to prevent sesamoiditis is to avoid overusing the tendons in the ball of the foot. Wear shoes that fit properly and have adequate cushion, warm up the feet before engaging in strenuous activity, and rest and ice the feet if any signs of strain occur. With all forms of tendonitis, it is necessary to cut back on or completely stop the aggravating activities in order for the tendons to heal.

Sever's disease (calcaneal apophysitis) The heel bone is known as the calcaneous, and in children there is an area on the heel bone where the bone grows that is called the growth plate, or apophysitis. An inflammation of this growth plate in the heel, Sever's disease, or calcaneal apophysitis, is common in children, adolescents, and teenagers who overuse the foot with repetitive heel strikes. It is the common cause of heel pain in young people.

Causes

The pain and inflammation of Sever's disease comes from the Achilles tendon pulling excessively on the growth plate in the heel, particularly during running and jumping. The condition can be exacerbated by tightness in the hamstrings, quadriceps, and hip flexor muscles. In addition, wearing shoes with inadequate heel padding or arch support can also cause Sever's disease.

Diagnosis

A child who complains of acute or chronic heel pain, especially with running and jumping, should be examined for Sever's disease. In athletes, the heel pain normally improves with rest and worsens with prolonged running. A reduced range of motion in the ankle and pain associated with extending the knee are common symptoms. The doctor will check for tenderness in the bottom part of the heel and may order an X ray to ensure that there is no damage to the growth plate.

Treatment

Rest from aggravating activities and wearing shoes with appropriate padding and support will help. Extra heel pads can be placed in the patient's shoes and in some cases orthotics may be necessary to obtain the appropriate arch support. In some cases, anti-inflammatories may be prescribed.

The patient may return to normal activities when the pain is gone. Returning too soon may cause even more pain and could lead to permanent damage of the heel. If the pain returns, the child should rest for three to four days until the pain subsides before trying to resume normal activities.

If the heel hurts, the child needs to rest from his or her sport or activity. The child should rest for several days at a time and then go back gradually. Before returning, the child should be able to jog painlessly, then sprint painlessly, and be able to hop on the injured foot painlessly. If at any time during this process the child develops further heel pain, he or she should rest for three to four more days until the pain is gone before trying to return again.

Prevention

Wearing shoes that fit properly and have adequate cushion in the heel will go a long way toward preventing the development of Sever's disease. Check to be sure that the heel of the shoe is not too tight and that it has good padding. If there are any doubts, try putting extra heel pads in the child's shoes.

shin splints Shin splints is the name given to pain at the front of the lower leg. The most common cause is inflammation of the periostium of the tibia, which is the sheath surrounding the bone. Shin splints is an OVERUSE INJURY that occurs quite commonly in runners and in other athletes who overtrain.

Causes

Shin pain generally occurs from overuse. It can be caused by running on hard surfaces, running on tiptoes, and participating in sports where a lot of jumping is involved. The problem can also come from irritation of the muscles or other tissues in the lower leg or from a stress fracture. This injury is most common in runners who increase their mileage or the intensity of their running or who change the surface on which they are running. Overpronation, which is the flattening out of the foot while running, can contribute to shin pain as well. Several specific conditions can cause shin pain. These include STRESS FRACTURES, medial stress syndrome, and COMPARTMENT SYNDROME.

A stress fracture in the lower leg is a hairline crack in either the tibia or the fibula. Medial stress syndrome occurs when the muscles that attach to the inner side of the tibia are inflamed. Compartment syndrome occurs when the anterior compartment of the leg, which is the part of the leg containing the muscles responsible for pointing the foot and toes toward the body, is overused and painful.

Diagnosis

Patients with shin splints normally describe tenderness over the inside of the shin, lower leg pain, sometimes swelling in the lower leg, lumps and bumps over the bone, pain when the toes or foot is bent downward, and redness over the inside of the shin. If the pain is being caused by compartment syndrome, and the muscles in the compartment become swollen during exercise, they may irritate the nerves and blood vessels surrounding them and cause weakness, numbness, or coldness in the foot.

The diagnosis will involve a medical history as well as a physical examination. The medical history will focus on an exact description of where and when the pain occurs. The physical exam will include palpation of the lower leg and watching the patient walk or run to assess for overpronation problems. The doctor may also want to perform a test to check for pressure inside the lower leg if compartment syndrome is suspected.

Treatment

The first step in treatment of shin splints is rest from the offending activities. Ice should be helpful in the early stages to ease swelling and pain. Using shock-absorbing insoles in shoes may also help ease the pain. Patients do not need to be inactive but should completely avoid any activities that cause pain in the lower leg. Heat can be used as well to ease the discomfort. Anti-inflammatory medication will help with the swelling and pain. The ankle may also be taped to provide more stability and take some pressure off the lower leg. Sports massage techniques may be beneficial, too. If overpronation is a problem, the patient should be fitted for orthotics. Stretching exercises to relieve tight muscles will help the patient avoid shin splints in the future.

In some cases of compartment syndrome, surgery is necessary to relieve the pain. In this type of surgery, the tissues that form the covering of the compartments are opened up to reduce the pressure in the compartments. Certain types of stress fractures may also require surgery in order to heal.

It is vital that patients switch their activities during recovery from shin splints so that they do not further damage the lower leg. Runners may need to swim or bike, for example. It is safe to return to the primary sport when the following has been achieved:

- full range of motion in the injured leg compared to the uninjured leg
- full strength of the injured leg compared to the uninjured leg
- ability to jog straight ahead without pain or limping
- ability to sprint straight ahead without pain or limping
- ability to perform cuts and figure-eights while running without pain
- ability to jump on both legs without pain and on just the injured leg without pain

Prevention

Since shin pain usually occurs from overuse, be sure to return to activities gradually when recovering from shin splints. Always wear shoes with proper padding, and run on softer surfaces whenever possible. Runners should opt to run on dirt tracks and trails whenever possible. Pavement is softer than concrete, so in town run on the streets instead of the sidewalks. Athletes should always warm up properly and stretch the muscles in the front of the leg and in the calf.

shoulder dislocation The shoulder is the most commonly dislocated joint in the body, with nearly all of these dislocations caused by a traumatic injury.

A dislocation of the shoulder joint happens when the bones making up the shoulder joint are moved apart so that the joint no longer functions.

The shoulder is made up of two bones—the ball and the socket. The ball is the end of the arm bone, or humerus, and the socket is part of the shoulder blade, or scapula. When the ball part of the joint is dislocated in front of the socket, it is called an anterior dislocation. When it is dislocated behind the socket, it is called a posterior dislocation. In severe cases, ligaments, tendons, and nerves also can be stretched and injured. When a shoulder dislocates frequently, the condition is referred to as shoulder instability. A partial dislocation where the upper arm bone is partially in and partially out of the socket is called a subluxation.

Causes

Any sport that forces the shoulder joint into extreme positions may result in dislocation. In a typical case of a dislocated shoulder, a strong force that pulls the shoulder outward or causes an extreme rotation of the joint pops the ball of the arm bone, or humerus, out of the shoulder socket. Dislocation also commonly occurs when there is a backward pull on the arm that either catches the muscles unprepared to resist or overwhelms the muscles. Risk is increased if the athlete has a history of prior dislocation or subluxation or has looseness in the joint.

Violent collision sports, such as football and rugby, are most likely to cause shoulder dislocations, but any sport in which an athlete reaches high velocity and then subjects the shoulder to a sudden change in the direction of motion may dislocate the arm bone from the shoulder. Sports such as rodeo, downhill skiing, bicycling, and other sports that have the potential for falling accidents can make the athlete vulnerable to a shoulder dislocation.

A small number of shoulder dislocations result from atraumatic situations. They are associated with neuromuscular causes, such as cerebral palsy, and genetic predisposition, either of which can render the shoulder unstable.

Diagnosis

The shoulder can dislocate either forward, backward, or downward. Not only does the arm appear out of position when the shoulder dislocates, the dislocation also produces pain. Muscle spasms may increase the intensity of pain. Swelling, numbness, weakness, and bruising are likely to develop. Problems seen with a dislocated shoulder are tearing of the ligaments or tendons reinforcing the joint cap-

sule and, less commonly, nerve damage. Doctors usually diagnose a dislocation by a history of trauma and a physical examination that reveals signs of dislocation. X rays may be taken to confirm the diagnosis and to rule out a related fracture.

A dislocation of the shoulder joint is usually an obvious diagnosis. The medical history will focus on determining the exact cause of the dislocation and distinguishing the type of dislocation and the severity in order to determine the proper treatment. It is necessary that the doctor understand the position of the arm at the time the dislocation occurred because this will reveal the direction of the dislocation.

The doctor will also want to determine if there is any history or family history of general looseness in the ligaments. If a dislocation occurs with what seems like very little trauma, general looseness in the ligaments should be suspected. Any history of instability or dislocation from traumatic or nontraumatic events should be recorded.

There is usually severe pain with a shoulder dislocation, and the patient may be unable to move the joint. If it is possible, the doctor will want to palpate the head of the arm bone and test the limitations in the patient's range of motion. The doctor will check to see which way the arm is rotated and held and how the injured shoulder appears in comparison to the noninjured side.

If the patient has an anterior dislocation, which is the most common, the arm on the dislocated side will be held slightly away from the body with the opposite hand. This will keep the dislocated shoulder in the least uncomfortable position. The shoulder will have a large bump rising up under the skin in front of the shoulder, and the shoulder will look square instead of round.

If the patient has a posterior dislocation, the arm on the dislocated side will be held tight against the body. There will be a large bump on the back of the shoulder.

It is also important that the doctor complete a thorough neurovascular examination both prior to reduction and following reduction.

Lab studies are not necessary to diagnose shoulder dislocation injuries.

X rays are usually taken to confirm the diagnosis and to rule out fractures or other problems. The rotator cuff is at risk of tearing during a shoulder dislocation in middle-aged and older patients due to the decreased flexibility of the tendons that comes with aging. If a patient fails to show improvement in range of motion and function without pain following a reduction, a MAGNETIC RESONANCE IMAGING (MRI) scan may be used to check for ROTATOR CUFF TEAR.

Treatment

Shoulder dislocations are extremely painful events. The most important treatment of a shoulder dislocation is prompt reduction of the joint. This is a procedure in which the doctor puts the ball of the humerus back into the joint socket. There are numerous techniques for accomplishing the reduction that can be performed under conscious sedation. Several of the most common include the Hippocratic method, the Stimson technique, and the Milch maneuver. The shoulder muscles must be relaxed in order to successfully complete a reduction. The arm is then immobilized in a sling or a device called a shoulder immobilizer for several weeks. X rays should follow the reduction to ensure that it is complete.

Usually the doctor recommends resting the shoulder and applying ice three or four times a day. After pain and swelling have been controlled, the patient enters a rehabilitation program that includes exercises to restore the range of motion of the shoulder and to strengthen the muscles to prevent future dislocations. These exercises may progress from simple motion to the use of weights.

After treatment and recovery, a previously dislocated shoulder may remain more susceptible to reinjury, especially in young, active individuals. Ligaments may have been stretched or torn, and the shoulder may tend to dislocate again. A shoulder that dislocates severely or often, injuring surrounding tissues or nerves, usually requires surgical repair to tighten stretched ligaments or reattach torn ones.

Sometimes, the doctor performs ARTHROSCOPY through a tiny incision into which a small scope is inserted to observe the inside of the joint. After this procedure, the shoulder is generally immobilized for about six weeks and full recovery takes several months. Arthroscopic techniques involving the shoulder are relatively new, and many surgeons prefer to repair a recurrent dislocating shoulder by the time-tested open surgery under direct vision. There are usually fewer repeat dislocations and improved movement following open surgery, but it may take a little longer to regain motion.

Physical therapists usually instruct their patients with recently dislocated shoulders to "keep the hand in view" during the first three weeks following the injury. While looking forward, the patient never should let the hand be placed in a position outside the line of vision. After the initial period of immobilization, passive range-of-motion exercises should begin. The older population should begin performing range-of-motion exercises of the shoulder after one week of immobilization because they are prone to shoulder stiffness.

After about six weeks, most patients are ready for more vigorous therapy. This might include rotator cuff strengthening exercises. Since the rate of redislocation is so much higher in young adults, vigorous training and strengthening should wait until approximately three months after the injury. Swimming is an ideal exercise to regain shoulder strength and should be encouraged once strengthening exercises have begun.

When full range of motion and strength have been regained, athletes may return to their sports. Usually, the older adult can return to play within three months, while younger adults may have to wait longer due to their increased risk of experiencing another dislocation during the recovery. Younger adults are much more likely to experience a recurrence, and most redislocations occur within two years of the initial injury.

Prevention

Educating the patient on the importance of strength training following shoulder dislocation will help in preventing recurrence. Avoid situations that could lead to another dislocation. Athletes should take care to wear protective equipment for the shoulders whenever possible and to avoid violent contact sports that put them at increased risk of hurting the shoulder.

shoulder separation (AC [acromioclavicular] joint injury)   Acromioclavicular (AC) joint injuries, or shoulder separations as they are commonly called,

account for 40 to 50 percent of all athletic shoulder injuries. They occur in many different kinds of sports, but especially in collision sports such as hockey, rugby, football, and cycling, and are precipitated by a blow to the tip of the shoulder. Most common in males, due to their greater participation in collision sports, the shoulder separation injury is one that disrupts the group of ligaments that holds the clavicle to the portion of the scapula known as the acromion. The severity of the disruption can vary, resulting in different degrees of AC separation, from Type I to Type V, each requiring its own specific treatment.

Cause

A fall on, or hard blow to, the tip of the shoulder is the most common cause of shoulder separation, which is classified according to the severity of the damage to the ligaments, with Type I being a strain and Type V describing the most severe form of separation and disturbance of the ligaments.

Diagnosis

A patient who complains of acute or chronic shoulder pain, either in the front or back of the shoulder, will normally be considered a candidate for AC joint injury. Often there is acute pain, tenderness, and swelling around the shoulder right after the injury occurs. Once the generalized pain dissolves, the point over the AC joint remains tender. An abrasion or prominence may be visible at the clavicle. If patients are involved in weight training, they will usually experience pain with certain exercises, especially bench presses and dips. In addition, patients often report pain during the night, when they roll onto the shoulder while sleeping. Although not common, there is sometimes a popping noise or catching sensation associated with the shoulder separation.

The doctor will question the patient concerning the experience of pain. When there is pain and swelling over the joint, it may be difficult for a doctor to determine the stability of the AC joint. Asking the patient to stretch the injured arm across the chest will normally produce pain. If the ligaments are actually torn, as opposed to strained, it may be difficult to rule out a ROTATOR CUFF TEAR due to limitations in the movement of the shoulder.

Imaging studies, primarily radiographs, are used to evaluate the severity of the separation injury. A minimum of two views is necessary. In some cases, it may also be helpful to take a stress radiograph of the AC joint, in which the patient holds a certain amount of weight while moving the injured shoulder. Since this is usually painful, the test is not recommended unless it is the only way to determine if the ligaments have been completely torn.

Bone scans are not recommended as initial screening tools, but they have been proven extremely effective in demonstrating AC joint injury in patients whose plain radiographs returned negative results.

MAGNETIC RESONANCE IMAGING (MRI) scans are rarely used in diagnosing shoulder separations, but in a couple of cases they may be required. In middle-aged and older patients who have disabling shoulder pain after the acute pain of an AC injury subsides, an MRI may be useful to rule out a rotator cuff tear. In athletes with persistent pain over the AC joint, an MRI may help determine if there is irreversible damage to the cartilaginous disk or if OSTEOARTHRITIS has set in.

Treatment

During the acute phase of the injury, a conservative treatment may involve PHYSICAL THERAPY to help restore normal flexibility and range of motion. Exercises may also be prescribed to help strengthen the rotator cuff, which has been reported to improve the symptoms associated with the shoulder separation. Type I and Type II injuries are always treated conservatively, and there is little controversy about these treatments. In Type III injuries, there are conflicting opinions concerning the use of surgery. The complications involved in the surgery and the realization that the recovery time for surgery was as long as the recovery time of the conservative treatment have led many orthopedic surgeons to reconsider surgical approaches that were once common, especially in athletes such as baseball players, who use overhead movements. Type IV and V injuries require some type of reconstruction in order to prevent further complications. Surgeries for AC joint reconstruction may be done arthroscopically, which has the potential advantage of offering a shorter period of post-surgery symptoms and a quicker recovery of strength. One major risk involved in the surgical approach is failure to complete an adequate resection of the ligaments. This is the most common cause of post-surgery pain.

Patients are ready to return to their normal activities when there is an absence of significant symptoms. For those who have undergone surgery, healing of the wound and muscles, as well as a return of strength to the shoulder, dictate when normal activity may be resumed.

Prevention

Prevention is accomplished simply by avoiding the maneuvers that may cause the injury. In addition, proper diagnosis of the AC joint pathology from the start helps in the prevention of greater injury to the area. Those with osteoarthritis in the AC joint must refrain from engaging in the movements that cause pain in order to gain relief from symptoms.

skin cancer Skin cancer is the most common type of cancer in the United States. According to current estimates, 40 to 50 percent of Americans who live to age 65 will have skin cancer at least once. Athletes spend a great deal of time exercising outside in all kinds of weather conditions, which puts them at especially high risk for contracting skin cancer. The increased amount of time spent in the sun, the lack of protective clothing, and the constant sweating make the athlete more susceptible than the average person.

The largest organ in the body, the skin is the body's protection against heat, light, injury, and infection. It regulates body temperature and stores water, fat, and vitamin D. It is made up of two main layers—the outer layer, or epidermis, and the inner layer, or dermis. The epidermis consists mostly of flat, scalelike cells called squamous cells. Under these squamous cells are basal cells, and deep inside the epidermis are melanocytes, which are the cells responsible for producing melanin that gives the skin its color.

Cancer is a very general term that refers to a group of more than 100 diseases. Each type of cancer is different from the others, but they are all the same in that they are a disease of certain cells in the body. Healthy cells grow, divide, and replace themselves regularly. When cells lose their ability to do this, they can divide too rapidly and grow without any order. This produces too much tissue, which can result in the formation of tumors. Tumors can be benign, which means that they are not cancerous and do not present a significant threat to the body. Malignant tumors, however, are cancerous and can destroy healthy tissue and organs and spread to other parts of the body where they may form additional tumors.

Basal cell carcinoma and squamous cell carcinoma are the two most common kinds of skin cancer. Basal cell carcinoma accounts for more than 90 percent of all skin cancers in the United States. It is a slow-growing cancer that seldom spreads to other parts of the body. Squamous cell carcinoma also rarely spreads, but it does so more often than basal cell carcinoma. However, it is important that skin cancers be found and treated early because they can invade and destroy nearby tissue.

Basal cell carcinoma and squamous cell carcinoma are sometimes called nonmelanoma skin cancer to differentiate them from melanoma, which is a very serious type of cancer that begins in the melanocytes.

Causes

Ultraviolet (UV) radiation from the sun is the main cause of skin cancer. Artificial sources of UV radiation, such as sunlamps and tanning booths, can also cause skin cancer. Consequently, the risk of developing skin cancer is affected by how much exposure a person has to the sun, which is, in part, determined by where a person lives. People who live in areas that get high levels of UV radiation from the sun are more likely to contract skin cancer than people who live in areas with lower levels of UV radiation. In the United States, people who live in Texas, for example, are exposed to more UV radiation than people who live in North Dakota, where the sun is not so strong. Skin cancer is also related to age because exposure to the sun accumulates over one's lifetime. Most skin cancers appear after the age of 50, although the damage that causes the cancer begins at an early age. Protection from the sun's damaging radiation should thus begin in infancy.

Additional factors that increase the risk of skin cancer include fair skin, red or blond hair, and a

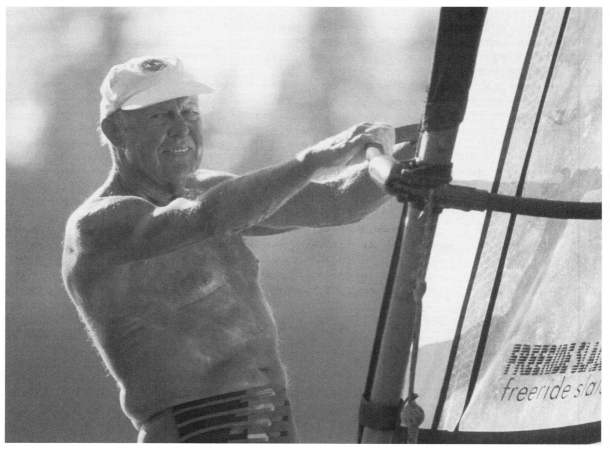

The most common form of cancer in the United States, skin cancer occurs more frequently in people over the age of 50 since they have accumulated more total exposure to the sun. When exercising outside, athletes of all ages should limit their exposure to the sun, wear sunscreen and protective clothing, and check themselves regularly for skin changes that might be early signs of cancer. *(Fogstock, LLC)*

history of sunburns, especially as a child. Those who freckle or sunburn after only short exposure to the sun are at greater risk.

Diagnosis

The most common warning sign of skin cancer is a change on the skin, especially a new growth or a sore that does not heal. Skin cancers do not all look the same. For example, the cancer may start as a small, smooth, shiny, pale, or waxy lump. Or it can appear as a firm red lump. Sometimes, the lump bleeds or develops a crust. Skin cancer can

also start as a flat, red spot that is rough, dry, or scaly.

When an area of skin does not look normal, the doctor may remove all or part of the growth in what is called a biopsy. The tissue from this growth is checked under a microscope by a pathologist who can determine if the cells are cancerous.

When diagnosing someone with skin cancer, a doctor will normally classify the cancer as either local or metastatic. Local skin cancer is affecting only the skin. Metastatic skin cancer has spread beyond the skin. Because skin cancer rarely spreads, a biopsy is most often adequate to determine the extent of the cancer. In cases where the growth is very large and has been present for a long time, the doctor will check the nearby lymph nodes, and the patient may need to have additional tests, such as special X rays, to determine if the cancer has spread to any other parts of the body.

Treatment

In treating skin cancer, the doctor's main goal is to remove or destroy the cancer completely with as small a scar as possible. To plan the best treatment for each patient, the doctor considers the location and size of the cancer, the risk of scarring, and the person's age, general health, and medical history.

It is sometimes helpful to have the advice of more than one doctor before starting treatment. It may take a week or two to arrange for a second opinion, but this short delay will not reduce the chance that treatment will be successful.

Treatment for skin cancer usually involves some type of surgery to remove the growth, although sometimes the biopsy completely removes the cancer and no further treatment is needed. If additional surgery is needed, there are several options. These include curettage and electrodesiccation, Mohs' surgery, cryosurgery, and laser therapy. Grafting of skin is sometimes necessary to close the wound when a large cancer is removed. Radiation therapy and chemotherapy are other options for treating cancer and may be used in conjunction with surgery or alone. A number of other treatments for skin cancer are currently in clinical trials and may be widely available in the near future.

Skin cancer is usually cured by the prescribed treatment, but the disease can recur in the same place. In addition, people who have developed skin cancer in one place have a greater chance of developing skin cancer in another place. It is essential that patients examine themselves regularly, visit the doctor for regular check-ups and do everything possible to protect their skin from further damage by the sun.

Prevention

The best way to prevent skin cancer is to avoid long exposure to the sun's ultraviolet rays. Try to do outdoor workouts before 10 A.M. or after 4 P.M., when the sun's rays are less intense. Workout clothing should also be chosen for its sun-protective features. A tightly woven, white fabric that covers the back, shoulders, and neck is best. It is also a good idea to wear a hat or helmet and sunglasses.

Sunscreen protects the body from the sun's normal rays, but it only reduces the amount of exposure to UV rays and thus cannot prevent skin cancer. Some people even argue that sunscreen contributes to the incidence of melanomas by lulling people into feeling safe about their exposure to the sun. Athletes who stay out in the sun longer because they are wearing sunscreen might not burn but are still exposing themselves to higher levels of UV radiation.

Skin cancer, if caught early, responds well to treatment so it is important to check the body for signs of early cancers. Any changes in the skin, including moles and lesions, should be viewed suspiciously. Asymmetry in a mole or lesion, inconsistent color, and irregularity in the border of a mole or lesion are all potential signs of skin cancer that should be checked by a doctor. In addition, if a skin mole or lesion is larger than the eraser head on a pencil, it should be examined.

slipped capital femoral epiphysis   Slipped capital femoral epiphysis (SCFE) is the most common hip disorder among young teenagers. SCFE happens when the cartilage plate (epiphysis) at the top of a child's thighbone (femur) slips out of place. In a growing child, the plate is what controls the way the top of the thighbone grows. It is also a pivotal part of the hip's ball and socket joint, so slippage of the epiphysis may severely deform the child. Children aged 10 to 18 are at risk for SCFE, particularly African-American boys and all children who are overweight or athletic. More than one-third of the time, children with SCFE in one hip develop the same condition in the other hip.

Causes

The underlying cause of this condition is not well understood. Athletic children are at greater risk, however, than those who do not participate in sports.

Diagnosis

SCFE is normally diagnosed as either stable or unstable. A child with stable SCFE may first have stiffness in the hip, which may get better after rest. After a while, the stiffness may turn into a limp, and the child may have pain that comes and goes. The pain is often felt in the groin, the thigh, or the knee and not necessarily in the hip itself. In the later stages, the child may lose some ability to move the involved hip. This leg will usually twist out. It may look shorter than the other leg. The child may not be able to play sports or do simple tasks such as bending over to tie shoes. The symptoms may change gradually or rapidly.

A child with unstable SCFE has extreme pain. The pain is similar to what might be felt with a broken bone. The child probably won't be able to move the injured leg. It is important not to force the leg to move because that could cause the thighbone to slip even more.

This condition most often occurs in adolescent males between the ages of 10 and 16. The left hip is more commonly affected than the right. Obesity may be a factor. The doctor will want to get an exact idea about the duration, location, and radiation of the pain, as well as the patient's ability to bear weight. It is important to note any family history of the problem because genetics may play a role. In addition, any prior diagnosis of metabolic endocrine disorders, such as hypothyroidism or growth hormone disorders should also be noted since these are sometimes associated with the condition. The doctor should be sure to rule out any traumatic event that may have caused the hip pain as well.

The physical examination will focus on the patient's gait pattern and ability to bear weight, the range of motion in both hips and knees, and determination of any deformities in the lower legs, such as external rotation of the lower leg or shortening of the leg.

Lab studies are generally not needed unless surgery is going to be performed, in which case routine blood work is done. Patients with the condition in both hips, however, may need to be tested for metabolic disorders.

X rays are normally taken of the hips. COMPUTERIZED AXIAL TOMOGRAPHY (CAT) SCANS are not performed routinely but may be helpful in confirming the diagnosis if some doubt exists or if the amount of displacement needs to be more accurately measured.

Treatment

Surgical repair of the hip is the primary means of treatment. This surgery involves stabilizing the child's hip with pins to stop the SCFE from getting any worse. The pins help the growth plate fuse into place and become stable. The doctor may also want to pin the child's other hip to prevent it from developing the same problem.

Following surgery, the patient is given crutches and instructed to allow only partial weight bearing for six to eight weeks. However, most patients are noncompliant and discontinue the use of crutches after a few weeks once they have achieved an acceptable comfort level. Most children return to play once the pain has resolved. Recurrence is rare.

Prevention

This condition cannot be prevented, but it is important to recognize it early and get the proper treatment to ensure the best outcome for the child. Surgery is less complicated and the outcome is better with quick diagnosis. If left untreated, the child's deformities will worsen and arthritis is likely to set in.

sports nutrition   Sports nutrition is the specialist application of the science of nutrition to enhance performance in sport. The nutritional demands of training and competition vary according to sporting discipline and the individual requirements of athletes, but everyone agrees that nutrition plays an essential role in athletic performance. Accredited sports nutritionists are trained in both the science of nutrition and its practical application. They help athletes achieve the nutrient intake necessary to maintain maximum physical condition for top efficiency and performance. Sports nutritionists may serve the athletic community as consultants, lecturers, or advisers in many different settings.

Training

Sports nutritionists are trained to help their clients meet their nutrition and fitness goals. A sports nutritionist usually completes a four-year curriculum in the field of food sciences. Students often study topics such as the impact of daily nutrition and wellness practices on long-term health and wellness; physical, social, and psychological aspects of healthy nutrition and wellness choices; planning for wellness and fitness; selection and preparation of nutritious meals and snacks based on USDA Dietary Guidelines including the Food Guide Pyramid; safety, sanitation, storage, and recycling processes and issues associated with nutrition and wellness; impacts of science and technology on nutrition and wellness issues; and nutrition and wellness career paths. Laboratory experiences, which emphasize both nutrition and wellness practices, are required components of this field of study.

The sports nutritionists' education enables them to utilize theories from the natural sciences, social sciences, exercise physiology, and nutrition to assist individuals at all stages of life to attain and maintain optimal physical fitness and nutritional status. Sports nutritionists demonstrate the ability to assess, implement, and evaluate the fitness and nutritional needs of well individuals and groups. They recommend the proper nutrition and exercise protocol for those who wish to develop or maintain healthy lifestyles. They work with other health care professionals to assess the fitness and nutritional needs of individuals with chronic illnesses. They collaborate with health professionals and consumers to support changes in overall health behaviors for the welfare of society. Finally, they must demonstrate accountable and ethical behavior in compliance with established standards as nutritional recommendations are made for athletes of all ages and fitness levels.

Careers

There are a variety of career opportunities for graduates with sports nutrition degrees. These include positions with corporate wellness centers, fitness centers, professional sports teams, collegiate sport teams, high school sport teams, amateur sports teams, sports training camps, health clubs, and sports clinics.

Treatment by a Sports Nutritionist

Sports nutritionists may work with athletes to develop an optimum diet for performance in their sport, or they may work with athletes who have specific nutritional problems, such as eating disorders or diabetes that make it difficult for them to meet their nutritional goals. Athletes who want to lose or gain weight may also consult with a sports nutritionist so that the diet they choose is not harmful to their athletic performance.

sports psychology   Sport psychology is the study of the psychological and mental factors that influence and are influenced by participation and performance in sport, exercise, and physical activity, and the application of the knowledge gained through this study to everyday settings. Many sports psychologists work with competitive athletes at various levels to help them maximize their performance.

An athlete's state of mind can significantly affect performance or the eventual outcome of competition, so developing strong mental skills can help athletes of all levels who are searching for a competitive advantage. Some of the factors affecting an athlete's state of mind include the pressure and desire to win; past success or failure in competition; injuries or rehabilitation issues; expectations of coaches, parents, sponsors, or other interested parties; and the pressures of a busy competition and training schedule.

Training

Sports psychologists normally have at least a master's degree in psychology if not a doctorate and are certified by the Association for the Advancement of Applied Sport Psychology (AAASP) and/or the

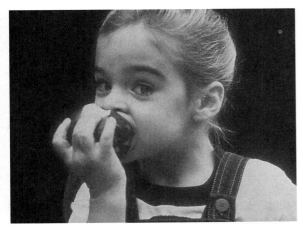

Proper nutrition is important for athletes of all ages.
(Courtesy Public Health Image Library)

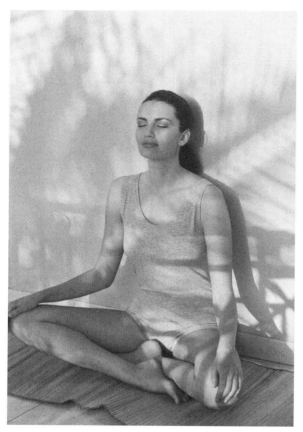

Yoga and meditation can improve an athlete's state of mind and make it easier to manage the stress of competition. *(Fogstock, LLC)*

Individuals working in this area come from sub-specialties within psychology, such as developmental, educational, clinical, counseling, industrial, comparative, physiological, social, personality, hypnosis, motivation, human factors, ergonomics, and health psychology. Although professionals and students in this area represent numerous specialties within psychology, they are bonded together by a common interest in sport and exercise.

Some individuals are concerned with research issues and applications involving competitive athletes, and some even restrict their attention to elite athletes who perform at the national and international levels. However, an equal number focus on the study and application of exercise and sport in noncompetitive settings. These individuals, for example, study exercise and sport from the perspective of motor development and motor learning; compliance recidivism; the aging process; prevention of various psychic and somatic disorders; personality structure and high-risk occupations such as firefighting, and high-risk recreational pursuits such as skydiving; and cellular adaptations at both the peripheral and central levels.

Sports psychologists may work in a number of different settings, including private practice, working for an athletic team or school; and working at a sports medicine clinic.

Treatment by a Sports Psychologist

Sport psychology is often focused on helping athletes to prepare mentally for competition, manage emotions affectively following competition, improve dedication and commitment; increase enjoyment of the sport; optimize self-confidence; respond better to adversity; avoid burnout in the sport; and increase ability to cope with the stress of competition.

Many athletes work regularly with sports psychologists to help focus their minds on delivering consistent athletic performances while balancing sport within the context of their lives.

Services offered by sports psychologists often include individual and team counseling; team-building and group facilitation; coaching consultation; goal setting and motivational counseling; precompetitive stress management instruction; emotional and cognitive regulation techniques; concentration and confidence methods; positive

American Psychological Association. Only those individuals with specialized training and appropriate certification or licensure may call themselves a sport psychologist.

Sports psychologists who are certified by the AAASP are designated as certified consultants and have met a minimum standard of education and training in the sport sciences and in psychology. They have also undergone an extensive review process.

Careers

Sport psychology professionals are interested in how participation in sport, exercise, and physical activity may enhance personal development and well-being throughout the life span.

SPORTS PSYCHOLOGY TIPS

Tips for Athletes

Stay committed. To succeed in competition, commit to being the best athlete. Maintain that commitment through specific, performance-oriented goals. Write them down and keep them on hand as a constant reminder.

Control emotions as well as play. The ups and downs of a season can have a dramatic effect on confidence and emotions. Remember that mistakes, losses, and setbacks are a part of sports. Don't hang it up just because things get difficult. In fact, practice how to react to these adversities before they occur.

Keep it realistic. Being the best player on the team doesn't mean that everything will always go perfectly during competition. Sometimes, expecting perfection during competition can turn into disappointment and frustration. During competition, athletes should play in the present, always try to do their best, and leave the expectations for perfection on the practice field.

Tips for Coaches

Don't forget the fun. As a coach to student athletes and young adults, it is important to keep the atmosphere around a team positive and enjoyable, finding a good balance between working hard and having fun. One of the most commonly given reasons by kids for quitting their sport is that they no longer enjoy it. Coaches should try to find positives in every competitive experience and reward effort from their players.

Bag the pre-game pep talk. Although they have their time and place, pre-game pep talks solely for the purpose of getting a team "fired up" may actually push adrenaline levels too high for some athletes. This emotional charge can even disrupt players' coordination and concentration. A better tactic may be to focus on specific, competitive goals and game plan visualization instruction; and sport-specific mental training techniques.

strategies during a pre-game talk. If the team isn't ready to play, getting them "fired up" moments before the game probably won't help.

Don't play favorites. A coach's interaction with each player is important to those individuals as well as the entire team because it affects team chemistry, cohesion, and morale. Back-up players should be treated with as much respect as star players, and rules about conduct should apply equally to every member of the team. Remember, back-ups are one injury away from being starters.

Tips for Parents

Stay in control. While everyone wants their children to perform well and beat the other team, it is important to stay in control of emotions and keep the sport participation experience in perspective. Children look to their parents as role models of appropriate behavior and how to handle emotions maturely.

Remember why you are there and why they are playing. Through sport participation, children often learn and practice important life lessons. Boys and girls can develop physical fitness, emotional maturity, and a healthy lifestyle by playing competitive sports. They can also learn to overcome individual and team challenges, work as a member of a team, and make a personal commitment to being the best they can be. These lessons are often more important than whether the child's team wins or loses.

Sometimes it's better to listen. Children may not always want (or need) to hear what their parents think of their backhand, but they will always need their support and encouragement for their competitive efforts. Sometimes, this means simply listening after a bad performance or a losing game instead of saying anything.

strength training   Weight training to strengthen the muscles is the natural complement to flexibility conditioning, or stretching the muscles. It is an important component of any balanced exercise plan.

Weight training means adding resistance to the body's natural movements in order to make those movements more difficult, which in turn encourages the muscles to become stronger.

How It Works
Weight training increases fitness by:

- increasing muscle strength and endurance
- enhancing the cardiovascular system
- increasing flexibility

• maintaining the body's fat within acceptable limits

Weight training programs can be done with free weights or with weight machines. Free weights are less expensive than weight machines and are more easily adapted to smaller and larger body types. Machines are safer than most free weights because the weight is more controlled.

With multiple-purpose machines, several individuals can exercise simultaneously on the same piece of equipment within a small space. Those who use free weights should select a set of barbells

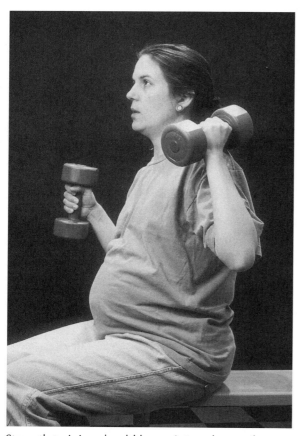

Strength training should be an integral part of everyone's fitness program, including pregnant women and senior citizens. *(Courtesy Public Health Image Library)*

or dumbbells and a weight bench for the upper extremities and barbells for the lower extremities.

For all lifting, it is helpful to use a weight belt. Some people think that weight gloves give them better grip strength, but they are not necessary. Good athletic shoes that provide firm floor traction are a must.

When beginning a new strength training program, it helps to first establish goals. One might exercise to obtain good muscular tone and cardiovascular endurance, to build muscle strength in a particular muscle group to improve sports performance, or to rehabilitate an injured muscle.

To improve muscle tone and cardiovascular performance, design a program along the lines of a circuit program. In such a program, exercises are done at least four times a week for approximately 20 to 30 minutes a session. Very short rest periods (30 seconds or less) are allowed between exercises. This program generally consists of 15 to 20 repetitions of an exercise for each major muscle group.

To build strength, exercise the muscle group to be strengthened until it is fatigued. This program incorporates fewer repetitions than circuit training. For example, do three sets of repetitions, but only eight to 10 repetitions per set, with a longer rest period of 60 to 90 seconds between each exercise. This may be done every other day, but not so frequently as a circuit program because the fatigued muscles need longer to recover.

To rehabilitate an injured muscle, use a program similar to the circuit training program of higher repetitions and lower weights. However, a rehabilitation program, unlike a circuit training program, focuses on working the injured muscle group.

An exercise professional, like a certified athletic trainer, a sports physical therapist, an exercise physiologist, or a strength and conditioning coach can help design a program that's suitable for any individual's needs.

Be Aware

To avoid injury when weight training, it is important to use the following guidelines:

• Wear appropriate clothing.

• Keep the weight training area clean and free of debris.

- Stay well hydrated while lifting.
- Get adequate rest.
- Eat sensibly.
- Stretch after warming up but before lifting.
- Always use a spotter when doing bench presses and squats.
- Lift with a buddy, whenever possible.

Weight Training and Aging

It is extremely important to check with a doctor before beginning a weight training program, particularly for those over 30 or who have any physical limitations. Those who have musculoskeletal problems, check with an orthopedist to make sure that the program will not aggravate those problems.

stress fracture A spontaneous hairline crack that can occur in bones as a result of overuse or accumulated stress, stress fractures appear most commonly in the foot bones (metatarsals), shinbone (tibia), outer leg bone (fibula), thighbone (femur), and back bones (vertebrae). Originally called "March fractures," stress fractures were first described about 1855 by a physician in the Prussian army who observed fractured metatarsals in otherwise healthy soldiers following long marches. Now they are commonly seen in runners and dancers, as well as in athletes whose activity involves a lot of jumping.

Stress fractures are extremely common. Five to 10 percent of all sports-related injuries involve stress fractures, and the incidence of the injury is on the rise due largely to an increase in the number of persons who participate in sports. The most common type of metatarsal injury is a stress fracture involving the second, third, or fourth metatarsals.

Causes

Stress fractures are caused by overuse. They may occur anywhere in the body. The majority of stress fractures involving the legs are caused by activities such as running and jumping, but there are also stress fractures of the bones in the hand that boxers experience.

Diagnosis

Pain associated with activity is usually involved in a stress fracture. Specifically, most athletes will describe pain that increases progressively and correlates with a change in activity, footwear, training, playing surface, or equipment. Patients usually report that the pain is worse when they jump or land on the injured foot or leg.

A physical examination may reveal bruising or swelling, and the point just over the affected body part may be tender if pressure is applied. Walking on the toes or running in place may be a good way to reproduce the symptoms experienced with activity.

The doctor may order an X ray, although X rays often miss stress fractures. For this reason, if a stress fracture is suspected, a bone scan may be more appropriate since it is more effective at showing stress fractures. MAGNETIC RESONANCE IMAGING (MRI) scans can also be used.

Treatment

Rest is the most important step in treating a stress fracture. In addition, ice packs should be applied to the injury for 20 to 30 minutes every three to four hours for two to three days until the pain subsides. Anti-inflammatory medication may help with the pain. In addition, patients should refrain from participating in the activity that caused the fracture until there is no pain at all associated with the activity.

In some cases, patients will need to wear a cast for three to six weeks until the bone has time to heal, and in rare cases surgery may be necessary if conservative therapy fails to heal the bone. In addition, surgery should be considered an option only if the fracture is located in a bone in which a complete fracture causes serious complications.

Rehabilitation can begin when the bone has healed. The length of time required for this healing varies depending upon the severity of the fracture. Usually, the longer one waits to begin treatment after experiencing symptoms, the longer it will take for the bone to heal. The patient should remember that everyone recovers from injury at a different rate.

It is fine to participate in sports and activities that do not cause any pain, but with stress fractures especially, it is extremely important not to continue the activity that causes the pain because this will likely cause further injury. Patients should vary their activities, changing every week. With stress fractures, it is advisable to implement a cross-training program so that overuse of the same injured body parts becomes less of a problem. In other words, for a runner accustomed to running six days a week, it is advisable to consider cycling and swimming in addition to running as part of regular training. This will reduce the repetitive stress placed on feet and legs with running.

Once the patient feels no pain with the activity that caused the stress fracture, he or she may begin to participate in the activity again for limited periods of time, gradually increasing the length and intensity of the workouts.

Prevention

The best way to avoid stress fractures is to pay attention to the way the body feels and temporarily discontinue activities that cause pain. Cross training in a various complementary sports is a good way to prevent overuse of any one body part.

stretching Stretching has been promoted for years as an integral part of fitness programs to decrease the risk of injury, relieve pain associated with stiffness, and improve performance in sports. In addition to increasing the athlete's flexibility, stretching brings with it a host of other potential benefits that are part of the reason it is a crucial part of any training program.

How It Works

A good stretch should start with isolating a particular muscle to stretch. The stretch should be held at least 30 to 45 seconds without bouncing. In an ideal stretch, the athlete should feel a small tension and hold the stretch against that tension. Each stretch should be repeated in sets of two to five repetitions with 15 to 30 seconds rest in between.

Proper breathing control is also important for a successful stretch. The athlete should take slow, relaxed breaths, trying to exhale as the muscle is stretching. The proper way to breathe is to inhale slowly through the nose, expanding the abdomen, not the chest; hold the breath a moment; then

exhale slowly through the mouth. With proper breathing, the body can relax and blood flow can increase throughout the body.

A regular program of stretching increases the muscles' tolerance to stretch, which means that athletes feel less pain for the same force applied to the muscle. The result is increased range of motion, even though true stiffness does not change. This could occur through increased tissue strength or through the painkilling effects of the exercise, but this is not completely understood.

It is important to remember that heat, ice, and warming up all increase the effectiveness of stretching to increase range of motion, but only warm-up is likely to prevent injury.

Although one 30-second stretch per muscle group is sufficient to increase range of motion in most healthy people, it is likely that longer periods or more repetitions are required in some people, injuries, and/or muscle groups.

Individuals should determine a strategy for themselves by simply holding a stretch until no additional benefit is obtained.

Side Effects

When done properly, stretching can do more than just increase flexibility. Other benefits include enhanced physical fitness; enhanced ability to learn and perform skilled movements; increased mental and physical relaxation; reduced risk of injury to joints, muscles, and tendons; and reduced muscular soreness and tension.

Unfortunately, even those who stretch do not always stretch properly and hence do not reap some or all of these benefits.

Be Aware

Some of the most common mistakes made when stretching are improper warm-up and overstretching. For example, it is better to stretch one hamstring at a time than both hamstrings at once. Isolating the muscle gives greater control over the stretch and allows easier change in intensity. New evidence suggests that stretching immediately before exercise does not prevent overuse or acute injuries. It is recommended that athletes warm the muscles a bit before stretching in order to receive the maximum benefit of the stretch.

sudden death Although lack of regular exercise is considered the fourth major risk factor for coronary heart disease, it is clear that there are occasions when apparently healthy athletes, who are considered fit and in shape, die suddenly during exercise. A graphic example of this misfortune is that of a 57-year-old American master's runner who collapsed and died within one minute after setting a regional master's record for the 3,000-meter indoor run. There had been no previous cardiac symptoms reported by the athlete, and a maximal exercise test performed on him less than two years prior to his death did not reveal any cardiac problems. It is a bit of a conundrum that regular exercise can be essential in preventing heart disease yet also be implicated as an important risk factor in sudden death.

Causes

Although there has been much debate over the actual causal relationship between exercise and sudden death, many studies have shown that almost all of the people who die suddenly during exercise have a serious disease, usually of the heart, that adequately explains the cause of death.

Many cardiac conditions have been associated with sudden death during exercise, but the most common is coronary artery disease, which is the major cause of death in people over the age of 40.

Athletes under the age of 40 who die suddenly during exercise are more likely to have hypertrophic cardiomyopathy, which is the overgrowth of heart muscle that may impede blood flow in and out of the heart. Some athletes, however, may have severe coronary artery disease as a result of inherited high levels of blood cholesterol.

Other causes of sudden death during exercise include genetic anomalies of the coronary arteries, mitral valve prolapse, right ventricular dysplasia, aortic rupture associated with Marfan's syndrome, sickle cell trait, coronary artery dissection, and various types of arrhythmia. Anabolic steroid use and cocaine abuse have also been associated with instances of sudden death during exercise. These conditions linked to sudden death are not caused by exercise, and there is no evidence that exercise accelerates the progression of any of these cardiac conditions.

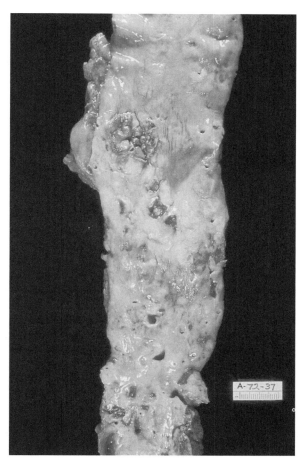

This autopsy specimen of an aorta studded with arteriosclerosis graphically illustrates the damage that takes place with heart disease, which may lead to sudden death in some athletes. *(Courtesy of Centers for Disease Control, Dr. Edwin P. Ewing, Jr., Public Health Image Library)*

The exact mechanism of sudden death during exercise in people with cardiac disease is not known, however. In the general population, plaque rupture or thrombosis are by far the most common occurrences in sudden cardiac deaths, but in sudden deaths that occur during exercise, the incidence of these appears to be lower. It is possible that ischemia, which is narrowing of the coronary arteries caused by decreased blood flow to the heart, or coronary spasm may more often be the mechanism involved in cardiac death in people who are exercising.

Diagnosis

Patients are not diagnosed with sudden death. Rather, an autopsy is usually done to try to determine the exact cause of death in people who die suddenly during exercise.

Patients can, however, be diagnosed with heart disease, and people who die suddenly during exercise frequently do have warning signs of heart disease that they ignored. Warning signs include pain in the chest, abdomen, and/or arm. Risk factors include a history of cigarette smoking, a family history of heart disease, elevated levels of cholesterol in the blood, and high blood pressure.

Treatment

There is no treatment for sudden death since the condition is one that causes immediate death. Treatment for patients with diagnosed heart disease varies depending upon the exact diagnosis but may include an organized exercise program, medication to lower blood cholesterol and/or blood pressure, and dietary changes, among other things.

Prevention

Because athletes who die suddenly most often have advanced cardiac disease, they are at high risk of dying suddenly whether or not they exercise. Quite a few studies have attempted to determine whether or not exercise increases the risk that persons with advanced heart disease will die suddenly during exercise instead of at rest. Some of these studies have found that moderate exercise does not increase the risk of sudden death. Other studies have found that more vigorous forms of exercise, such as cross-country skiing or running, are associated with a five- to seven-fold greater risk of sudden death. The studies do indicate that there is an increased likelihood that those persons who have heart disease in spite of their regular exercise will die during the short period that they spend exercising. However, if these people avoided all exercise, their overall risk of sudden death would be increased, not decreased. The higher the level of coronary risk, the greater the degree of benefit from exercise.

Nevertheless, it is advisable that all persons over 50 should undergo cardiovascular screening before starting any type of exercise program. Younger persons (under 50 years of age) who are either already participating or who wish to start exercising should first be interviewed for a family history of conditions associated with sudden death and screened for symptoms and clinical signs of cardiovascular disease, and for risk factors for heart disease. When either the family history is suggestive, or clinical suspicion is raised, or risk factors are present, subjects should undergo maximal exercise testing for measurement of exercise performance and the electrocardiographic response to exercise. This will help a doctor advise the patient on an exercise program.

When an athlete is diagnosed with heart disease, there is debate over whether the individual should be advised to refrain from strenuous exercise such as running in favor of more moderate exercise. A person with latent heart disease is best advised to continue running since this exercise helps provide protection from the disease. A person with heart disease that predisposes one to sudden death is best advised to refrain from running and other strenuous forms of exercise since these greatly increase the risk of sudden death. The difficulty comes in distinguishing between latent heart disease and heart disease that predisposes the person to sudden death during exercise.

superior labrum lesion A superior labrum lesion is an injury to the cartilage in the shoulder, specifically to the labrum, which is a liplike piece of cartilage that deepens the socket of the shoulder joint. It functions to help stabilize the shoulder. The labrum is divided into superior, inferior, anterior, and posterior parts. A tear of the superior labrum from anterior to posterior, causing the shoulder to dislocate forwardly, known as a SLAP lesion, or a superior labrum anterior-posterior lesion.

Causes

Superior labral tears can occur when a person falls onto an outstretched hand or shoulder. They may also occur in association with ROTATOR CUFF TENDONITIS and TEARS, which means that they occur commonly in athletes involved in overhead activities, such as throwing and swimming. Oftentimes, however, the exact cause of the superior labral tear is not known.

Diagnosis

A patient with a superior labral tear usually complains of a clicking sound in the shoulder that is associated with a vague pain at the front or top of the shoulder. The patient will often describe pain with overhead activities, and weakness, stiffness, or pain while lying on the affected shoulder and arm. A medical history may reveal a traumatic injury during a fall on an outstretched hand or shoulder, but this is not always the case. Sometimes, the patient does not recall the exact moment of injury.

The physical exam involves a thorough examination of the patient's neck, shoulder girdle, and upper arm. The doctor will want to test the shoulder's range of motion, stability, muscular strength, and nerve functioning. The compression rotation test, biceps tension test, and active compression test may be positive with a superior labrum lesion, but there is no single physical sign or test that is specific for diagnosing a superior labrum lesion.

A MAGNETIC RESONANCE IMAGING (MRI) scan may reveal the tear, but shoulder ARTHROSCOPY is the only definitive way to confirm a superior labral tear.

Treatment

Many superior labral tears can be treated with anti-inflammatory medications, activity modification, and physical therapy to restore strength and range of motion in the shoulder once the pain has resolved. If conservative measures fail to establish stability in the shoulder joint, then arthroscopic surgery is advised. During this procedure, the doctor will smooth the labrum and either remove or reattach the torn pieces.

Most patients with surgically repaired superior labral lesions can expect to return to sports activities within four to six months of the surgery. Overhead athletes, such as swimmers or throwers, may require a longer period of time in PHYSICAL THERAPY since these actions require highly conditioned rotator cuff and scapula-stabilizing muscle function.

Prevention

Prevention of superior labrum tears is best achieved by maintaining strong shoulder and upper back muscles. Some of these tears may be unpreventable since they happen in accidents.

swimmer's ear (otitis externa) Swimmer's ear is inflammation, irritation, or infection of the outer ear and ear canal. It is found in individuals who swim frequently or extensively while vacationing and in people who are chronic Q-tip abusers. The ear is normally protected from developing infection by its slightly acidic pH, but people who scrape away the wax in the canal with Q-tips disturb this pH balance and render the ear more susceptible to infection. The ears also become susceptible to problems when they remain immersed in water for long periods of time. This immersion causes the skin to swell and lose its natural acidic protection.

Causes

Swimming in polluted water, staying in any water for long periods of time, or undergoing some type of mechanical trauma to the ear, such as in overuse of a Q-tip, may cause swimmer's ear to develop. The presence of moisture predisposes the ear to infection from fungus or water-loving bacteria. Chronic otitis externa may occur as a result of inadequate treatment, or may suggest the presence of disease in underlying bone, a complication described as malignant otitis externa. Eczema may also be an underlying cause of swimmer's ear.

Diagnosis

Symptoms of swimmer's ear include ear pain that worsens with pulling on the external ear, itching of the ear or ear canal, persistent drainage from the ear, which may be yellow or yellow-green and have a foul odor, and finally hearing loss.

Diagnosis is made primarily based on the findings of the physical exam. The ear may be red and swollen, including the ear canal. The ear canal may appear to have eczemalike symptoms, with scaly shedding of the skin inside the canal. Patients normally complain of pain that increases when the outer ear is touched. In advanced cases, the outer ear may also become infected and appear red or swollen.

Doctors must be careful in diagnosing swimmer's ear in diabetics since there is another potentially fatal condition, pseudomonas osteomyelitis of the temporal bone, that diabetics sometimes develop and that looks like swimmer's ear in a physical examination.

Treatment

The goal of treatment is cure of the infection, and consists of topical application of ear drops containing antibiotics to fight infection and corticosteroids to reduce itching and inflammation. Swimmer's ear usually responds to treatment, but about 1 percent of cases do become chronic.

The treatment involves application of one of a number of commercial eardrops. Placing a dosage of one, two, or three drops into the external canal two, three, or four times a day, depending on the exact prescription, will normally cure the condition. It may also be advisable for the patient to take some kind of painkiller until the symptoms resolve since the ear canal can be quite painful. Heat applied to the ear will help relieve some of the discomfort as well. Certain drops contains antibiotics and will be prescribed when infection is present.

Chronic swimmer's ear, which usually occurs in daily swimmers, is easily treated with an eardrop that should be used following every session in the pool.

Prevention

It is always important to dry the ear thoroughly after exposure to moisture. Individuals who swim frequently should use earplugs. Otitis externa should be treated completely, and treatment should not be discontinued sooner than recommended by the health care provider. Those with chronic problems should use acidifying drop following every swim. In addition, it is a good idea to avoid using any kind of cotton-tipped swab since improper use can easily cause damage to the ear canal that makes the ear more vulnerable to infection.

swimmer's shoulder   Also known as shoulder impingement syndrome, swimmer's shoulder is a general term used to describe an overuse shoulder injury occurring primarily in swimmers. It represents a chronic irritation of the soft tissues of the shoulder, including the tendons, muscles, and ligaments.

Causes

Repetitive microtrauma to the soft tissues of the shoulder often due to biomechanical problems or training errors can result in swimmer's shoulder.

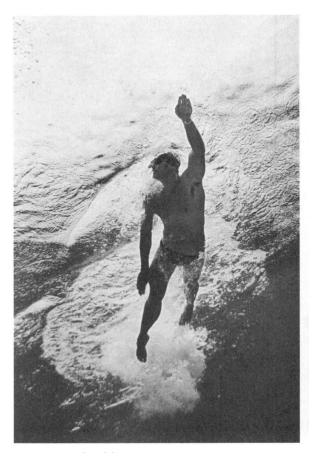

Swimmer's shoulder is a common overuse injury. Determining which part of a stroke causes the most pain will help the doctor diagnose the exact source of the pain. In addition, videotaping the athlete during the stroke may reveal problems in stroke mechanics that could be causing the injury. *(Fogstock, LLC)*

Most often swimmer's shoulder results from muscle imbalance in the shoulder. The shoulder is relying too heavily on either the large internal rotator muscles or the smaller, weaker external rotators, otherwise known as the rotator cuff muscles. The problem may be with either group of muscles, but it is more common to have trouble with the rotator cuffs.

Other causes of swimmer's shoulder include biomechanical problems and improper technique in certain strokes, as well as simple overtraining. Many different scenarios can cause excessive wear and tear on the tendons that eventually leads to shoulder impingement when inflammation hinders the normal range of motion in the shoulder.

Diagnosis

The symptoms vary depending on the exact cause. However, there are some general trends. Usually, the pain is the worst in the backstroke and at its best during breaststroke. Pain may occur at any phase of freestyle. If the athlete experiences pain that is worse during the recovery phase of the stroke, then the rotator cuffs are most likely to be the culprit. If the pain is worst during the initial pull of the stroke, the biceps tendon may be involved. In most cases of swimmer's shoulder, sleeping on the involved side aggravates the pain. When the problem is fairly advanced, the swimmer will also experience shoulder pain when not swimming and the shoulder becomes progressively more tender to the touch.

The shoulder exam should include inspection, palpation, and testing of passive and active range of motion, strength, instability, and impingement. It is vital to completely examine both shoulders as well as the neck and elbows. Inspection of posture, muscle groups, and bones for asymmetry will help evaluate atrophy, muscle imbalance, and evidence of traumatic injury.

In addition, the swimmer's form should be closely assessed for abnormal mechanics. It is useful to consult an experienced coach to assess and correct form.

Swimmer's shoulder is not an exact diagnosis. In order to determine exactly which muscles and tendons are involved, a doctor or other specialist who understands the mechanics of swimming will need to assess the shoulder in all types of movement for the presence of pain and weakness. This should be done with and without resistance.

Treatment

In order to determine the best treatment plan, it is necessary to know exactly which muscles and tendons are involved. Treatment will focus on reducing the inflammation and resting the injured shoulder. Various therapeutic techniques, including ultrasound, massage, and chiropractic adjustment may be used. Rehabilitation exercises aimed at strengthening the weak muscles will be part of the treatment approach as well. The swimmer will likely need to modify training to avoid developing the problem again in the future. The swimmer should have the mechanics of the stroke checked thoroughly by a coach so that problems in stroke mechanics can be identified and changed to prevent problems in the future.

Prevention

The primary way to prevent swimmer's shoulder is to avoid overtraining. In addition, it is vital that swimmers correct any problems in stoke mechanics. Stretching and controlled warm-up exercises will help, as will STRENGTH TRAINING that emphasizes development of the rotator cuff muscles.

tennis elbow (lateral epicondylitis) Tennis elbow, also known as lateral epicondylitis or wrist extensor tendonitis, is the name for a condition in which the bony bump at the outer side of the elbow is painful and tender due to overuse or repetitive stress. The elbow joint is made up of the bone in the upper arm, called the humerus, and one of the bones in the lower arm, the ulna. The bony bumps at the bottom of the humerus are called epicondyles. The bump on the outer side of the elbow, to which certain forearm muscles are attached by tendons, is called the lateral epicondyle.

Causes

Tennis elbow results from overusing the muscles in the forearm that straighten and raise the hand and wrist. When these muscles are overused, the tendons are repeatedly tugged at the point where they attach, the lateral epicondyle. As a result of this tugging, the tendons become inflamed. Repeated, tiny tears in the tendon tissue occur and cause pain. Among the activities that can cause tennis elbow are tennis and other racket sports, carpentry, machine work, typing, and knitting.

Diagnosis

The doctor will take a complete medical history, asking about the patient's daily and recreational activities. The physical examination will focus on the elbow and arm and will include having the patient do movements that may cause pain in the outer part of the elbow. The doctor may also order X rays of the elbow.

The most common symptoms of tennis elbow include the following:

- pain or tenderness on the outer side of the elbow
- pain when straightening or raising wrist and hand
- pain made worse by lifting a heavy object
- pain when making a fist, gripping an object, shaking hands, or turning door handles
- pain that shoots from the elbow down into the forearm or up into the upper arm
- forearm muscle tightness
- insufficient forearm functional strength

Treatment

In most cases, conservative treatment of tennis elbow is successful. However, occasionally severe cases require surgery.

Conservative treatment includes the following:

- Put an ice pack on the elbow for 20 to 30 minutes every three to four hours for two to three days or until the pain goes away.
- Massage the elbow with ice by freezing water in a Styrofoam cup. Peel the top of the cup away to expose the ice and hold onto the bottom of the cup while rubbing the ice over the elbow for five to 10 minutes.
- Wear a tennis elbow strap. This strap wraps around the forearm below the elbow, acting as a new attachment site for the forearm muscles and keeping them from pulling on the painful epicondyle.
- Take anti-inflammatory medication as prescribed by the doctor.
- Do the exercises recommended by the doctor, which may include attending PHYSICAL THERAPY. These strengthening exercises, both with and without weights, will go a long way in helping the patient avoid a recurrence of tennis elbow. Be sure not to do any exercise that produces pain.

- If the above measures do not alleviate the pain, the doctor may recommend an injection of a corticosteroid medication around the lateral epicondyle to reduce the inflammation.

During the recovery period, it is important for the patient to avoid any repetitive motion of the elbow and to change usual sports or activities to ones that do not make the condition worse. For example, tennis players may need to try running for a while.

The patient may return to the usual sport or activity when able to forcefully grip the tennis racket, bat, or golf club, or do activities such as working at a keyboard without producing pain in the elbow. In sports such as gymnastics, it is important that the patient be able to bear weight on the elbow painlessly. It is also important that there is no swelling around the injured elbow and that it has regained its normal strength compared to the uninjured elbow. Full range of motion must also be present in order for the elbow to be considered healed.

If the patient is a tennis player and has healed enough to return to tennis, it may be advisable to switch to a racket that has a larger grip. In addition, the doctor may want to observe the way the patient holds and swings the racket to make sure the techniques are not aggravating the elbow. Finally, the patient should try to lift objects with the palm facing up to keep from overusing the lateral epicondyle.

Prevention

The following are good guidelines for preventing tennis elbow:

- Use proper form during activities, whether they are sports or job-related. For instance, be sure the tennis stroke is correct and that the tennis racket has the proper grip size and is properly strung. A medium head size is preferable since it does not allow for as much increased torque from shots hit off-center.

- Warm up before playing tennis or doing other activities that involve the elbow or arm muscles. Gently stretch the elbow and arm muscles before and after exercise.

- Ice the elbow after exercise or work.

- In job-related activities, be sure posture is correct and that the position of arms during the work does not cause overuse of the elbow or arm muscles.

testicular injury   Since the testicles hang in a sac outside the body, bones and muscles do not protect them, which makes it easier for them to be injured during sports. However, their loose attachment to the body and the fact that they are made of a spongy material do give them the ability to absorb some shock without being permanently damaged. Two types of injury commonly occur to the testicles. These are testicular trauma and testicular torsion. Testicular trauma is defined as any injury sustained by the testicle. These injuries can be blunt, penetrating, or degloving, which occurs when the scrotal skin is sheared off when it becomes trapped in heavy machinery. Quite often, testicular injury is an associated complication of a larger trauma.

Causes

Testicular trauma is caused by the testicles being struck, hit, crushed, or kicked, such as in baseball when the ball hits the testicles, or in lacrosse when the athlete is struck by the stick. A rare form of testicular trauma is called testicular rupture, which occurs when the testicles receive a direct blow or are crushed against the public bone by an external force, causing blood to leak into the scrotum.

Testicular torsion occurs suddenly when the testicles become twisted, cutting off the blood vessels that supply blood to the testicle. Testicular torsion might occur as the result of trauma to the testicles, strenuous activity, or it might develop while a man is sleeping. It occurs frequently in males between the age of 12 and 18.

Diagnosis

The diagnosis of testicular injury is usually quite obvious due to the extreme amount of pain associated with injuries of the testicles. Patients may experience nausea, light-headedness, dizziness, and sweating in addition to the pain. For minor testicular injuries, the pain should gradually subside in less than an hour and the other symptoms should go away.

The signs and symptoms of testicular torsion are more severe and usually affect only one testicle, usually the left testicle. A patient with testicular torsion might experience rapid swelling and extreme pain in the scrotum, which does not go away, nausea, vomiting, and abdominal pain. Testicular rupture also causes extreme pain and swelling in the scrotum, as well as nausea and vomiting.

Doctors will first assess the degree of pain in a patient with a testicular injury. In a physical examination, the testicles will be evaluated for swelling, discoloration, thickening of the skin, puncture wounds, or any other abnormality. The doctor may also want to examine the abdomen and groin in order to rule out a hernia.

In cases of testicular torsion, the doctor will want to check the reflexes in the genital area by stroking or gently pinching the skin of the upper thigh while watching the muscles of the scrotum. Absence of this reflex is a good indication of testicular torsion.

The doctor may want to do a urinalysis to rule out the possibility of infection since urinary tract infection can cause testicular pain. Ultrasounds may also be helpful in evaluating the scrotum.

Treatment
Mild testicular injuries are treated with rest and analgesics to help deal with the pain. Patients should lie down, gently support the testicles with supportive underwear, and apply ice packs to relieve swelling and pain.

In the case of a twisted testicle, the doctor may try to manually rotate the testicle, but usually surgery is required to repair a testicular torsion. This surgery involves a small incision in the scrotum that allows the doctor to examine the testicle for any signs of problems, untwist it, and anchor it so that twisting cannot occur in the future. Testicular rupture requires surgery as well to drain and repair the ruptured testicle.

Following surgery, patients should not resume normal sports activities until the genitals are completely healed. This can take several months.

Although the testicles are extremely sensitive, they bounce back from injury quite well. Minor injuries and major injuries treated within the first six hours after the pain starts usually do not have any lasting effects. In some cases of testicular torsion, however, the testicle eventually has to be removed. This is most likely when treatment is delayed. Removal of one testicle does not impede normal sexual functioning, and since both testicles produce sperm, fertility is not totally impaired.

Prevention
Athletes should always wear an athletic cup or supporter when playing sports or doing any other strenuous activity that might affect the genital area. It is important, too, that the cup or supporter fit properly. Safety equipment that is too small or large will not protect effectively against injury. Athletes should always discuss any testicular pain with their doctor since this may be an indication of something that makes them more vulnerable to testicular injury. Those who play lacrosse or baseball and those who ride horses should be especially careful about protecting themselves from injury since these are the sports with the highest incidence of testicular injury.

thigh bruise (quadriceps contusion) A thigh bruise is a bruise, or contusion, to the quadriceps, which are a large group of muscles in the front of the thigh that help straighten the leg. A thigh bruise is also sometimes called a charley horse.

Causes
A direct blow to the muscles of the thigh causes a thigh bruise.

Diagnosis
With a thigh bruise, there is pain in the middle of the thigh and difficulty walking or running. There may also be difficulty in bending or straightening the leg or lifting the knee. The area where the injury occurred may appear swollen and discolored as well. In addition to the bruise, patients should be aware of the possibility of a hematoma. A hematoma develops when a large bruise bleeds into the muscle. The hematoma may become calcified and form a hard lump in the quadriceps. The stiffness or "bump" in the muscle that results from this calcification may last a very long time, so it is important to receive appropriate treatment if a hematoma occurs.

The doctor will take the patient's history to determine what caused the bruise. There will also be a physical examination of the thigh. If the doctor has any reason to suspect an area of calcification, an X ray may be ordered.

Treatment

Immediate treatment for a thigh bruise involves wrapping the knee in a bent-leg position and placing ice over the thigh. This position ensures that the quadriceps are stretched to their maximum length so that they do not become stiff during the healing process.

Other treatment may include:

- placing ice packs on the thigh for 20 to 30 minutes every three to four hours for two or three days or until the pain goes away
- lying down and elevating the thigh by putting a pillow under it
- taking an anti-inflammatory medication to ease the swelling and discomfort
- wearing an elastic thigh wrap when returning to sports
- participating in prescribed physical therapy, including rehabilitation exercises and deep tissue treatments such as ultrasound or electrical stimulation

It is important to participate in activities that do not aggravate the condition until the thigh has had a chance to heal completely. Running, for example, with a thigh bruise is not advisable, so a runner may need to switch to swimming. The following conditions should be present in order for the patient to return to normal activities:

- full range of motion in the injured leg compared to the uninjured leg
- full strength of the injured leg compared to the uninjured leg
- no pain or limping when jogging straight ahead, sprinting straight ahead, performing cuts and figure-eights, and jumping on both legs or just on the injured leg

Prevention

A thigh bruise usually occurs from a direct blow to the thigh, which may not be preventable. However, in contact sports such as football it is always important to wear the proper protective equipment.

thoracic outlet syndrome   Thoracic outlet syndrome affects the shoulder, arm, and/or hand. The thoracic outlet is the space between the rib cage and clavicle through which neurovascular structures pass from the neck and thorax into the arm. Thoracic outlet syndrome (TOS) refers to the symptoms that develop when these blood vessels and nerves are compressed. Often seen in swimmers, thoracic outlet syndrome occurs most often in patients who engage in repetitive motions that place the shoulder in extreme rotation positions. Freestyle, breaststroke, butterfly, and backstroke all do this.

Causes

A history of repetitive trauma to the head or neck, a fracture of the first rib or clavicle, poor posture, and subluxation of the cervical vertebrae are the primary causes of thoracic outlet syndrome. Swimming is a common cause of thoracic outlet syndrome, since the extreme shoulder positions involved in swimming freestyle, backstroke, breaststroke, and butterfly can cause the accumulation of microtraumas that contribute to the development of the condition. Other sports that put athletes at risk of developing thoracic outlet syndrome include water polo, baseball, and tennis. Genetic predisposition is another common cause of thoracic outlet syndrome. Some people have congenital bands, which are fibrous thickenings of muscle that compress the blood vessels and nerves in the thoracic outlet.

Diagnosis

Patients with thoracic outlet syndrome normally complain of hand pain that is most severe in the fourth and fifth fingers. The pain gets worse with use of the arm, and there is often significant fatigue in the arm. When a swimmer complains of tightness and pain about the shoulder, neck, and clavicle as a hand enters the water, one should suspect the presence of thoracic outlet syndrome.

Other common symptoms of this condition include hand, arm, shoulder, and neck pain;

numbness and tingling of the neck, arms, and hands; muscle weakness; reflex loss; sensations of hot and cold; and swelling. Headaches are sometimes reported.

Most patients have normal findings in a physical examination, but poor posture may be observed, especially in overhead athletes, such as swimmers and baseball players. This slouching posture may contribute to the compression of nerves. Other findings may include coolness of skin, lower blood pressure, and blue fingers on the affected side. There may be swelling in the veins, and the veins of the shoulder and chest may be distended.

X rays of the cervical spine and chest may be used to identify bony abnormalities. Ultrasound may be useful in quantifying changes in blood flow in both the arteries and veins. MAGNETIC RESONANCE IMAGING (MRI) scans are used only to rule out other possible causes of the symptoms suggestive of thoracic outlet syndrome. Other tests that may be used include an elevated arm stress test, also called a Roos test, an Adson maneuver, a Wright test, and a costoclavicular maneuver.

Treatment

The vast majority of patients with thoracic outlet syndrome improve with just physical therapy. Exercises normally include neck stretching, abdominal breathing, and postural exercises. Medications are often prescribed for swelling, pain relief, and muscle relaxation.

When conservative therapies fail to produce improvements after several months, surgical decompression of the vessels and nerves is necessary. Following surgery, it is essential that patients undergo PHYSICAL THERAPY to strengthen the muscles and improve range of motion. The patient may return to normal activities approximately four to six weeks after surgery. It should be understood, however, that a good surgical outcome means improvement of the symptoms, but there is rarely a complete cure. Patients must be educated in prevention techniques to avoid frequent problems with thoracic outlet syndrome.

Prevention

To prevent recurrence of thoracic outlet syndrome, the patient should avoid any repetitive or overhead actions that may have caused the original symptoms. This includes sleeping with the arms overhead.

The patient should also avoid repetitive motions, stressful lifting, and overhead work. Performing a regular exercise program for improving flexibility and strength is beneficial.

tibialis posterior syndrome   The tibialis posterior muscle comes from behind the shinbone (tibia) and runs into a tendon that passes behind the bony protrusion on the inside of the ankle, which is technically called the medial malleolus. Inflammation can occur around the medial malleolus and farther down under the foot where the tendon attaches. Athletes who overpronate are more vulnerable to this injury than others. In addition, athletes who are involved in sports that require the foot to roll a lot, such as speed skating or basketball, are also more prone to this injury.

Diagnosis

An athlete with tibialis posterior syndrome usually has pain over the attachment of the tendon to the navicular bone in the foot. During exercise, the athlete will experience pain when the tendon slides in the sheath during the stretching and rolling of the foot. Swelling around the medial malleolus is another common symptom.

A doctor will make a diagnosis based on a medical history of the patient and an examination of the foot that includes palpating the area of the tendon as it passes through the inside of the ankle. Swelling and tenderness there will suggest the diagnosis.

Treatment

Initial treatment involves resting the foot for a couple of weeks until the pain and swelling have had a chance to resolve. Ice should be applied for 20 minutes every two to three hours during the first three days following the injury. The doctor may recommend anti-inflammatory medication such as ibuprofen. If the injury is severe, the doctor may apply a plaster cast to the ankle for three weeks and/or give the athlete a steroid injection directly into the tendon sheath to reduce the swelling. In cases where the tendon is completely ruptured, surgery is necessary to repair the tendon because this tendon is extremely important in supporting the arch of the foot.

Prevention

As with other OVERUSE INJURIES, proper stretching before and after activity and appropriate rest between workouts will help prevent tibialis posterior syndrome from developing. Once it has begun to be a problem, it is important to give the foot adequate rest so that the tendon can heal. Many athletes continually reinjure the tendon by never allowing it enough rest to fully heal. A conservative approach initially will pay off in the long run by helping the athlete avoid a painful condition that can become chronic if not properly treated in the beginning.

trigger finger (stenosing tenosynovitis) Trigger finger is a condition in which it is difficult to straighten a finger once bent. The medical term for trigger finger is stenosing tenosynovitis. It is most often an OVERUSE INJURY that affects the tendons of the finger. When trigger finger develops as a result of repeated trauma, the tendon's sheath and the tendon itself thicken, making it difficult for the tendon to get through the sheath. The flexor muscles of the finger are able to pull on the tendon and bend the finger, but the extensor muscles are not strong enough to bend it back. The finger ends up in a chronically bent position that is the same position of a finger that is pulling a trigger on a gun. The only way to straighten out the finger is to pull on it with the other hand.

Causes

Trigger finger is caused by repeated trauma to the palm of the hand that injures the tendons of a finger. The resulting inflammation or swelling of the fibrous sheath that encloses the tendons makes it difficult for the tendon to move through the sheath. A tennis racket repeatedly jamming into the palm or a baseball repeatedly hitting the catcher's mitt can cause this kind of damage to the tendon.

Diagnosis

Patients with trigger finger often describe a snapping sensation in the affected finger or fingers. The condition is characterized by an inability to extend the finger smoothly or at all. It may stay locked in a bent position. The patient often describes tenderness to the touch over the tendon, usually at the base of the finger or palm and soreness in the affected finger or fingers. Diagnosis is usually made on the basis of these physical findings.

Treatment

Rest and ice to relieve the swelling are the first steps in treating trigger finger. If these do not produce relief of symptoms, the doctor may recommend an injection of a local anesthetic to reduce the pain and a corticosteroid injection to reduce the swelling of the tendon sheath.

In rare cases, surgery is necessary to remove the thickened part of the tendon sheath that is causing the tendon to get stuck. When the finger no longer catches or locks, it is safe to return to normal sports activities, but the patient should be careful to protect the palm of the hand from aggravating situations.

Prevention

Protecting the palm of the hand from repeated blows is the best way to prevent trigger finger.

turf toe Turf toe is pain at the joint where the big toe attaches to the rest of the foot. It has become a more common injury in recent years with the increase in use of artificial surfaces.

Causes

A jammed big toe or overuse of the big toe in pushing off and jumping activities can result in turf toe. In addition, wearing lightweight, flexible shoes with poor support can make athletes vulnerable to this injury.

Diagnosis

If the patient complains of difficulty in bending and straightening the big toe and pain where the big toe attaches to the foot, a diagnosis of turf toe will probably be considered. On examination, the toe joint may be swollen, and the condition may look like gout, which is a type of arthritis in the big toe. Tests may be ordered to ensure that the patient does not have gout, and an X ray may be taken to rule out the possibility of a broken toe.

Treatment

Resting the foot, icing the toe, and keeping the foot elevated at a level above the heart to reduce the swelling are all parts of the initial treatment for turf toe. Anti-inflammatory medications will also likely be prescribed. The most important factor in treatment of turf toe is ensuring that the big toe does not move too much. To aid in restricting movement, the doctor may tape the big toe and place a special insole in the shoe that will reduce movement of the toe.

Rehabilitation may involve exercises to strengthen the foot. Patients may resume normal activities when they again have full range of motion in the toe and can run, jump, and perform pushing off activities without pain.

Prevention

Turf toe is best prevented by wearing good shoes that fit properly and provide adequate cushion and support. In addition, avoiding any activity that jams the big toe into a hard surface will help in preventing turf toe.

weight training   Weight training to strengthen the muscles is the natural complement to FLEXIBILITY conditioning, or stretching the muscles. It is an important component of any balanced exercise plan.

Weight training means adding resistance to the body's natural movements in order to make those movements more difficult, which in turn encourages the muscles to become stronger.

Benefits of Weight Training
Weight training increases fitness by:

- increasing muscle strength and endurance
- enhancing the cardiovascular system
- increasing flexibility
- maintaining the body's fat within acceptable limits

Special Equipment Needs
Weight training programs can be done with free weights or with weight machines. Free weights are less expensive than weight machines and are more easily adapted to smaller and larger body types. Machines are safer than most free weights because the weight is more controlled.

With multiple-purpose machines, several individuals can exercise simultaneously on the same piece of equipment within a small space. Those who use free weights should select a set of barbells or dumbbells and a weight bench for the upper extremities and barbells for the lower extremities.

For all lifting, it is helpful to use a weight belt. Some people feel that weight gloves give them better grip strength, but they are not necessary. Good athletic shoes that provide firm floor traction are a must.

How to Begin a Weight Training Program
First, it helps to establish goals for the program. Decide if the goal is to obtain good muscular tone and cardiovascular endurance, to build muscle strength in a particular muscle group to improve sports performance, or to rehabilitate an injured muscle.

To improve muscle tone and cardiovascular performance, design the program along the lines of a circuit program. In such a program, exercises are done at least four times a week for approximately 20 to 30 minutes a session. Very short rest periods (30 seconds or less) are allowed between exercises. This program generally consists of 15 to 20 repetitions of an exercise for each major muscle group.

To build strength, exercise the muscle group to be strengthened until it is fatigued. This program incorporates fewer repetitions than circuit training. For example, do three sets of repetitions, but only eight to 10 repetitions per set, with a longer rest period of 60 to 90 seconds between each exercise. This may be done every other day, but not so frequently as a circuit program because the fatigued muscles need longer to recover.

To rehabilitate an injured muscle, the program would be similar to the circuit training program of higher repetitions and lower weights. However, a rehabilitation program, unlike a circuit training program, focuses on working the injured muscle group.

An exercise professional, such as a certified athletic trainer, a sports physical therapist, an exercise physiologist, or a strength and conditioning coach can help design a suitable program.

Cautions About Weight Training
To avoid injury when weight training, it is important to use the following guidelines:

- Wear appropriate clothing.
- Keep the weight training area clean and free of debris.

- Stay well hydrated while lifting.
- Get adequate rest.
- Eat sensibly.
- Stretch after warming up but before lifting.
- Always use a spotter when doing bench presses and squats.
- Lift with a buddy, whenever possible.

Weight Training and Aging

It is extremely important to check with a doctor before beginning a weight training program, particularly for people over 30 or those who have any physical limitations. Those with musculoskeletal problems should check with an orthopedist to make sure that the program will not aggravate those problems.

whiplash (neck sprain)   Whiplash is a common injury for those involved in contact sports injuries that include a hard fall, as is common in football. There are seven cervical vertebrae in the neck that are connected to one another by ligaments. Whiplash occurs when these ligaments are stretched or torn beyond their ability to flex. Often this happens with a sudden movement that causes the neck to extend, or snap back, in an extreme position with extreme force.

Causes

A hard fall in contact sports is often the cause of whiplash. Car accidents that cause the neck to suddenly snap back with violent force are another common cause of whiplash.

Diagnosis

Patients with whiplash commonly complain of pain in the back of the neck that worsens with movement. There is often delayed pain that does not develop until a day or so after the injury. Muscle spasms and pain in the upper shoulders are frequently reported as well. Headache, sore throat, numbness in the arm or hand, stiffness and decrease in range of motion in the neck, tingling and weakness in the arm, and increased fatigue and irritability are other common symptoms.

Treatment

All sprains or strains, no matter where they are located in the body, receive basically the same type of treatment. Usually, neck sprains, like other sprains, will gradually heal, given time and appropriate treatment. Patients may need to wear a soft cervical collar to help support the head and relieve pressure on the neck so the ligaments have time to heal.

Anti-inflammatory medications may be prescribed to help reduce the pain and any swelling. If muscle spasms occur, muscle relaxant medication may be prescribed as well. Patients should ice the neck 15 to 20 minutes at a time, several times a day, for the first two or three days after the injury to help reduce inflammation and discomfort. Although heat, particularly moist heat, can help loosen cramped muscles, it should not be applied until the swelling has subsided.

Most symptoms will resolve in four to six weeks, although severe injuries can take longer to heal completely. Return to normal activities takes place when the neck is completely healed. For those who participate in contact sports, it is crucial that the neck and shoulders be properly rehabilitated before returning to competition. An athlete must have full range of motion in the neck, which means being able to turn the head fully to look over both shoulders, extend the head backward as far as possible, flex the neck forward until the chin touches the chest, and bend the head sideways in each direction so that the ear touches the shoulder. If the patient experiences burning or muscle spasms in the neck or shoulder with any of these actions, the neck is not completely healed, and he or she should not return to sports.

Prevention

Having strong and supple neck muscles best prevents whiplash. People who stay in one position for long periods of time in their sport or occupation should be sure to rest the head and neck periodically and do stretching exercises.

wrist injuries   The wrist, also called the carpus, is a complex joint. The most common injuries involving this joint are fractures and dislocations that occur from accidents and OVERUSE INJURIES that lead to tendonitis or other injuries to the tendons and muscles responsible for wrist movement.

When someone breaks the wrist, any of a number of bones may also be broken. The most common types of wrist fractures are those involving ones of the wrist bones, but a wrist fracture can also involve breaking one of the bones at the end of the forearm, where the arm and wrist connect.

Causes

Most commonly seen in the very young, ages six to 10, and in senior citizens, wrist injuries occur from accidents and from overuse. Sports such as rollerblading and gymnastics can easily lead to falls that injure the wrist, since it is instinctual to stretch the hand out to catch the fall, and this is what often puts the wrist in the position of receiving the force of the fall and becoming injured in the process.

Sports such as golf, tennis, and baseball contribute to overuse injuries involving the wrist since they rely on repetitive motions of the wrist, often at high speeds, in the golf swing, tennis serve, and baseball throw.

Women with osteoporosis experience wrist fractures much more commonly than the general population due to the weakening that has occurred in their bones. Women with osteoporosis should therefore be especially cautious about protecting the wrist.

Diagnosis

The patient with a fracture or dislocation will likely have significant pain and some type of deformity. Such fractures and dislocations of the joint that occur in accidents are diagnosed through a physical examination and a medical history to determine the source of injury. The doctor will want to hear how the injury happened and what the history of pain has been since the injury occurred. In most cases, some type of diagnostic test will be ordered to confirm the doctor's suspected diagnosis following the physical examination. This may be a simple X ray or may involve a COMPUTERIZED AXIAL TOMOGRAPHY (CAT) SCAN or a MAGNETIC RESONANCE IMAGING (MRI) scan if there is suspected soft tissue damage as well.

With overuse injuries, such as tendonitis, the patient will normally describe localized pain along the course of the tendon or muscle. In severe tendonitis, there may be pain whenever the wrist is moved. Swelling, grinding, and a creaking sensation may also accompany wrist movement in more severe cases.

Treatment

Treatment for tendonitis usually consists of ice, anti-inflammatory medication, bracing, stretching, and strengthening, and occasionally corticosteroid injections to relieve the inflammation and pain. Surgery is rarely indicated for wrist tendonitis.

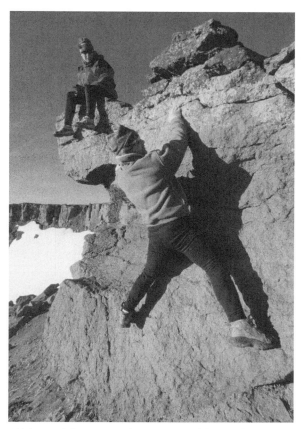

All four of the grip techniques used by rock climbers make them vulnerable to a number of different hand injuries since they transmit extremely high forces through the tissues of the fingers, hands, and forearms, resulting in a variety of possible acute and chronic injuries. These include tendonitis, wrist fractures, trigger finger, and torn ligaments, among others. *(Fogstock, LLC)*

Treatment for a fracture or dislocation may include repositioning bones and immobilization using a splint or cast. Fractures with three or more pieces of broken bone, known as a comminuted fracture, may require pins or other devices to hold the bones in proper position while they heal. Recovery from fractures and dislocations of the wrist takes a surprisingly long time—anywhere from six to 12 months is common. Often there will be some continuing pain and loss of grip strength following a wrist fracture.

PHYSICAL THERAPY is usually very helpful in preventing wrist and finger stiffness following a wrist fracture. It can also help the patient to recover a strong grip and become pain-free.

Prevention

A combination of strengthening and stretching can help prevent wrist injuries. The golf swing, for example, requires more wrist motion than most daily (and vocational) activities. Stretching should be performed before practice and play as well as after a round is completed. Stretching can also be performed during a round as needed.

Exercises to strengthen the wrist are equally important. Emphasis must be placed on proper technique as faulty exercise mechanics can lead to injuries of the wrist, elbow, and shoulder. Athletes in any type of sport that requires gripping a racket or club will want to find a grip that is comfortable, incorporates proper positioning, and is neither too strong or too weak so that the wrists are allowed maximum flexibility. An excessively strong or weak grip will result in improper hand position that limits wrist flexibility and arm rotation as well. Amateurs often grip too tightly, making them more vulnerable to wrist injuries. In addition, slippery or excessively narrow grips may increase wrist tension, making the wrists more vulnerable to injury.

yips Yips is a condition that affects the performance of many amateur and professional golfers. It refers to involuntary motions of the hand or wrist that can make putting all but impossible, even for the most experienced and talented of golfers. A golfer with yips experiences a mild spasm, usually on putts that are shorter than five feet and usually just as the putter is about to make contact with the ball. These twitches or jerks, as they are sometimes called, occur less frequently during a tee or iron shot and thus appear to be related to the precision of the golf shot being undertaken.

Causes

There is considerable debate about the cause of yips. Some researchers suggest that it is a neurological problem called focal dystonia. Others attribute the yips to performance anxiety. Still others say it can result from a combination of these two conditions.

Although the exact cause of the yips is yet to be determined, some researchers think that the condition may result from biochemical changes in the brain that accompany aging. Excessive use of the involved muscles and intense demands of coordination and concentration may make the problem worse.

Diagnosis

Diagnosis of the yips is usually fairly straightforward, and based on the patient's reported medical history, but determining the underlying cause is quite complex.

Studies have shown that golfers who experience the yips have anxiety levels similar to golfers who do not have the yips, but there are some differences in these players. Those who experience the yips appear to have faster than average heart rates and increased muscle activity in the wrists. In addition, they tend to grip the putter with greater force.

Golfers who experience the yips normally report that the condition comes and goes, occurring more frequently in situations of greatest stress, such as tournament play. In a minority of golfers, the yips affects more than one hand, spreading to the other hand and sometimes to other parts of the body, including the arms, shoulders, legs, feet, neck, jaw, and even the eyelids.

Although the condition is most common in golfers, it occurs to other athletes and professionals as well, including baseball players, dentists, and musicians.

Focal dystonia may be a possible diagnosis in those who are forced to repeatedly assume a prolonged, abnormal posture. There are numerous kinds of focal dystonia, including spasmodic torticollis, which causes intermittent or continuous spasms on one side of the neck that may cause the head to tilt or turn. This condition is commonly known as wryneck. Other types of focal dystonia include blepharospasm, which occurs when the eyelids spasm continuously and force themselves shut, and writer's cramp, which is a spasmodic contraction of the muscles in the hand and forearm. Such focal dystonias are task-specific, meaning that they occur only when performing a specific task. In golfers, the yips may be a task-specific disorder tied to the act of putting or swinging a golf club. As with other forms of focal dystonia, anxiety and stress may make this symptom worse.

Performance anxiety may also be a factor in the yips. A doctor examining a patient with complaints of yips will want to take a thorough medical history that addresses the patient's feelings of anxiety or tension in addition to the physical symptoms of the condition.

Treatment

Treatment for the yips commonly involves participation in a sports psychology program that uses techniques such as conscious relaxation, hypnosis, and guided imagery to help the patient control the yips. In addition, it is advisable that patients with the yips cut back on caffeine consumption and participate in activities that alleviate anxiety, such as running or other aerobic activity.

youth participation in sports Participating in sports is a fundamental part of life. Athletic activities can contribute to healthy growth and development and should be regarded as an extension of the child's playtime, a way to channel youthful energy in a positive, safe direction. The participation of children in organized athletic activities, however, raises many concerns. The appropriate age for participation in organized sports and the risk of injury with particular sports are two of the most common concerns.

Most children are ready to begin participating in organized sports between the ages of six and 10. Before age six, children do not comprehend competition per se. They are interested in playing and are usually difficult to organize. Sports activities for children under six should be opportunities to play.

Between the ages of six and 10, children come to appreciate interaction with their peer groups but, psychologically, still do not compete in the adult sense. Play and fun are the primary goals for these youngsters, with structure, organization, and scoring of secondary importance. Children in this age group generally have very short attention spans and generally cannot perform in the adult-imposed structure of most sports activities. They are ready for group interaction but not for many restrictive rules or too much structure.

Between age 10 and the onset of puberty, a youth develops increasing awareness of the goals, structure, and discipline required for team sports. The prime motivation of children this age is still joining in and having fun with their teammates. However, they will accept increasing amounts of structure and are becoming more goal-oriented.

During and after puberty, the aspiring athlete develops an increasingly sophisticated perspective on the structure and organization of team sports.

In some budding athletes, this evolves into a readiness for the discipline required to perform well in competitive sports.

In terms of physical capabilities of the young athlete, participating in sports depends upon both chronological age and physiological maturity. The positive effects of sports activity or training on the body are measurably less prior to puberty. There are benefits, however, at every age in conditioning the heart and lungs, but this becomes more significant after puberty. Lifting weights can have a positive effect on younger athletes if done in a well-controlled setting, but the most important results occur following puberty when hormonal changes occur and permit the body to begin muscle bulking.

It should be noted that no matter what the form of specific training or sport activity, STRETCHING and FLEXIBILITY drills should be included in any sports program, even in the very young.

Given the limitations outlined above, young children can still benefit immensely from athletic activities. They develop motor skills, proper training habits, and a work ethic, which can carry over to life in general. They also benefit from proper training with weights, cardiovascular conditioning, and from working with adults other than their parents.

The young athlete should participate in a variety of sports activities. Psychologically, the sports goal for a child under 10, and perhaps even the older child, should be fun. Physically, the young athlete should be encouraged to acquire basic individual skills. Sports participation by these younger athletes should be an opportunity to develop motor skills and to have fun. These limited goals will give the child a healthy mental attitude as well as a healthy body, both of which will give benefit throughout life.

Above all, a young athlete must not become the focus of the personal athletic dreams or wishes of a parent or coach. While parental and coaching guidance is of immense value, the young athlete should not be pressured to swim or play football, for example, when another sport better fits his or her emotional and/or physical makeup. The post-pubescent athlete will usually select athletic endeavors based on a personal skill or through associations with a particular role model or peer group.

Risk of Injury

The question is not whether injuries accompany youth sports, but whether there is undue risk. Many studies have documented a very low incidence of injury in the total spectrum of youth sporting endeavors. Interestingly, the occurrence of injury in the pre-pubescent athlete has been documented as being much lower than in the post-pubescent athlete, and lower in the post-pubescent than in the young adult.

This is probably because the younger athlete has less speed and power with which to do damage. Since the magnitude of injury is almost always directly related to energy expended in a traumatic event, the younger athlete is less likely to get injured than his older counterpart. The athletic injuries that do occur are usually minor contusions and sprains. Fractures, dislocations, and major ligament injuries can happen, but are more common in older age groups.

Parents have expressed concern about the potential for injuries to the growth areas of developing bones and muscle in the growing athlete. This concern has proven to be more perceived than real. Only in extreme cases, such as young gymnasts in intense training for long periods of time, is there some risk of growth-plate injuries.

Young people have definite physical and emotional energies, and it is probably less hazardous to release these energies in directed endeavors than through alternative means.

Types of Injuries

In youth sports, the biggest distinction is made between contact sports and noncontact sports when discussing types of injuries.

The most notable examples of contact sports practiced in the United States are football, ice hockey, wrestling, and basketball. In each of these sports, the athlete's body is used to physically control the opponent and, thus, to influence the play of the game. Using the body in this manner creates the opportunity for injury.

Fortunately, the majority of injuries in these contact sports are bruises and scrapes. The more significant injuries such as fractures, dislocations, and major ligament damage occur in the post-pubescent athlete. Parents should be responsive to complaints of pain and discomfort from athletes in all age groups and be aware that any athlete who is not playing up to skill level may be suffering from a significant injury.

In noncontact sports, major fractures, dislocations, and ligament injuries are usually associated with accidental rather than intended collisions. Minor sprains, strained muscles, blisters, and OVERUSE INJURIES are commonly seen in noncontact sports.

The overuse syndrome is usually related to sports requiring repetitive, high-stress motion, such as tennis, swimming, track, golf, and baseball. However, there are overuse injuries that can occur in every sport. Injury occurs as a result of constant repetition of a particular movement. STRESS FRACTURES, SHIN SPLINTS, and LITTLE LEAGUE ELBOW are examples of overuse injuries.

The treatment in each case is early recognition of the problem followed by abstinence from competition and at least a decrease or change in training until the affected area is totally free of symptoms. Training intensity and duration can then increase again. Return to the previous level of training should be gradual and well planned. If the symptoms of overuse persist beyond a few days of rest or if they recur, a physician should evaluate the athlete.

While very few athletes participate on organized teams beyond high school, and even fewer beyond college, sports activity creates a physical fitness discipline and a positive learning experience that carries through to an active, healthy adult life. Although participation does carry some risk of injury, the risk in most cases is reasonable considering the benefits of participation.

The following list of sports commonly played by young athletes is intended to provide helpful guidelines to parents and coaches who want to be aware of risk factors and use all preventive measures possible.

Football

Common injuries and locations: bruises, sprains, strains, pulled muscles, soft tissue tears, broken bones, internal injuries (bruised or damaged organs), back injuries, sunburn; knees and ankles the most common injury sites

Protective equipment and tools: helmet; mouth guard; shoulder pads; athletic supporters for males; chest/rib pads; forearm, elbow, and thigh pads; shin guards; proper shoes; sunscreen; water

Prevention: proper use of safety equipment, warm-up exercises, proper coaching and conditioning

Basketball

Common injuries and locations: sprains, strains, bruises, fractures, scrapes, dislocation, cuts, dental injuries. Ankles, knees (injury rates are higher in girls, especially for the ANTERIOR CRUCIATE LIGAMENT, the wide ligament that limits rotation and forward movement of the shin bone), shoulder (ROTATOR CUFF TEARS and strains, where tendons at the end of muscles attach to the upper arm and shoulder bones)

Protective equipment and tools: eye protection, elbow and knee pads, mouth guard, athletic supporters for males, proper shoes, water; if playing outdoors, a hat and sunscreen

Prevention: STRENGTH TRAINING, particularly for the knees and shoulders; aerobic exercises that develop the strength and endurance of heart and lungs; warm-up exercises; proper coaching; and use of safety equipment

Soccer

Common injuries and locations: bruises, cuts and scrapes, ankle sprains, concussions, headaches, sunburn

Protective equipment and tools: shin guards, athletic supporters for males, cleats, sunscreen, water (The importance of using helmets is currently being debated among soccer coaches, players, and others.)

Prevention: aerobic conditioning and warm-ups; proper training in "heading" the ball

Baseball and Softball

Common injuries and location: impact injuries that include fractures due to sliding and being hit by a ball, LITTLE LEAGUE ELBOW, ABRASIONS, sunburn

Protective equipment and tools: batting helmet, shin guards, elbow guards, athletic supporters for males, mouth guard, sunscreen, cleats, hat, breakaway bases

Prevention: proper conditioning and warm-ups; following guidelines for resting the pitcher's arm; use of protective gear

Gymnastics

Common injuries and locations: ANKLE SPRAINS, other soft tissue sprains and strains, carpal bone injuries, athletic amenorrhea, ANOREXIA, OVERTRAINING SYNDROME

Protective equipment and tools: athletic supporters for males, safety harness, joint supports such as neoprene wraps, water

Prevention: proper conditioning and warm-ups; appropriate rest between workouts; proper nutrition

Track and Field

Common injuries and locations: strains, sprains, ABRASIONS, PIRIFORMIS SYNDROME, RUNNER'S KNEE, JUMPER'S KNEE, OVERTRAINING SYNDROME

Protective equipment and tools: proper shoes, athletic supporters for males, sunscreen, water

Prevention: appropriate footwear; proper rest between workouts; proper conditioning and coaching

APPENDIXES

I. Safety Tips by Sport
    A. Baseball Safety Tips
    B. Basketball Safety Tips
    C. Bicycling Safety Tips
    D. Gymnastics Safety Tips
    E. Running Safety Tips
    F. Skiing Safety Tips
    G. Soccer Safety Tips
    H. Swimming Safety Tips
    I. Volleyball Safety Tips
    J. Wrestling Safety Tips

II. Nutrition by Sport
    A. Nutrition for Basketball Players
    B. Nutrition for Cyclists
    C. Nutrition for Golfers
    D. Nutrition for Long-Distance Runners
    E. Nutrition for Middle-Distance Runners
    F. Nutrition for Soccer Players
    G. Nutrition for Sprinters
    H. Nutrition for Swimmers
    I. Nutrition for Tennis Players
    J. Nutrition for Triathletes

III. Common Sports Injuries
    A. Five Commonly Misdiagnosed Sports Injuries
    B. Common Ankle Injuries
    C. Common Back Injuries
    D. Common Elbow Injuries
    E. Common Foot Injuries
    F. Common Hand Injuries
    G. Common Shoulder Injuries
    H. Common Injuries by Sport

IV. Training Tips for Running a First Marathon or Riding a First Century

V. Associations and Organizations

VI. Sports Medicine Schools

VII. Sports Medicine Journals

VIII. Sports Medicine Web Sites

APPENDIX I
SAFETY TIPS BY SPORT

A. BASEBALL SAFETY TIPS

Each year, almost 500,000 baseball-related injuries are treated by doctors. The following tips are designed to help athletes avoid becoming one of the injury statistics.

- Always take time to warm up and stretch. Research studies have shown that cold muscles are more prone to injury. Warm up with jumping jacks, stationary cycling, or running or walking in place for three to five minutes. Then slowly and gently stretch, holding each stretch for 30 seconds.

- Be sure equipment fits properly and is worn correctly.

- Wear a batting helmet at the plate, when waiting a turn at bat, and when running bases.

- Wear facial protection devices whenever available. These can help reduce the risk of a serious facial injury when hit by a ball.

- Follow the guidelines about the number of innings pitched as specified by one's baseball league (usually four to 10 innings a week).

- While there is no concrete guideline for the number of pitches allowed, a reasonable approach is to count the number of pitches thrown and use 80 to 100 pitches as a maximum in a game, and 30 to 40 pitches in a practice.

- Wear the appropriate mitt for one's position. Catchers should always use a catcher's mitt.

- Wear a helmet, face mask, throat guard, long-model chest protector, protective supporter, and shin guards when catching behind the plate.

- Wear molded, cleated baseball shoes that fit properly.

- Inspect the playing field for holes, glass, and other debris.

- Be knowledgeable about first aid and be able to administer it for minor injuries, such as facial cuts, bruises, or minor tendonitis, strains, or sprains.

- Be prepared for emergency situations and have a plan to reach medical personnel to treat injuries such as CONCUSSIONS.

B. BASKETBALL SAFETY TIPS

Each year, more than 1.6 million basketball-related injuries are treated by doctors. The following tips can help athletes avoid some of the most common injuries.

- Always take time to warm up and stretch. Research studies have shown that cold muscles are more prone to injury. Warm up with jumping jacks, stationary cycling or running or walking in place for three to five minutes. Then slowly and gently stretch, holding each stretch for 30 seconds.

- Play only the position assigned and know where other players are on the court to reduce the chance of collisions. Don't hold, block, push, charge, or trip opponents. Use proper techniques for passing and scoring.

- Select basketball shoes that fit snugly, offer support, and are nonskid. Cotton socks can absorb perspiration and also give added support to the foot. Ankle supports can reduce the incidence of ankle sprains.

- Wear protective knee and elbow pads as protection from bruises and ABRASIONS.
- Use a mouth guard to protect teeth and mouth.
- For those who wear glasses, use safety glasses or glass guards to protect the eyes.
- Do not wear jewelry or chew gum during practice or games.
- Check outdoor courts to be certain they are free of rocks, holes, and other hazards. Inside courts should be clean, free of debris, and have good traction.
- Avoid playing outside in extreme weather conditions or on courts that are not properly lit after dark.
- Be sure that baskets and boundary lines are not too close to walls, bleachers, water fountains, or other structures.
- Be knowledgeable about first aid and be able to administer it for minor injuries, such as facial cuts, bruises, or minor tendonitis, strains, or sprains.
- Be prepared for emergency situations and have a plan to reach medical personnel to treat injuries such as CONCUSSIONS, dislocations, elbow contusions, wrist or finger sprains, and fractures.

C. BICYCLING SAFETY TIPS

The bicycle as it is known today has been around since the late 1800s. It was used first for recreation, and then quickly became an important mode of personal travel in many areas of the world. Its form changed little until demand-driven innovations began pouring out of the bicycle industry, enhancing a broader use and attracting a larger market of users. Disregarding the stationary bicycle, there remain three general categories of bikes.

CHOOSING THE RIGHT BIKE

Racing Bike
The road bike or "racing bike" consists of a diamond-shaped frame with gears. Because of road-racing rule restrictions, the basic design has changed little since its initial development. It features a tighter geometry

to enhance "stiffness" and a response to the energy imparted by the cyclist. This has been the prototype bought by most American consumers, but with a more aerodynamic forward-leaning body position and a relatively harsh ride, it has always been best accepted by the subset of riders interested in training and road racing.

Touring Bike
The touring bike is similar in design to the road bike, but has a more relaxed geometry for a comfortable ride, and more gear combinations to accommodate the long-distance touring cyclist possibly carrying baggage. The bike is generally somewhat heavier and has a third chain ring, or set of sprockets, at the pedal end of the chain; the freewheel or gear cluster on the hub of the rear wheel has often seven to eight gear selections.

Mountain Bike
The mountain bike, or more appropriately, the all-terrain bike makes up the third category of bikes. In its original conception, it was designed to be sturdy enough to climb up and plunge down rocky foot trails, but has become popular for even casual street riding because of the more upright body position, the multiple gear combinations similar to the touring bike, and the presence of comfortable front and, sometimes, rear shock absorbers. They are also available with less heavy-duty frames and tires that are better suited for the roads than for the trails.

With all of these variations, many people are discovering the enjoyment of riding for pleasure and exercise; however, the streets are not user-friendly for the biker. Cyclists must use proper bike-handling skills and a healthy dose of caution when they ride, since designated bike lanes and trails are still infrequent in most areas. Cycling skills are best mastered by riding with more experience cyclists; group rides are often organized or promoted by bike shops and can be a good opportunity to learn from more experienced riders.

Ensuring a Proper Fit
For personal comfort and injury prevention, it is important that cyclists select a bike that fits them well. The first consideration should be proper

frame size. Frame size is important because one's upper body should feel comfortable when leaning forward and grasping the handlebars. In addition, the size of the bike needs to match the length of the cyclist's legs. The seat should be adjusted so that when one leg is fully down and the foot is flat on the pedal, there is a 15 to 20 degree bend in the knee. If there is a question, err on the high side to protect the knees. When pedaling, the cyclist should be able to maintain a level pelvis. If there is rocking from side to side with pedal strokes, the seat must be lowered in small increments until that disappears. The staff at a local bike shop should be helpful in fitting a cyclist on a bike.

Special pedals with clip-in devices attached to the rider's shoes optimizes pedaling efficiency by generating power not only in the push-down phase but in the pull-up and transition phases as well. However, becoming comfortable while tethered to the bike usually takes some getting used to.

The handlebars most commonly seen on racing bikes have been the standard until recently when the more upright position permitted by the straight handlebar of the mountain bike became popular. This allows a more relaxed body position for the recreational rider and is often found to be easier on the back. Additional bar end extensions can give the rider a choice of hand positions. The most comfortable and efficient hand position will change with variations in terrain and incline. Newer handlebar designs for better aerodynamic position on the bike have become popular in triathlons and time trial bike races. However, with these aerobars one sacrifices some stability and quick response. Rearview mirrors have been attached to handlebars, helmets, and even eyeglasses, and remain very important in assessing the traffic, which may be developing behind when riding on the road.

Many training techniques can help maximize the use of a bike for fitness. It is important to acquire a sense of cadence. Learning to keep pedal speed with a certain range, despite the terrain, by using different gear combinations can minimize some of the injuries that come from "cranking." Riders will be best served by learning to maintain a pedal rate of 80 to 100 strokes per minute. For the beginning rider who is comfortable on a bike, trying to ride two to three times per week will help to build a base of training that can later be expanded with ease. Select a terrain and a pace that result in comfortable fatigue in 20 to 30 minutes of relatively steady riding then expand the riding time gradually to an hour or more depending on interest. This might satisfy a need for basic fitness, but if harder workouts are desired, develop at least a good two- to three-month base of riding before seeking out the hills and hard-pushed workouts. Though highly trained riders might ride up to 500 miles a week, both enjoyment and fitness can be gained on a fraction of this, and without nearly the risk of injury.

CYCLING ETIQUETTE AND SAFETY EQUIPMENT

The standard when biking on the road is to ride with the flow of traffic, not against it, and to stay to the right. Cyclists must obey the same rules of the road as those driving a car. This means stopping at all stop signs and stoplights, giving the appropriate turn signals, and following right-of-way rules.

The bicycle safety helmet has become standard since the data overwhelming supports its effectiveness in reducing injury. Two rating services, ANSI and Snell, approve helmets based on their safety performance, and cyclists should be careful to wear an approved helmet. Reflective vests and gear for bikes are critical for the safety of those choosing to ride in the early morning or late evening.

STATIONARY BIKES

Perhaps the most common bike for training purposes is the stationary bike. The necessity of fit on a stationary bike is just as important to injury prevention as it is on a road bike, but few people consider this seriously. To safely use the stationary bike, consider how the seat or saddle feels, whether the height can be adjusted appropriately, whether foot straps or toe clips can be added later if desired, and how smoothly the bike creates resistance as the pedals spin. Many people simply record the miles that they ride, but in reality a better gauge of effort is the combination of pedaling speed, time pedaled, and the amount of resistance. The manufacturers of the more expensive bikes provide these facts, and these bikes tend to be more durable over time.

When using the bike primarily for fitness, learn to monitor pulse rate at the wrist or neck. Those who are basically healthy and are not on medications that alter pulse rate should strive to maintain a pulse level between 60 and 80 percent of predicted maximum pulse rate. That number can be determined accurately by undergoing a maximum aerobic test under supervision. It can also be approximated by simply subtracting one's age in years from 220. The more efficient one becomes on the bike, the more effort will be required to maintain a heart rate in this range, thereby verifying the training effect of cycling.

PREVENTING INJURIES

The injuries that occur while cycling can be categorized into extrinsic injuries, such as those that occur from a fall, and intrinsic injuries, such as those that relate to overuse or overstress of a body part. Developing good bike handling skills, avoiding dangerous situations, and wearing the proper protective clothing are the best ways to avoid the extrinsic injuries.

The most common intrinsic injuries are those to the hands and knees. Sustained pressure on the palms from resting on the handlebars can cause an injury to either the median or ulnar nerves of the hands. The earliest perception of this is a tingling or numbness. This injury can be averted by using bike gloves, which now are generously padded, and by frequently changing hand position on the handlebars.

Knee injuries are best avoided by proper seat height. However, if the knee is a problem in spite of proper seat height, consider the foot position on the pedal (usually toeing in slightly will help with this). It also helps to concentrate on spinning rather than pushing down hard with each revolution. This is not natural, but rather a learned skill and will require some discipline initially. There are few intrinsic injuries that result in permanent damage, but it is not worth pushing through pain. Find a local sports physician who is knowledgeable about cycling. It is a great sport for fitness, and a special enjoyment comes from knowing one is riding the most efficient machine yet devised by humans.

Other common injuries include the following:

- a degeneration of cartilage behind the kneecap, called chondromalacia, caused by using inappropriately high gears or by overextending the knee because a seat is too high
- ACHILLES TENDONITIS caused by side-to-side movement of the ankle or by simple overexertion
- muscle strains in the hamstrings, quadriceps, and lower back

Important injury prevention tips include:

- wearing a helmet and other protective gear as necessary
- proper stretching, especially for the back, Achilles tendon, and hamstring
- shifting hand and back positions frequently while riding
- STRENGTH TRAINING to develop the muscle strength necessary to handle the demands of the sport
- following a conditioning program that allows for gradual increases in mileage and intensity of workouts

D. GYMNASTICS SAFETY TIPS

Doctors treat more than 86,000 gymnastics-related injuries each year. Following are some guidelines for avoiding the most common injuries.

- Always take time to warm up and stretch. Research studies have shown that cold muscles are more prone to injury. Warm up with jumping jacks, stationary cycling or running or walking in place for three to five minutes. Then slowly and gently stretch, holding each stretch for 30 seconds.
- Always spot gymnasts and be sure to be spotted when performing complex routines.
- Check the equipment to make sure it is properly maintained.
- Arrange equipment to avoid the accidental collision of gymnasts with equipment or other athletes during workouts.
- Be sure the training facility has appropriate floor padding to help reduce the force from a landing.
- Check to make sure that mats are placed under the equipment and secured properly.

- Be knowledgeable about first aid and be able to administer it for minor injuries, such as facial cuts, bruises, or minor tendonitis, strains, or sprains.
- Be prepared for emergency situations and have a plan to reach medical personnel to treat injuries such as CONCUSSIONS, dislocations, elbow contusions, wrist or finger sprains, and fractures.

E. RUNNING SAFETY TIPS

Aerobic exercise has become one of the most popular forms of endurance training today. In the United States, running and jogging are the most popular forms of aerobic exercise, with an estimated 15 percent of the American population participating in running, jogging, or walking exercise on a regular basis.

The aim of aerobic conditioning is to improve the function and efficiency of the cardiovascular system. To be effective, exercise must be at a pace great enough to reach 75 to 80 percent of one's maximum heart rate and continued for least 25 minutes. It is not necessary to exercise every day to obtain the maximum aerobic effect. Three to four time per week is sufficient.

Benefits of regular running and jogging include prevention or postponement of coronary disease, personal gratification and enjoyment, and enhanced appearance due to increased muscle tone and loss of excess weight, which sometimes accompanies a regular program of running or jogging. In addition, running is a low-cost sport, requiring only a good pair of shoes.

Causes of Running Injuries

An unfortunate by-product of this increased interest in running has been an increase in the number of injuries that result primarily from inadequate shoes, training errors, poor conditioning, and anatomic abnormalities that predispose the runner to certain injuries. The vast majority of running-related injuries can be prevented with adherence to the following guidelines.

Shoes

An appropriate running shoe is very important in training and may help prevent running injuries. Shoes should provide shock absorption, motion control, and stability for the runner. When selecting a running shoe, the athlete should look for a style that will provide all of the above benefits as well as fit comfortably. Fortunately, all of the major brands make a shoe appropriate for the vast majority of runners.

Laboratory studies that analyzed an athlete's gait (pattern of walking or running) have determined that during running on level surfaces, the forces exerted on the lower extremities are two to three times body weight. Under this heavy pounding, shoes will lose approximately 60 percent or more of their shock absorption capability after 250 to 500 miles of use. A runner who puts in 10 miles per week, therefore, should consider buying new shoes after nine to 12 months. When a shoe's mileage exceeds 500 to 600 miles, it should be discarded for running purposes. Resoling will not revitalize the "dead" shoe. Sole wear should also be checked regularly because it can be an indicator of other problems.

Training Errors

Too much, too fast, too soon, and too little rest appear to be the hallmarks of training errors. Every runner has a physiologic limit, and trying to exceed that limit can lead to injury. The mileage one runs should be gradually increased, on an individual basis. A good rule of thumb is to increase mileage no more than 10 percent per week. Overall, injuries are most likely to occur in one or more of the following situations:

- running too far without adequate stretching
- increasing distances too quickly
- increasing hill training too quickly
- beginning interval training too abruptly (going from slow speeds over long distances to fast speeds covering less ground)
- allowing insufficient rest between training sessions

Anatomic Abnormalities

Preexisting structural or biomechanical problems such as a high foot arch, a limb length discrepancy, scoliosis (curvature of the spine), or excessive muscle tightness may increase a runner's susceptibility to injury during intense training. The athlete can compensate for these abnormalities by following special training guidelines, incorporating a stretching regimen into the conditioning program, and using semi-rigid orthotics, or shoe inserts. Following are some common physical abnormalities that can lead to running injuries.

Joint instability in the ankle can lead to frequent ankle sprains and pain. Beneficial treatment includes muscle strengthening to increase stability, shoe modification to alter gait, and change of a running surface.

Knee joint and kneecap injuries are common sites of overuse injuries. A 20-minute ice massage to the involved area, stretching of the hamstring and quadriceps muscles, a program of strengthening exercises, and a short course of an over-the-counter anti-inflammatory medication may also be added.

Foot problems in runners are related to foot types. Nonoperative treatment such as orthotics and shoe modifications should be used if necessary.

Hip and back injuries account for a smaller but growing number of running injuries and should be treated on an individual basis.

Environmental Factors

Running is a flexible exercise that can be done anywhere and anytime. However, the runner is often faced with a variety of environmental factors—such as terrain, altitude, temperature, and air quality—that can adversely affect performance and physical health.

The same runner will recognize potential environmental problems and make adjustments in training routines, terrain, clothing, and fluid intake to reduce the risk of injury.

In choosing a place to run, keep in mind that the ideal surface for running is flat, smooth, resilient, and reasonably soft. Avoid concrete or rough road surfaces. If possible, use community trails that have been developed specifically for jogging and running; they usually have the appropriate surface and are isolated from vehicular traffic and poor air quality.

Hills should be avoided at first because of the increased stress placed on joints and muscles. The ankle and foot are stressed most by running uphill, while downhill running stresses the knee and lower leg. For the competitive runner, hills often

cannot be avoided, so care should be taken when running on such terrain.

Temperature variation, air quality, and altitude are significant environmental factors affecting the runner. During warmer, humid weather, take care to increase fluid intake, and in cool weather, dress appropriately. It is often helpful to be weighed before and after running on a hot, humid day. One pint of water should be consumed for every pound of weight lost. Avoid running during temperature extremes—both hot and cold—or when the air pollution levels are high. The entire body is stressed by exercising in these conditions, and the risk of injury is increased. When running at higher altitudes, the runner should gradually acclimate to the lower oxygen levels by slow, steady increases in speed and distance.

Common Running and Jogging Injuries

Following are abbreviated descriptions of some of the most common running injuries. See the complete entries on these injuries in the main body of the book.

METATARSALGIA—Pain in the region of the five long bones (metatarsals) of the foot (ball of the foot). Its causes may be excessive pressure on the ball of the foot, abnormality in foot type or metatarsal phalangeal joint, and stress fractures. Treatment includes use of orthotics if necessary, activity modification, and change to a softer running surface.

PLANTAR FASCITIS—Inflammation of the fibrous connective tissue of the sole of the foot. It is a common cause of low-grade, insidious heel pain. Treatment consists of activity modification, nonsteroidal anti-inflammatory medications, stretching exercises to the heel and foot, ice massage, and use of a soft heel pad.

POSTERIOR TIBIAL TENDONITIS—Inflammation of the tendon behind the inner heel. Treatment consists of activity modification, ice massage, aspirin, and, occasionally, shoe appliance.

STRESS FRACTURE—A complete or incomplete hairline break in a foot bone resulting from abnormal stress to normal bone. It usually occurs in the heel and forefoot/midfoot bones and results from fatigue or stress produced by frequent, repeated physical activity (overuse). It constitutes 10 percent or more of all running injures. Treatment consists of rest or immobilization. Running should be resumed gradually after four to six weeks.

Back

Lumboscral strain—Abnormal strain of the lower back muscles. This condition produces pain, spasms, and tenderness in the lower back. It can be relieved by rest, stretching, and ice massage.

SCIATICA—Sharp, burning pain and numbness that radiates down the sciatic nerve into the buttock and down the back of the leg. It may indicate a ruptured disk and should be evaluated and treated promptly by a physician.

Spinal stenosis—Gradual narrowing of the spinal canal in the lower back causing back and hip pain particularly in the older runner. Lying down usually relieves the symptoms within minutes. It can be treated by activity modification and stretching. Occasionally, cortisone injections or surgery are required for the condition.

Knee

PATELLOFEMORAL PAIN SYNDROME—As one of the most common injuries that affect runners, it centers on the kneecap (patella). Its onset is usually insidious and related to increased mileage, a change in terrain, or a change in running shoe. Treatment consists of anti-inflammatory medication, alteration in running terrain (avoidance of hills), and strengthening exercises for the quadriceps muscles (the four divisions of muscles at the front of the thigh).

Tendonitis of the knee—Inflammation resulting in pain and tenderness in one of the tendons surrounding the knee. Tendonitis is usually caused by overuse. Treatment includes rest until the acute symptoms subside, icing, stretching, and anti-inflammatory medication. The conditions can become chronic if not treated.

Leg

ACHILLES TENDONITIS—Inflammation of the heel tendon producing pain and tightness in the calf of the leg is caused by repetitive overuse of the Achilles tendon typically from running up hills. The condition may become incapacitating particularly to the competitive athlete. Treatment includes rest until acute inflammation subsides, Achilles stretching, ice massage, anti-inflammatory medication, and shoe appliance such as heel lifts to relieve tension on the tendon.

COMPARTMENT SYNDROME—Caused by overuse of leg muscles resulting in decreased blood supply to a particular group (compartment) of muscles. Treatment consists of rest or, in severe cases, surgery to relieve the pressure constricting the leg muscles.

Medial tibial stress syndrome (SHIN SPLINTS)—Pain in the lower leg due to inflammation of the lining surrounding the shinbone. This is usually caused by an imbalance in calf muscle strength. Treatment consists of discontinuing exercise until the athlete is able to resume without pain, icing of the affected area, stretching, and occasionally taping of the leg to relieve tension on the lining of the bone.

STRESS FRACTURE—A complete or incomplete hairline break in the fibula or tibia. It results in localized pain over the affected bone. Treatment includes activity modification, use of an orthotic with a stirrup or possible immobilization with a cast or brace. Gradual return to running or jogging, after four to six weeks, will allow the fracture to heal.

Thigh and Pelvis

BURSITIS—Inflammation of a bursa (fluid-filled sac between a tendon or muscle and a bony prominence) of the side of the hip. Bursitis occurs when a bursa becomes inflamed as result of chronic, repetitive use. Treatment includes rest until acute symptoms subside, icing, and anti-inflammatory medication.

HAMSTRING TENDONITIS—Pain, tenderness, and swelling in the hamstring muscle in the back of the thigh. Treatment consists of rest, ice massage, and non-steroidal anti-inflammatory medication.

Guidelines for Managing Running Injuries

General guidelines.   The basic principle of treatment for running injuries includes rest or modification of activity to allow healing and reduction of inflammation. A gradual return to running (10 percent increase in mileage per week) can be allowed after flexibility, strength, and endurance have returned.

Mild Injuries

Minimal pain occurs at onset or during running and decreases as running progresses. There is no limitation of motion. Stretching, reducing mileage, and icing can manage this type of injury.

Moderate Injuries

Moderate pain is present throughout the running session or occurs just after running starts. This type of injury can often be managed by activity modification and use of anti-inflammatory medication.

Severe Injuries

Severe pain, swelling, loss of motion, and/or alterations in running form are indicative of more significant injuries. Immediate medical treatment is advised.

Rehabilitation

There are no definite guidelines for determining when an athlete may resume activity following an injury. However, runners should remember that there are four periods of time when they are most likely to break down:

- during the initial four to six months of running
- upon returning to running after an injury
- when the quantity of running is increased (distance)
- when the quality of running is increased (speed or terrain)

The goal of rehabilitation of injuries suffered by runners and joggers is to return safely to the desired level of running. Remember, training errors constitute the most common cause of injuries. A well-planned program prevents injury while benefiting the athlete.

F. SKIING SAFETY TIPS

The sport of alpine skiing continues to grow in popularity. People of all skill levels—from expert to beginner, from highly conditioned athlete to the physically challenged—enjoy snow skiing.

Despite vastly improved equipment, stronger training regiments, and better skiing facilities, skiers continue to suffer injuries. Most of these injuries occur as a result of falls or collisions. However, hypothermia can also cause injury, especially when skiers fail to take the proper precautions while skiing in severely cold weather.

The majority of ski injuries are preventable, and the following guidelines are designed to help skiers understand the risks and to take steps to avoid situations that often lead to injury. The causes of skiing injuries can be grouped into the following categories:

Experience and Ability

Skiers with more experience seem to suffer few injuries.

Perhaps the single most important factor affecting ski injury rate is skier ability. Less-skilled skiers suffer more injuries than advanced skiers. Ski lessons are the best tool for improving skiing techniques as rapidly as is practical. With increased ability, the number of falls decrease, improving skiing pleasure as well as safety. Ski lessons are also strongly recommended for anyone returning to the slopes after recovering from an injury. This is especially true after knee anterior cruciate ligament (ACL) reconstruction. Lessons can help build not only strength and endurance, but also overall confidence.

There is widespread evidence, however, that unless ski lessons are combined with lots of practice time, there will be no improvement in skiing safety. If inexperienced skiers learn too rapidly, they may be overconfident and attempt skiing terrain that is more difficult than they would otherwise attempt until much later.

Therefore, relatively inexperienced skiers should avoid skiing too long (especially on difficult terrain) and in poor snow conditions.

Ski Equipment

The type of ski bindings have a direct effect on the overall injury rate in skiers.

During the past several years many sports medicine researchers have observed a significant reduction in binding-related injuries. This type of injury occurs when the ski binding fails to release properly or releases at the wrong time. Evidence shows that better function of ski-boot binding systems is the single most important factor contributing to this favorable trend. However, nearly 50 percent of all injuries remain related to improper binding performance. Thus, the binding is the single most important piece of equipment in terms of safety. The binding is designed to release before reaching the point where stresses are passed from the ski through the binding and boot to the leg where an injury can occur. It should not, however, release under normal forces that are generated by skiers as they maneuver to control their skis.

In theory, this goal seems quite simple. In practice, it becomes quite difficult. When designing the binding, the manufacturer must decide in which direction the binding should release. The choice may be to achieve multidirectional release, so that the binding will release in any direction the skier might fall. Unfortunately, the more flexibility desired, the more difficult it is to construct a binding that will consistently hold the ski and boot together during normal skiing maneuvers.

Most manufacturers opt to produce bindings with a side-to-side, or twist, release capability at the toe and a forward-lean mechanism at the heel. Most falls result in forces that allow this release system to protect the leg. However, backward falls and those requiring twists at the heel, and rolls from the top of the ski, will still produce injuries with this type of binding.

A few bindings incorporate several of these modes, but they are sometimes criticized for their tendency to release inadvertently. However, when a binding of this type is correctly mounted, set, and maintained, it is not very likely to release in unwanted situations.

Choosing the right binding. The first decision skiers make when picking out ski equipment is which type of binding to use. Beginners who tend to fall frequently should consider choosing bindings that release in as many directions as possible. Those who have previously sustained lower leg injuries should also choose this type of multi-mode release binding, especially in the case of a

knee ligament sprain. The multidirectional release binding will have a good chance of releasing no matter which way a skier falls.

Whether a multidirectional release binding or some other type, most recent models of all major brand bindings are markedly improved over those of the past. These newer bindings are mounted, maintained, and functionally tested with machines capable of measuring force and movements that could result in injury. For this reason, skiers should avoid old or used equipment; it is not only outdated in mechanical design, but it often has been poorly maintained.

Once a skier has purchased equipment, it is important to keep it maintained from season to season. Binding function changes with time and wear, and it is advisable to have a complete mechanical check by a reliable ski shop at least once before each ski season begins. An active skier may need more frequent evaluations.

Cleaning equipment is also important to preventing injury. Avoid wearing ski boots on surfaces other than snow. Dirt, mud, and sand ground into the sole increase friction and, with wear, may alter the shape of the boot and impair proper binding function.

Skiers should get in the habit of performing self-release checks on their bindings each day before heading to the slopes. The skier should test the binding by doing slow twisting and leaning motions, using muscle control instead of sudden thrusts, to force the binding to release. If the skier feels leg pain before the binding releases, then the binding needs to be adjusted before skiing. Such self-release checks confirm that the binding mechanism is not jammed and that the release settings have not varied.

Skiers should also avoid setting their bindings tighter if they experience a premature release of the binding. This can greatly increase the risk of injury since usually a premature release occurs because of incompatibility between the boot and binding, poor binding design, mechanical failure of the binding, or failure to clear snow, ice, or mud from the boot or binding. Premature releases rarely occur due to the binding being set too low.

Boots. Boots also play a role in safe skiing. Skiers need to be aware of a few simple guidelines in order to choose boots that provide reasonable safety. Boots should be comfortable enough to be worn for long periods of time. If pressure points develop while skiing, it is best to go to the ski shop and see if someone can help adjust the boot to fit better. Ski shop experts may be able to provide inserts or make a custom orthotic to help the boot fit better. Loosening the boot to relieve the pressure may result in a boot that is too loose to allow proper control of the skis.

Skis. Beginning skiers may want to use skis with ski brakes. They should also use relatively short skis, since they are easier to control than longer ones. In addition, skiers need to be aware that the ski's sharp edge causes between 7 and 15 percent of all skiing injuries in the form of lacerations, mainly to the head and face.

Ski poles. Ski poles contribute to the most common upper body injury suffered by skiers—skier's thumb. This injury, which involves strained or torn ligaments in the thumb, occurs most often when a skier takes a fall and lands on the thumb because the hand is attached to the ski pole and cannot be easily released.

One way to reduce the risk of thumb injury is to avoid placing hands through the straps of the ski pole so that poles can be easily discarded during a fall.

Ski clothing. Ski clothing is important for its role in helping to prevent injury from exposure to the cold. Hypothermia and frostbite can occur while skiing, so it is important to dress appropriately for the conditions.

Sex

Female skiers have a greater tendency toward lower extremity injuries than males. They also have more knee injuries.

Age

Younger skiers are more likely to be injured than older skiers, but they receive fewer serious knee injuries.

Fatigue

Skiing for too long a time increases vulnerability to injury.

Although sports medicine physicians have no direct evidence that good conditioning through preseason training programs prevents injury, it is reasonable to consider that well-trained recreational skiers are less likely to sustain injury than those who tire significantly during the course of a skiing day. Many injuries occur later in the day when fatigue sets in. Many injured skiers admit that they noted fatigue, but wanted one "last run." It's best to listen to the body and stop sooner rather than later.

Skiing requires sustained muscle contractions; quick bursts or powerful but finely coordinated muscle contractions; general flexibility; and cardiopulmonary fitness. Ideally conditioning programs should be year-round. At a minimum, one should begin conditioning at least eight to 12 weeks before the ski season begins.

To meet the physical challenges required of alpine skiing and to reduce the chance of injury, a well-rounded training plan should be followed; such a plan would include endurance work (jogging, biking, cross-country skiing, or swimming) as well as cardiovascular and STRENGTH TRAINING, as well as proper nutrition and hydration. Also, a regular program of stretching will improve FLEXIBILITY and joint range of motion.

Even well-conditioned skiers may have difficulty when skiing at higher altitudes. Care should be taken especially on the first few days at a higher altitude. It is important to decrease the intensity and duration of skiing, to remain well hydrated, and to minimize alcohol intake.

To develop an appropriate conditioning program, consult a sports medicine physician or an athletic trainer. Popular ski magazines often feature preseason-training programs.

Snow Conditions

The type of snow conditions do have a bearing on lower extremity injuries. Ice decreases the incidence of these injuries while packed powder leads to an increase in lower leg injuries.

Skier Attitudes

This is an intangible factor in ski injuries. Skiing attracts people who find the risk exhilarating and who are looking to constantly challenge their abilities. Although skiers of this type tend to be highly skilled, they can still have accidents, and when they do, the injuries sustained tend to be worse than those sustained by less-aggressive skiers.

At the other end of the spectrum are those skiers who are intimidated by the challenge and consequently ski with excess caution, resulting in slow-speed falls that rarely cause the bindings to release. Failure of the binding to release can be the cause of injuries for these skiers.

For all skiers, exercising common sense when judging conditions and being alert and in control when skiing contribute greatly to safety.

G. SOCCER SAFETY TIPS

Each year, more than 477,500 soccer-related injuries are treated by doctors. The following tips are designed to help soccer players avoid some of the most common causes of injury.

- Always take time to warm up and stretch. Research studies have shown that cold muscles are more prone to injury. Warm up with jumping jacks, stationary cycling or running or walking in place for three to five minutes. Then slowly and gently stretch, holding each stretch for 30 seconds.

- Wear shin guards to help protect the lower legs. Soccer tournament records have shown that most players who sustained lower leg injuries were not protected by adequate shin guards.

- Wear shoes with molded cleats or ribbed soles. Shoes with screw-in cleats often are associated with a higher risk of injury. However, shoes with screw-in cleats should be worn when more traction is needed, such as on a wet field with high grass.

- Use synthetic, nonabsorbent balls on wet playing fields. Leather balls can become waterlogged and very heavy when wet, putting players at high risk for injury.

- Do not crawl or sit on the goal or hang from the net. Injuries and deaths have occurred when goals have fallen onto players.

- Make sure soccer goals are well padded and properly secured. Padding the goal decreases the incidence of head injuries when the goalie and other team members collide with the posts.

- Check to be sure the playing surface is kept in good condition. Holes on the playing field should be filled, bare spots reseeded, and debris removed.

- Be knowledgeable about first aid and be able to administer it for minor injuries, such as facial cuts, bruises, or minor tendonitis, strains, or sprains.

- Be prepared for emergency situations and have a plan to reach medical personnel to treat injuries such as CONCUSSIONS, dislocations, elbow contusions, wrist or finger sprains, and fractures.

H. SWIMMING SAFETY TIPS

Almost 150,000 swimming-related injuries are treated by doctors each year. The following tips will help swimmers avoid some of the most common hazards and injuries.

- Always take time to warm up and stretch. Research studies have shown that cold muscles are more prone to injury. Warm up with jumping jacks, stationary cycling or running or walking in place for three to five minutes. Then slowly and gently stretch, holding each stretch for 30 seconds.

- Learn how to swim and do not swim alone. Swim in supervised areas where lifeguards are present. Inexperienced swimmers should wear lifejackets in the water.

- Do not attempt to swim if too tired, too cold, or overheated.

- Avoid diving into shallow water. Each year approximately 1,000 disabling neck and back injuries occur after people go headfirst into water that is shallow or too murky to see objects.

- Swim in a pool only if the bottom at the deepest point is visible; check the shape of the full diving area to make sure it is deep enough.

- Dive only off the end of a diving board. Do not run on the board, try to dive far out, or bounce more than once. Swim away from the board immediately after the dive, to allow room for the next diver. Make sure there is only one person on the board at a time.

- Never run and enter the waves headfirst when swimming in open water. Make sure the water is free of undercurrents and other hazards.

- Do not swim in a lake or river after a storm if the water seems to be rising or if there is flooding because currents may become strong. The clarity and depth of the water may have changed, and new hazards may be present.

- Check weather reports before going swimming to avoid being in the water during storms, fog, or high winds. Because water conducts electricity, being in the water during an electrical storm is dangerous.

- Remember that alcohol and water do not mix. Alcohol affects not only judgment, but it slows movement and impairs vision. It can reduce swimming skills and make it harder to stay warm.

- Be knowledgeable about first aid and be able to administer it for minor injuries, such as facial cuts, bruises, or minor tendonitis, strains, or sprains.

- Be prepared for emergency situations and have a plan to reach medical personnel to treat injuries such as CONCUSSIONS, dislocations, elbow contusions, wrist or finger sprains, and fractures.

I. VOLLEYBALL SAFETY TIPS

More than 187,000 volleyball-related injuries are treated by doctors each year. The following tips are designed to help volleyball players avoid some of the most common injuries in the sport.

- Always take time to warm up and stretch. Research studies have shown that cold muscles are more prone to injury. Warm up with jumping jacks, stationary cycling or running or walking in place for three to five minutes. Then slowly and gently stretch, holding each stretch for 30 seconds.

- Use knee pads to prevent injury when falling or diving onto the court.

- Wear defensive pants, which are padded from hip to knee, to prevent floor burns and bruises.

- Wear lightweight shoes that provide strong ankle and arch support and offer good shock absorption.

- Be sure the volleyball court has at least 23 feet of overhead clearance. Objects such as portable basketball goals, lighting fixtures, and tree limbs should be cleared from the space above the court.

- Check to make sure that wires supporting the net are covered with soft material.

- Do not grab the net or hang onto supports, which can cause the net to overturn and fall.

- "Call" the ball to reduce the chance of colliding with another player.

- Be knowledgeable about first aid and be able to administer it for minor injuries, such as facial cuts, bruises, or minor tendonitis, strains, or sprains.

- Be prepared for emergency situations and have a plan to reach medical personnel to treat injuries such as CONCUSSIONS, dislocations, elbow contusions, wrist or finger sprains, and fractures.

- Before playing an outdoor volleyball game, always check the ground for sharp objects and glass.

J. WRESTLING SAFETY TIPS

Wrestling is one of the world's oldest sports and is offered at various levels of competition, including the Olympics, the American Athletic Union, the U.S. Wrestling Federation, and high school and college-sponsored tournaments. Although it is often associated with big burly physiques, wrestling is a sport for people of all sizes. Competition rules require that athletes be paired against one another according to their weight class. Some competitions require that contestants be matched by age, experience, and/or gender. This not only allows more people to participate but also decreases the risk for injury. Nevertheless, injuries do occur during the course of a wrestling season. The knee, shoulder, skin, and head are particularly at risk.

Common Wrestling Injuries
The face and head are the most common areas injured during wrestling. However, knee injuries occur with more severity than all other frequent injuries and are responsible for the most lost time,

surgeries, and treatments. Specifically, pre-patella bursitis and ligament sprains are among the most common injuries.

Pre-patella bursitis occurs as a result of the nature of the sport. Since two-thirds of an average wrestling match is spent with the athlete down on the mat on the knees, the bursas around the kneecaps can become inflamed. Once pre-patella bursitis has occurred, it is best treated by anti-inflammatory medication, rest, and knee pads.

Collateral ligament injuries can occur to the inside or outside of the knee. These injuries are the result of a stress to the knee that causes strain on the ligament. These strains vary in severity. First-degree strains can be treated with RICE (rest, ice, compression, and elevation) and the athlete can return to wrestling when the pain subsides. Second- and third-degree strains need to be treated by a physician, but they rarely need surgical intervention. ANTERIOR CRUCIATE LIGAMENT (ACL) strains are injuries that cause instability of the knee, and in most cases require surgery for the athlete to compete at the same level. The wrestler can expect to return to competition in six to nine months after this surgery.

Bruises and scrapes are common to all sports, especially contact sports. In wrestling, they are especially prevalent because of the constant rubbing of a competitor's skin against the mat or an opponent. In no other contact sport is so much skin exposed.

Skin-to-skin contact can also result in skin infections. Epidemics of skin infections have been known to spread through a team and from one team to another. The three most common infections contracted by wrestlers are herpes simplex, ringworm, and impetigo. The best way to prevent such infections is to maintain high standards of cleanliness. Thorough showers both before and after practices and matches should be routine. Clean clothing should be worn at every practice session, and the mats should be washed with antiseptic solution after each practice.

If an infection does develop, a doctor should treat it promptly. To prevent infecting other team members, the infected athlete should not practice with them until the infection is cleared up. Wrestlers may continue to drill or participate in conditioning workouts but should avoid bodily contact until the infection is resolved.

Weight Control
Wrestlers are also at risk of developing injuries that result from improper methods of attempting to control their weight. Extreme tactics of weight reduction, such as utilizing rubber suits and a sauna to sweat off weight, pose a health hazard to the wrestler and definitely weaken the wrestler just before a match. Severe DEHYDRATION and food deprivation diminish muscle strength and endurance, leading to a weakened physical condition. Entering a bout under these conditions will make wrestlers more susceptible to injury as they tire and more susceptible to illnesses such as the common cold. The practice of "making weight" through food deprivation and then overeating, with weight swings of 10 pounds or more, also weakens the body and deprives it of necessary energy at crucial times.

Injury Treatment
An injury, no matter how trivial, should be treated as soon as possible. A small cut or scrape may not be of much consequence in hockey, football, or track athletes, but even a minor infection can keep a wrestler out of a match. Any injury should be reported to the coach, trainer, or personal physician as soon as possible so that proper care can be started. Rehabilitation after an injury is an important part of preventing further injury, since a large number of all injuries result from aggravation of an old injury.

Injury Prevention
Prevention of injuries should be a primary goal of all participants, coaches, and trainers. This requires using good-quality equipment, including mats, uniforms, headgear, and pads. It also requires adequate room for practice and competition. The wrestler should be coached and supervised at all times, with emphasis placed on using proper technique and discipline to avoid injury. Proper officiating can also do much to prevent injuries. Finally, a well-structured strengthening program conducted under proper supervision will also do much to prevent injury and enhance the athlete's performance.

the freezer or fridge for the busy days. Players will appreciate coming home after a tiring game or practice and being able to zap up a meal in minutes.

- A household of young players without cooking skills is a high-risk situation for nutritional problems. Consider the services of a sports dietitian to arrange supermarket tours and cooking lessons.
- When energy needs are high, increase the frequency of meals and snacks, rather than trying to overeat at a few meals. This means being organized to have snacks available throughout the day. Things that can be carried around and eaten throughout the day include cereal bars, fruit, dried fruit and nut mixes, and muffins. If refrigeration is available, the options can expand to include yogurts, flavored milks, prepacked sandwiches, or a bowl of breakfast cereal and milk.
- Action-packed drinks such as fruit smoothies, liquid meal supplements, and sports drinks provide a low-bulk carbohydrate and energy boost.
- If games or practices are scheduled for late at night, make sure the meal plan for the day takes account of this. To stick with the tradition of having the main meal at night, have it prepared before the game or practice so that it can be ready within minutes of arriving home. Although it is important to refuel and recover after the workout, many people feel uncomfortable going to sleep on a very full stomach. An alternative is to restructure the day to make lunch the main meal, and then refuel after the session with a lighter meal or snack before going to bed.

Iron status.   Iron is an important nutrient for growth. Impact against other players or the floor may increase iron losses through increased red blood cell destruction. Some players may have problems with low iron status, especially females with low iron intakes. Iron levels should be checked regularly when in heavy training. Iron-rich foods such as lean red meat and breakfast cereals fortified with iron should be included regularly in the diet. Iron-rich plant foods such as wholegrain cereals, spinach, and legumes should

be combined with animal iron sources (e.g. whole wheat pasta and meat sauce) or vitamin C sources (a glass of juice consumed with breakfast cereal) to improve iron absorption. A sports dietitian will be able to provide specific dietary help.

The pre-event meal.   The pregame meal should fuel and hydrate players, but leave them feeling comfortable for the game. Ideally, the menu calls for a high-carbohydrate meal eaten at least two to three hours before a game. Pasta with low-fat sauces, rolls or sandwiches, baked potatoes with low-fat fillings, creamed rice, and fruit salad with yogurt, are all examples of suitable choices. Each player should experiment to find the routines that work best for his or her situation.

Fluids during training and games.   High-intensity exercise in a controlled atmosphere stadium can lead to dehydration through sweat loss—especially in large players. The good news is that basketball offers plenty of opportunities to hydrate during the game—time-outs, half-time breaks, and time spent on the bench. Coaches should also organize frequent drink breaks during practice. Players should have their own drink bottle courtside, so that they can keep track of how much they are drinking. In professional teams, the job of refilling bottles is often left to the team manager or other support staff member. Water is a suitable fluid, but a sports drink may promote better performance by topping up fuel stores for both the muscle and brain. Remember that basketball is not only a game of high-intensity running, but of skill, concentration and decision making. These last factors are impaired both by dehydration and lowering of blood glucose levels. Sports drinks top up carbohydrate needs during the game, but may also encourage players to drink more fluid.

Note that fluid losses are still high during winter sessions when it is chilly outside and many players do not think they need to bring a drink. Remember that the stadium is kept warmer than the outside conditions, and the players are working hard and producing their own heat. In addition, some players drink well without much encouragement; others need to be constantly reminded.

Postgame recovery. Effective recovery begins with the intake of fluid, carbohydrate, and other important nutrients. Left to chance, recovery eating may take a back seat to the postgame meetings, stretching and injury treatment, drug testing, media interviews, or the trip back to home or the team hotel. Many teams organize postgame recovery snacks that can be consumed simultaneously with these activities—sports drinks, liquid meal supplements, fruit, sandwiches, and cereal bars are some of the many quick options. Depending on the time of the game and the athlete's appetite, this postgame snack may be supplemented by a later meal.

Tournament nutrition and road trips.   As soon as the match schedule is known, plan a meal routine that schedules appropriate pre-event meals and recovery strategies. When several games are played in succession over as many days, proactive recovery techniques will be important in maintaining performance right through the end of the schedule. When playing away from home, plan where meals will be eaten, and organize the menus in advance. Similarly, take control of meals eaten on planes, buses, and other travel options. Always carry some high-carbohydrate snacks such as cereal bars, fruit, and yogurt for emergencies.

The following tips may help when traveling:

- Be clear about nutritional goals and stay committed while traveling.

- Do some investigation to find out what to expect upon arrival.

- Plan accommodations with meals in mind. Organizing an apartment with cooking facilities offers more control over meals and can keep food costs down. Those who choose not to cook should make sure the accommodation is conveniently located near shops and restaurants.

- Take a supply of snacks along to always have access to something suitable. Cereal bars, sports drinks, breakfast cereal, and rice cakes are good options to pack.

- Make good choices in restaurants. Beware of hidden fat in restaurant meals. Do not be afraid to ask the waiter about cooking methods and ingredients and request changes if necessary. Add carbohydrate to meals with plain bread, plain rice, and fruit or juice if necessary.

B. NUTRITION FOR CYCLISTS

Characteristics of the Sport

Road cycling involves both team and individual events. Races may be held over a number of stages or as single days. Other events include time trials (both team and individual) and criteriums (a race of varying number of laps around a circuit of roads). Races vary in distance from a few kilometers for some criteriums, to individual stages of 250 kilometers or more. Road cycling primarily requires strength and endurance, although anaerobic capacity may be called upon in breakaways, hill climbing, and all-out sprints to the line. Cycling is a sport that is heavily influenced by folklore. It is common to hear of cyclists adopting quite bizarre nutrition practices based on anecdotal evidence and hearsay.

Training.   Road cyclists do most of their training on the road, and training distances vary with the time of the year. At the elite level, training involves at least daily sessions, with weekly distances tallying 400 to 1,000 kilometers. Wind-trainer sessions and weights may also be included. Even at the recreational level, cyclists often undertake a serious commitment to training. Distances of 300 kilometers per week are common for a committed recreational rider.

Competition.   At the height of the elite season, cyclists race almost daily, leaving little time for training. Serious recreational cyclists tend to race one to two times per week. Occasionally, two to three day tours are scheduled. Road cycling is physically and nutritionally challenging. Meeting fuel and fluid needs becomes increasingly difficult as the duration of races increases. Elite cycling is very technical, and teams utilize a system of support vehicles to ferry food and fluid to team riders. At the recreational level, riders usually have to carry their own supplies from the start of the race or rely on friends or family to provide support along the way.

event and then by another 50 percent over the last three days.

- Consume eight to 10 grams of carbohydrate per kilogram body weight for the 72-hour taper period.

- Be extra careful with fat intake. This is not an excuse to binge. Overconsumption of food may cause gastric problems in the short term and weight gain in the long term.

Multistage races—the challenge of recovery. Some cycling events require days of successive riding with individual stages around 200 kilometers or longer. These events place enormous stress on the fuel and fluid reserves of athletes. Riders need to look after needs during each race and undertake strategies to assist recovery between days. Recovery of fuel stores is enhanced when a snack that provides carbohydrate and other nutrients such as protein and vitamins is consumed immediately after exercise. If there is more than an hour before the next meal, choose from the following options:

C. NUTRITION FOR GOLFERS

Characteristics of the Sport

Golf is a game of skill, which can be played at a number of levels from the weekend hacker to the professional. Competitive golf is played at both amateur and professional levels. Golfers can turn professional either through an apprenticeship or by attending player's school. Some professional golfers become attached to golf associations and concentrate on providing golf tuition and running golf clubs. Others spend their time competing on the professional circuit.

Training. Recreational golfers practice their golf simply by playing. Professional golfers can spend up to eight hours a day on the golf course, practicing specific skills, playing practice rounds, or playing actual competitions. Even during a competition, many players will conduct a practice session at the end of the day's play. Most modern players also include STRENGTH TRAINING, aerobic conditioning, and FLEXIBILITY in their training schedule to strengthen the muscles involved in golf, improve endurance, and minimize the risk of injury.

Competition. Competition golf is played in rounds of 18 holes. Tournaments are conducted as a single round on one day or as multiday competitions of two or four rounds on consecutive days. A round typically takes between three to five hours to play, depending on the skill level of the player and the number of players on the course. The average golf course is seven kilometers from first to last hole, although a player may walk 10 to 20 kilometers in a game depending on the accuracy of the shots.

In Australia, winter is the pro-am competition season and professional players typically travel on a circuit between club tournaments. During this season, a pro golfer could play in 10 tournaments, for a total of 15 days of competition each month. The major international tournaments in Australia are played from January to March and from October to December, flanking the major season overseas between April and October. At the top level, golfers are almost continually on tour.

Physical traits. Golf is primarily a game of skill, therefore top golfers come in many shapes and sizes. In recent times, there is a tendency for top golfers to be fitter and leaner than ever before. Theoretically, carrying excess weight may make a player more susceptible to physical fatigue and thus more likely to suffer loss of skill and mental concentration. Being overweight may also make a golfer suffer greater heat intolerance in hot conditions. As golf is a repetitive sport, carrying excess body fat may also make a golfer more susceptible to injury.

Common Nutrition Issues

Training nutrition. Golfers of all levels require a diet that provides a wide variety of foods. The diet should focus on carbohydrates and be balanced with moderate amounts of protein and smaller amounts of fat. The following are key points:

- Enjoy a variety of foods each day. It is easy to fall into the trap of having the same or very similar foods day after day. Different foods contain different nutrients and chemicals, so eating a variety of foods ensures exposure to all required substances. Priority should be given to nutrient-rich foods. However, there is room for all foods including those that are fun to eat or part of eating socially.

considerably higher at the beginning of the following season. Preseason training typically involves general conditioning work, WEIGHT TRAINING, and skill practice. During the season, two to four training sessions are generally scheduled between matches.

Competition. For most soccer teams, the competitive season involves a weekly match played during the day on weekends, or in the evening midweek. At the elite level, extensive travel is usually required and some double-headers may be scheduled. Tournaments of one to several weeks may also be played in addition to regular competition.

Soccer is a fast game of intensive play with light activity between bursts. While tackling rules are strict, significant body contact occurs with the potential for contact injuries. Time-motion studies of soccer have determined that the average national and international player covers about 10 kilometers in a match. Goalkeepers typically cover about four kilometers.

Soccer matches challenge fuel and fluid stores. One to two kilograms of fluid loss have been reported during standard soccer matches. Losses may be double this during humid conditions.

Physical traits. Soccer players must be skilled, agile, and fast. Players vary widely in body size, but most players tend to be well muscled with a low body fat level to maximize speed and agility.

Common Nutrition Issues

Body fat levels. It is important for soccer players to be aware of seasonal changes in energy requirements. For year-round weight control, it may be necessary for players to reduce food intake to match the decrease in training output during the off-season. Alternatively, players may choose to take up some activity to give them a head start in the next season.

Training nutrition. Soccer players require a high carbohydrate intake on a daily basis to replenish muscle stores after each training session. On average, players will require between five and eight grams of carbohydrate per kilogram each day. This requires making carbohydrate foods such as bread, breakfast cereal, fruit, pasta,

rice, vegetables, yogurt, and flavored low-fat milk the focus of meals and snacks. Players who fail to consume sufficient carbohydrate may suffer midweek slumps and progressive fatigue over the season. Players in heavy training need to start recovery nutrition tactics immediately after each training session. Ideally, players should aim to have 50 to 100 grams of carbohydrate within 30 minutes of finishing training. Recovery snacks should be combined with fluid to replace any fluid lost during the session.

Precompetition meal. Ideally, a light, high-carbohydrate meal should be eaten at least two hours before a match. Breakfast cereal plus fruit, pasta with tomato sauce, rolls or sandwiches, baked potatoes with low-fat fillings, and fruit salad with yogurt are all good options. Experiment to find the best one. Many clubs like to organize the pre-event meal as a team activity, especially when they travel to games away from home. Eating together can be a good way to raise team morale and get focused on the match, as well as making sure that all players are well fueled.

Fuel and fluid intake. Soccer matches place reasonable demands on both fluid and carbohydrate stores of players. Studies have reported low muscle glycogen levels in players after a match—sometimes with significant depletion occurring by half-time. Players with depleted muscle glycogen stores had a lower average speed and covered less ground than their teammates in the second half of the match. Studies show that strategies to increase carbohydrate supplies—both eating a high-carbohydrate diet in the days before a match and drinking sports drink during the match, keep players running faster and farther in the second half. In one study, high-carbohydrate tactics helped the players to make fewer errors.

Some studies have shown that soccer players during hot weather lose twice the amount of fluid in sweat as they take in during game play. It has been suggested that fluid intake during competition is limited by the rules of the game, which allow players to drink only at halftime, when they leave the pitch. However, players seem to become dehydrated at training sessions when these rules do not apply.

Tips for better drinking during soccer are:

- Drink sports drinks that encourage better fluid intake because of their taste, as well as supplying extra fuel for the match.
- Drink well during warm-up and half-time breaks.
- In hot weather especially, be creative in finding ways to grab a drink during halves. Some players leave their bottles around the side of the pitch and dash for a drink whenever there is a stoppage in play.
- Use pre- and post-weighing activities to monitor fluid losses over the game and try to keep these under one kilogram.
- Practice good drinking strategies in training sessions.

Post-competition recovery.   A team approach to recovery is the best way to ensure all players replace fuel and fluid immediately after matches. Organize to have suitable drinks and snacks available after the match as a team activity so that everyone can enjoy the benefits. A postmatch spread of sandwiches, fruit, soup, and carbohydrate drinks can get recovery off to a good start.

Alcohol intake.   There is a tendency in team sports to celebrate or commiserate at the end of a competition with alcohol intake, and unfortunately this often means excessive amounts of alcohol. The decision to drink alcohol is the personal right of each athlete. Sensible use of alcohol does not impair health or performance. However, alcohol intake can interfere with postexercise recovery. Alcohol acts a diuretic and may slow down the process of rehydration after the match. Despite what athletes may have heard about beer and carbo loading, alcoholic drinks are low in carbohydrate content and will not fuel up muscle glycogen stores. After exercise, the soccer player should concentrate first on rehydration and refueling goals. Rehydrate and refuel with carbohydrate-rich foods and fluids before having any alcoholic drinks. Then set a limit and be aware of how much was consumed. Avoid any alcohol for 24 hours post exercise if any soft-tissue injuries or bruising have occurred. The injured athlete who consumes alcohol immedi-

ately after the match may cause extra swelling and bleeding and delay recovery.

G. NUTRITION FOR SPRINTERS

Characteristics of the Sport

At Olympic-level competition, sprint events include the 100 meter, 200 meter, 400 meter, 4 × 100 meter relay, and 4 × 400 meter relay. The 100 meter, and 400 meter hurdles can also be considered as sprint events. Sprint and hurdle events rely primarily on the development of power through anaerobic energy, and this is what makes the sprinter's nutritional needs different from other runners.

Training.   Elite sprinters train all year round with the base or off-season involving around 11 sessions per week. Off-season training usually involves a considerable commitment to WEIGHT TRAINING, with about one-third of the total training load being carried out in the gym. In addition, off-season training focuses on refining technique with a combination of sessions on the track and drill work to improve aspects such as leg speed or knee lift. Stretching sessions, yoga, and Pilates are often included to aid in recovery. As the competitive season approaches, track work increases to include more intervals and sprints, although technique work and weight training are still maintained. Junior and recreational sprinters spend fewer hours training, and training is usually seasonal.

Competition.   Major competitions for elite sprinters are the Olympic games, world championships, and Grand Prix Circuit. At junior and recreational levels, competitions are usually held on a weekly basis during the school year.

Physical traits.   Power-to-weight ratio is important for sprinters, therefore maximizing muscle mass and maintaining low body fat levels is desirable.

Common Nutrition Issues

Training nutrition.   Sprinters need to consume sufficient carbohydrate to fuel training needs; however, carbohydrate requirements do not reach the level of endurance-type athletes. Sprinters need to be mindful of maintaining low body fat levels but still need to eat a sufficient variety and quantity of food to meet nutritional requirements and allow for the development of muscle mass. Diets need to be nutrient-dense. This is best achieved by including a wide variety of nutrient-dense carbohydrate sources such as bread, cereal, fruit, vegetables, and sweetened dairy products in the diet. Moderate portions of lean sources of protein such as lean meat, skin-free chicken, eggs, low-fat dairy foods, lentils, and tofu should also be on the menu. Energy-dense foods such as cakes, pastries, soft drinks, chocolate, and alcohol should be used sparingly. Appropriate snacks need to be included before and after training to maximize performance during training and to promote recovery. Snack foods such as yogurt, fresh fruit, low-fat milk, and sandwiches are all nutritious fuel foods and make good snacks.

Body fat levels. Sprinters require low body fat levels while also being strong and muscular. Low body fat levels usually occur naturally for male athletes, thanks to the cumulative effect of training and the right genetic stock. Male sprinters, however, often need to reduce total body mass leading into the competition phase. Some of the additional muscle mass gained in off-season weight training is not sport specific, and therefore needs to be trimmed to achieve an ideal racing body composition. Female sprinters sometimes need to manipulate their food intake and training to achieve their desired body fat levels. Sprinters needing to reduce their body fat level should target excess calories in their diet. In particular, excess fat, sugary foods, and alcohol can add unnecessary calories and would be better replaced with more nutrient-dense foods.

Precompetition meal. Sprint events do not deplete glycogen stores, therefore strict carbohydrate loading before a competition is not necessary. The day of competition is best tackled with glycogen stores topped up to their usual resting level. With a high-carbohydrate diet already in place for training needs, glycogen levels can be restored before competition with 24 to 36 hours of rest or very light training.

Fuel and fluid during competition. Although sprint events only last seconds or minutes, competition can be a drawn-out affair. A typical competition day involves a number of heats and finals with variable amounts of waiting around in between. Nutritional goals should be to keep hydrated, to maintain blood glucose levels and to feel comfortable—avoiding hunger but not risking the discomfort of a full stomach. It makes sense to start the day with a carbohydrate-based meal. The type of meal will depend on the timing of the event and the runner's personal preferences. Experiment in training if an important competition is coming up in order to be confident on race day. Take care to drink plenty of fluid when competing in hot weather.

Traveling. Elite sprinters are required to travel regularly to find quality competition opportunities. While this can be exciting, it can also be stressful. It is often hard to meet nutritional needs in unfamiliar surroundings, especially when time and finances are limited. Unusual foods, different standards of food hygiene, limited food availability, and interference with usual routines can contribute to athletes either gaining or losing weight or failing to meet their nutritional requirements. The following tips may help:

- Be clear about nutritional goals and stay committed while traveling.

- Do some investigation to find out what to expect upon arrival.

- Plan accommodations with meals in mind. Organizing an apartment with cooking facilities offers more control over meals and can keep food costs down. Those who choose not to cook should make sure accommodations are conveniently located near shops and restaurants.

- Take a supply of snacks along to always have access to something suitable. Cereal bars, sports drinks, breakfast cereal, and rice cakes are good options to pack.

- Make good choices in restaurants. Beware of hidden fat in restaurant meals. Do not be afraid to ask the waiter about cooking methods and ingredients and request changes if necessary. Add carbohydrate to meals with plain bread, plain rice, and fruit or juice if necessary.

Iron. Sprinters who adopt restricted eating habits to maintain low body fat levels can be at risk of a poor iron status. If in doubt, have iron levels checked by a sports physician. In addition, a sports dietitian will be able to help athletes increase their intake of iron-rich foods that are well absorbed by the body. Plant-based iron foods such as green vegetables are poorly absorbed compared to animal-based iron foods such as meat.

Supplements. Some runners try to replace sound nutritional practices with vitamin pills, protein powders, and liquid formulas. Popping a pill is not a quick fix to feeling flat and run-down. Athletes must take the time to eat well and get adequate rest as their bodies are working extra hard to maintain their conditioning and performance during races. Some supplements can help in certain situations, but this is best assessed by a sports physician and sports dietitian.

H. NUTRITION FOR SWIMMERS

Characteristics of the Sport
Training. Competitive swimming requires a serious commitment to training. Typically, six to 12 sessions are undertaken each week, with the distance covered in each session ranging from 1,000 to 2,000 meters of quality work for a sprinter in taper phase to 10 kilometers for a distance swimmer in the base phase of training. At the elite level, workloads can involve two to three daily sessions adding up to six hours of training per day. In addition, swimmers may undertake some land-based aerobic training such as running or cycling as well as WEIGHT TRAINING sessions. Training commitments are usually smaller at the school or recreational level.

Competition. Olympic swimming events last from 20 seconds to 15 minutes. Swimming is therefore a highly anaerobic sport, with aerobic metabolism becoming more important as the race distance increases. Although each event may be brief, swim meets are usually held over three to seven days, with swimmers typically competing in heats in the mornings and finals in the evening. In minor competitions, swimmers may enter a large number of events and be required to swim two or three times in one day with 20 minutes to several hours between events.

Physical characteristics. Swimmers tend to be tall with pronounced upper body muscle development. Low body fat is an advantage, since swimmers need to move their body weight through water. However, some body fat in the right distribution may enhance flotation.

Other issues. Many top swimmers are in their teens. Male adolescence is a period of heavy growth and muscular development, requiring high-energy support. For males, the addition of an intense training program means male swimmers can have trouble eating enough calories to meet energy needs. Adolescence for females brings hormonal changes, which promote an increase in body fat. Despite heavy training loads, many female swimmers struggle to maintain low body fat levels. Long training hours restrict a swimmer's lifestyle. This can either reduce the opportunities to eat in a busy daily schedule or raise the importance of eating for comfort or entertainment. Access to food can also be an issue when competing and traveling to meets.

Common Nutrition Issues
Daily recovery. Strenuous daily training requires a high-energy, high-carbohydrate diet. Swimmers who fail to consume enough carbohydrates will fail to recover adequately between training sessions, resulting in fatigue, loss of body weight, and poor performance. Additional energy requirements for growth may compound the problem. Swimmers with high-energy requirements need to increase the number of snacks during the day and make use of energy-dense foods. It is good to have nutritious carbohydrate-rich snacks on hand to eat immediately after training to start the refueling process. This is especially important for swimmers who travel long distances from their pool to work or home and have to wait until the next meal can be consumed.

Fluid needs in training. High-intensity exercise in the steamy environment of a heated indoor pool, or outdoors in the sun, can lead to moderate sweat losses, which are not obvious when the swimmer is already wet. Smart swimmers bring water bottles to the pool deck and drink during rest periods or between sets. Sports drinks provide an additional fuel supply for long training sessions.

Iron status.   An iron imbalance may occur in swimmers undertaking heavy training who fail to consume sufficient iron. Female swimmers on weight-loss diets are particularly at risk. Iron levels should be checked regularly when in heavy training. Iron-rich foods such as lean red meat and breakfast cereals fortified with iron should be included regularly in the diet. Iron-rich plant foods such as wholegrain cereals, spinach, and legumes should be combined with animal iron sources, such as wholegrain pasta with meat sauce, and vitamin C sources, such as a glass of orange juice consumed with breakfast cereal, to improve iron absorption. A sports dietitian will be able to provide specific dietary help.

Immune status.   Swimmers often worry about getting sick during periods of heavy training. Many nutritional supplements and strategies have been suggested to keep the swimmer from catching coughs and colds. To date, the most important strategy emerging from immune studies of athletes is to keep well fueled during training sessions. Sports drinks during the workout and a recovery snack or meal afterward help to reduce the stress on the immune system experienced in the hours after the session.

Competition nutrition.   Muscle glycogen stores can be filled by 24 hours of a high-carbohydrate diet and rest. Swimmers who are undertaking a long taper may need to reduce total energy intake to match their reduced workload in order to prevent an increase in body fat. Fluid levels and carbohydrate stores need to be replenished between events and between heats. A carbohydrate-containing fluid such as a sports drink, fruit juice, or soft drink is appropriate when there is only a short interval between races. Snacks such as yogurt, fruit, cereal bars, or sandwiches are suitable for longer gaps between races or for recovery at the end of a session. Between day heats and evening final sessions, most swimmers eat a high-carbohydrate lunch and have a nap. On waking, a carbohydrate-rich snack is eaten before returning to the pool.

I. NUTRITION FOR TENNIS PLAYERS

Characteristics of the Sport

Tennis is a game of skill, speed, agility, concentration, and often endurance. It is played by both men and women, in singles and in doubles competition (same-sex and mixed-sex pairs). At an elite level, tennis is a fast and mobile game, characterized by bursts of intense exercise during rallies. The game is highly reliant on anaerobic energy systems, although a developed aerobic capacity is an advantage in terms of recovery between points, stamina, and tolerance to heat. Men's international matches are known to last four or five hours. While the exercise is not continuous for this duration, such a game is likely to challenge the carbohydrate fuel stores of the athlete.

Training.   For professional players, tennis is a full-time job. Between tournaments, 20 to 40 hours per week may be spent in training with the majority of this devoted to on-court practice. Most players will supplement this with about an hour per day of off-court conditioning work such as running, WEIGHT TRAINING, and agility work. At the recreational level, training varies significantly with some players using matches as their main form of training.

Competition.   A tennis match is played over the best of three or five sets for men, and the best of three sets for women. The length of a match varies greatly, from 30 minutes to three hours for a three-set match and from 80 minutes to more than five hours for a five-set match. The fuel and fluid demands of a match will vary accordingly. However, in tournament tennis, the nutritional focus is not so much on the effects of a single match, but on the cumulative effects from playing so many matches in succession.

Tournament tennis sets an extremely tough schedule for players, requiring many to play in a singles and doubles match each day until their outcome is decided. Most tournaments require four to six wins to take home the trophy. On average, an elite player participates in 20 tournaments each year. While muscle glycogen levels may survive one match, the continual daily schedule will challenge the athlete to fully recover stores between matches. Depleted muscle glycogen levels will interfere with both sprint and endurance components of performance and hinder the player's ability to perform at an optimum level.

Physical characteristics.   Having long arms and a relatively low center of gravity (short legs in proportion to trunk) can facilitate extra reach for playing strokes, greater height for serving, and greater mobility around the court. However, tennis players come in all shapes and sizes. Players adapt their game to make the most of their physical strengths. For example, tall, muscular players might use their height and power with an aggressive serve and volley game, while shorter, agile players may do better with a mobile, court-covering game. In general, the body fat levels of tennis players are relatively low, allowing greater stamina and heat tolerance.

Common Nutrition Issues
Training nutrition.   The training and playing schedules of many elite players require large energy and carbohydrate requirements. At a lower level of play, carbohydrate needs may not be so great, but may still be beyond the level supplied by the typical diet. Active tennis players need to make nutrient-dense carbohydrate foods such as pasta, rice, bread, cereal, vegetables, fruit, and dairy products the focus of meals and snacks. Players in heavy training need to start recovery nutrition tactics immediately after each training session. Ideally, players should aim to consume 50 to 100 grams of carbohydrates within 30 minutes of finishing training. Recovery snacks should be combined with fluid to replace any fluid lost during the session.

Body fat levels.   Many players do not automatically arrive at the body fat level that does them justice on the court. Being overweight will reduce speed and stamina, and increase suffering during hot days on the court. If a player needs to reduce body fat, the first step is to forget quick-fix diets and other methods claiming miraculous results in favor of adopting a consistent, long-term approach to body fat maintenance. The following tips are helpful for achieving and maintaining low body fat levels.

- Consult a dietitian to help determine exactly how much and what is needed to eat to meet nutritional demands.

- Avoid getting too hungry. A small but well-timed snack will prevent overeating later on.
- Eat slowly to enjoy food and recognize when one has eaten enough.
- Enjoy high-fiber foods as they are more filling.
- Drink water before and during a meal.
- Take care with high-energy fluids such as juice and soft drinks. It is easy to consume too many calories when using such beverages to quench thirst.
- Include all favorite foods in a diet, just eat smaller quantities if necessary.
- Cut back on intake of fat, alcohol, and sugar.
- Find nonfood rewards.

Fluid intake during matches and training.   Tennis is often played in sweltering conditions. Court surface temperatures can soar. When matches or training sessions drag on for three hours or more, players can lose a tremendous amount of water in their sweat. Players must be especially careful to take in adequate fluids.

Tips for better drinking during tennis are:

- Follow a plan of fluid intake before, during, and after matches to keep reasonable pace with sweat losses.
- Use pre- and post-weighing activities to monitor fluid losses over training.
- Be aware of sweat losses during a match, and be especially aggressive about drinking fluids on hot and humid days.
- Keep a supply of cool and refreshing fluids easily accessible at the courtside and grab a drink as appropriate. On some days it may be sufficient to drink between sets, but it is probably good practice to grab a quick drink as players change ends after every second game.
- While water is adequate to replace fluid losses, there are additional advantages in using a carbohydrate-electrolyte beverage such as a sports drink during long, intense matches.
- After the match, replace any remaining fluid deficit to prevent problems of chronic dehydration throughout the tournament.

Tournament tennis. Tournament tennis is challenging from many nutritional viewpoints. Apart from the considerations of being away from home, even for a weekend tournament, the tournament schedule places great demands on nutritional strategies for recovery and on a player's flexibility and ingenuity. Not only must players be committed to looking after fluid and carbohydrate needs between matches, but they must do so without the benefit of having a definite timetable of their day's activities.

Since each day's match draw is determined by the results of the previous day's play, players receive short notice about their daily schedule. Forward planning is also made difficult by the loose nature of the daily timetable. While the starting time for the first match of each session can be set, all other matches simply follow in succession. Given the great range of duration of matches, it is often difficult for a player to predict accurately the time of their matches. Tournament players must learn to be adaptable with their eating plans.

Life on the circuit. Elite tennis players can look forward to a life of traveling. While this can be exciting, it can also be stressful. It is often hard to meet nutritional needs in unfamiliar surroundings, especially when time and finances are limited. Unusual foods, different standards of food hygiene, limited food availability, and interference with usual routines can cause athletes either to gain weight or fail to meet their nutritional requirements. The following tips may help:

- Be clear about nutritional goals and stay committed while traveling.
- Do some investigation to find out what to expect upon arrival.
- Plan accommodations with meals in mind. Organizing an apartment with cooking facilities offers more control over meals and can keep food costs down. Those who choose not to cook should make sure accommodations are conveniently located near shops and restaurants.
- Take a supply of snacks along to always have access to something suitable. Cereal bars, sports drinks, breakfast cereal, and rice cakes are good options to pack.

- Make good choices in restaurants. Beware of hidden fat in restaurant meals. Do not be afraid to ask the waiter about cooking methods and ingredients and request changes if necessary. Add carbohydrate to meals with plain bread, plain rice, and fruit or juice if necessary.

J. NUTRITION FOR TRIATHLETES

Characteristics of the Sport

Triathlon, as the name suggests, involves the combination of three separate sports—swimming, cycling, and running, usually in that order. Triathlons are completed over various distances ranging from sprint triathlons that are completed in just about an hour by most competitors to Ironman-distance events that last all day. The table below outlines the various distances over which triathlons are completed.

Training. Triathletes range from full-time professionals to age-group competitors, and the time spent training varies considerably. Since there are three disciplines to master, most triathletes train twice each day to make sure all disciplines are trained regularly. Athletes will routinely combine disciplines in each session to ensure their bodies are well adapted for the stresses of competition. These workouts are commonly called "brick sessions" and usually involve two or more of the sports. For professional triathletes, it is not uncommon to train two to three times daily, with some professional Ironman triathletes clocking as many as 40 hours of training per week.

Special considerations. In most triathlons, drafting (riding directly behind or beside a fellow competitor) during the bike leg is prohibited because it provides a 10 to 15 percent advantage to the athlete drafting. The only exception to this rule is for professional sprint- and Olympic-distance competitors, where drafting is legal. This "drafting permitted" ruling tends to put heavy stress on the physique of the athletes who are successful at these distances. Much of the advantage of being a strong cyclist is lost in the sprint and Olympic-distance events. Many triathletes who are successful at these shorter distances have light and lean physiques, which enables them to run quickly.

Ironman triathletes, however, tend to be more strongly built since the bike leg plays a crucial role in determining the outcome of the race.

Common Nutrition Issues

Daily recovery. Routine training loads for elite triathletes increase daily energy, carbohydrate, and protein requirements. Many triathletes in the past have focused exclusively on replacing carbohydrates at the expense of other nutrients such as protein. It is important for triathletes to ensure that meals and snacks are well rounded to meet daily fuel and nutrient demands. Persistent fatigue, poor recovery, illness, and unwanted weight loss are common among triathletes who fail to adequately meet daily calorie and nutrient requirements.

Timing of meals and snacks around training sessions. As triathletes are required to train two to three sessions each day, recovery from one training session to the next is crucial to maximize training gains. Triathletes need to plan their daily food intake to ensure regular snacks and meals are consumed around training sessions. It is important to have nutritious high-carbohydrate snacks on hand immediately after training to initiate the refueling process. Men need an average of 60 to 80 grams of carbohydrate following a workout; women on average need about 40 to 50 grams of carbohydrate immediately following a workout. The following snacks are examples that provide sufficient carbohydrates to optimize recovery: yogurt, cereal bars, sports drinks, and fruit.

Carbohydrate loading. The concept of carbohydrate loading is popular among triathletes prior to competition. Carbohydrate loading is more than simply eating pasta for dinner the night before competition, but it does not mean gorging yourself with food for the entire week leading into a race. As training decreases prior to a race, calorie and carbohydrate requirements also decrease. It is important to taper food intake just as workouts are tapered. Athletes should be careful, however, to consume enough carbohydrates in the days prior to the race that their muscle glycogen (carbohydrate stored in the muscle) levels are sufficient to last the duration of the race.

Prerace eating. The majority of triathlons start early in the morning so there is the temptation to miss breakfast before race start. It is crucial to eat a prerace meal in order to top up muscle and liver glycogen stores prior to race start. A prerace meal should contain familiar carbohydrate-rich foods and fluids that are low in fat and fiber. Foods such as liquid meal supplements, sports bars, bananas, and juice are popular prerace meal choices.

For those who suffer early morning jitters, liquid meal supplements provide an easily digested alternative to foods. It is also worthwhile to sip on water or a sports drink during the hour before race start to top up fluid levels. The advantage of competing in triathlons is that one can always urinate during the swim after drinking too much beforehand.

Eating during training and competition. Eating food during long training rides and races is essential for triathletes to help provide carbohydrates to the working muscles, meet daily energy and nutrient requirements, and keep hunger at bay. Most Ironman triathletes complete "brick" sessions during their preparation for a triathlon. Brick sessions may consist of a five- to six-hour bike ride immediately followed by an hour of running. Eating during brick sessions is not only beneficial, but essential.

During sprint and Olympic-distance triathlons it is usually not necessary to eat foods while racing. Triathletes competing in these events usually rely exclusively on sports drinks and sports gels to meet fuel and fluid losses. However, during Ironman races, in which athletes are competing over several hours and consequently missing regular meals, eating food plays an important role in meeting hourly carbohydrate requirements.

Ironman triathletes should be encouraged to think of the bike leg as a "moving feast" since they really need to consume adequate fuel and fluid during this leg of the race to set themselves up for the run. The bike leg presents the greatest opportunity to consume adequate food and fluid, compared to the run and swim. Athletes should take a variety of food on the bike to ensure they maintain interest in what they are eating. Sandwiches, fruit bars, sports bars, bananas, sweet biscuits, dried fruit, and sports gels are all examples of foods commonly eaten by triathletes while biking. It is good practice to have a combination of regular food items and sports foods.

The run presents many more challenges than the bike in meeting carbohydrate requirements.

Most triathletes use fluids such as sports drinks and soft drinks to simultaneously meet fluid and carbohydrate requirements during the run. During Ironman events, athletes will also use sports gels as these are far more practical to consume than food while running.

Meeting fluid requirements during training and competition.   Since triathletes are required to train two to three times each day, sweat losses tend to be high, particularly when training in warm environments. Athletes need to make a conscious effort during the day to adequately replace fluid losses so that they do not run the risk of chronic dehydration. Having access to a drink bottle during training and carrying a drink bottle around during the day is the key to ensuring that athletes compensate for their daily fluid losses. Dehydration is the most common cause of medical treatment following triathlons, despite race organizers' providing fluids during the bike and run legs.

Body fat levels.   As with most endurance-based athletes, triathletes often have low body fat levels due to the stringent demands of training. Athletes who need to watch their consumption of food in order to maintain low body fat levels must be very careful to consume adequate calories and nutrients while avoiding high-fat, high-calorie foods that contribute little in the way of nutrition.

Travel.   Professional triathletes often spend time traveling and competing in other countries. Since most triathletes travel alone, without the support of a team, they rarely enjoy the benefits of a dietitian who arranges meals ahead of time. Triathletes in these situations must take extra precautions to plan where they will eat ahead of time and to carry plenty of snacks with them so that they do not go too long between refueling. Breakfast cereals, breakfast bars, sports bars, and liquid meal supplements are easy to carry and provide good nutrition.

H. COMMON INJURIES BY SPORT

Baseball
Abrasions
Achilles Tendonitis
Ankle Sprains
Baseball Finger
Elbow Sprains
Little League Elbow Syndrome
Rotator Cuff Tear
Rotator Cuff Tendonitis
Tennis Elbow

Basketball
Achilles Tendonitis
ACL Injury
Ankle Fracture
Ankle Sprain
Hamstring Tendonitis
Ilioitibial Band Syndrome
Jumper's Knee
Rotator Cuff Tendonitis

Cycling
Abrasions
Acute Mountain Sickness
Bicycle Seat Neuropathy
Iliotibial Band Syndrome
Lumbosacral Disk Injury
Muscle Cramps
Runner's Knee
Wrist Injuries

Football
ACL Injury
Burners and Stingers
Concussion
Fractures
Heat Cramps
Heat Exhaustion
Heat Stroke
Lumbosacral Disk Injury
Sciatica
Second Impact Head Injury Syndrome
Shoulder Dislocation
Shoulder Separation

Golf
Acromioclavicular Joint Injury
Golfer's Elbow

Rotator Cuff Tendonitis
Stress Fractures of the Ribs
Swimmer's Shoulder
Wrist Injury
Yips

Hockey
Ankle Fracture
Ankle Sprain
Burners and Stingers
Concussion
Facial Soft Tissue Injuries
Gluteal Strain
Hamstring Tendonitis

Rowing
Blisters
Lumbosacral Disk Injury
Overtraining Syndrome
Runner's Knee
Stress Fracture of the Ribs
Wrist Tendonitis

Running
Abrasions
Ankle Sprain
Femoral Neck Stress Fracture
Hamstring Tendonitis
Iliotibial Band Syndrome
Piriformis Syndrome
Plantar Fascitis
Runner's Knee
Shin Splints
Stress Fracture

Skiing
ACL Injury
Acute Mountain Sickness
Fractures
Hypothermia
Medial Collateral Knee Ligament Injury
Skiier's Thumb

Soccer
ACL Injury
Ankle Fracture
Ankle Sprain
Concussion
Hip Pointer

Muscle Cramps
Piriformis Syndrome
Thigh Bruise

Swimming
Athlete's Foot
Knee Bursitis (Breaststroker's Knee)
Lumbosacral Disk Injuries
Muscle Cramps
Overtraining Syndrome
Painful Plica
Rotator Cuff Tendonitis
Swimmer's Ear
Swimmer's Shoulder
Tendonitis
Tennis Elbow

Tennis
Abrasions
Achilles Tendonitis
Ankle Sprains
Blisters
Heat Cramps
Heat Exhaustion
Heat Stroke
Plantar Fascitis
Rotator Cuff Tendonitis
Shin Splints
Stress Fractures
Tennis Elbow

APPENDIX IV
TRAINING TIPS FOR RUNNING A FIRST MARATHON OR RIDING A FIRST CENTURY

Many runners and cyclists do not consider themselves fully initiated into their sport until they have completed a marathon or a century ride (100 miles in one day), respectively. Although such an endurance event may seem extreme to the outsider, it is doable for many novice athletes given the proper training and outlook.

The following guidelines can help athletes achieve this milestone, but whether by bike or by foot, remember that the goal is enjoyment and fitness.

ALTERNATE HARD DAYS WITH EASY DAYS

When beginning to build distance, speed, and endurance, it is sometimes tempting to follow a hard workout with another hard workout, but it is important to allow the muscles time to recover. For this reason, alternate hard training days with easier training days.

INCLUDE HILL TRAINING

For runners and cyclists, an important component of building strength and endurance is working out in hilly terrain. This may be especially true if the anticipated century ride or marathon takes place on hilly terrain.

GET GOOD SLEEP

Sleep is another necessary component of any training regimen. The recovery that takes place following a hard workout is greatly boosted by a good night's sleep, so consider getting to bed on time to be as important as completing the next day's workout.

DO NOT IGNORE PAIN

Pain is the body's way of saying that something is wrong. Athletes must listen to what their bodies say and respond appropriately. Take time off from training and any activities that aggravate the injury when pain develops. If the pain is severe or persistent, be sure to see a doctor. Ignoring a chronic problem can cause it to become more serious and ultimately more detrimental to long-term goals.

MAKE THE MOST OF YOUR EQUIPMENT

Runners must always wear good shoes with adequate cushion. Cyclists need good shoes, too, but more important, they need a good bike that fits well. Achieving the proper fit on a bike can sometimes be challenging, but it is worth the time spent because it will help prevent numerous injuries that can develop when a bike does not properly fit.

FOLLOW A TRAINING SCHEDULE

Mapping out a good training program is an essential part of meeting marathon or century ride goals. However, it is equally important to remember that a training schedule is not written in stone. If an athlete is exhausted on a morning scheduled for a 20-mile run, it is probably better to skip the run, get some extra sleep, and do the run another day, feeling more rested. If hill workouts on the bike are planned, but the temperature is 105°F in the shade, opt for an easier ride or maybe a swim instead, and do the hill climbing on a day when heat stroke is not a risk.

EAT, DRINK, AND BE MERRY

Proper nutrition between training sessions and proper refueling during long training sessions and competitions are essential for endurance athletes. If a workout lasts as long as 90 minutes, plan to refuel during that time with some sort of carbohydrate replacement food, such as energy gels, energy bars, fruit, and sports drinks. Some athletes even eat bagels, sandwiches, and other more substantial food during training. Use a long period of training to experiment and learn what works best, then use those foods and beverages on the day of the big event.

APPENDIX V
ASSOCIATIONS AND ORGANIZATIONS

ACA Sports Council
P.O. Box 400
380 Wright Road
Norwalk, IA 50211
(800) 261-1495
(515) 981-9340
(515) 981-9427 (fax)
http://www.acasc.org/

**American Alliance for Health, Physical
   Education, Recreation & Dance**
1900 Association Drive
Reston, VA 20191-1598
(800) 213-7193
http://www.aahperd.org/

American College of Sports Medicine
401 West Michigan Street
Indianapolis, IN 46202-3233
(317) 637-9200
(317) 634-7817 (fax)
http://www.acsm.org/

American Massage Therapy Association
820 Davis Street
Suite 100
Evanston, IL 60201-4444
(847) 864-0123
(847) 864-1178 (fax)
http://www.amtamassage.org/

**American Osteopathic Academy of
   Sports Medicine**
7600 Terrace Avenue
Suite 203
Middleton, WI 53562
(608) 831-4400
(608) 831-5185 (fax)
http://www.aoasm.org/

American Physical Therapy Association
1111 North Fairfax Street
Alexandria, VA 22314-1488
(703) 684-2782

(800) 999-2782
(703) 683-6748 (TDD)
(703) 684-7343 (fax)
http://www.apta.org/

American Physiological Society
9650 Rockville Pike
Bethesda, MD 20814
(301) 634-7164
http://www.the-aps.org/

American Society of Exercise Physiologists
The College of St. Scholastica
1200 Kenwood Avenue
Duluth, MN 55811
(218) 723-6297
http://www.css.edu/asep/

American Academy of Orthopaedic Surgeons
6300 North River Road
Rosemont, IL 60018-4262
(847) 823-7186
(800) 346-AAOS
(847) 823-8125 (fax)
http://www.aaos.org/wordhtml/home2.htm

**American Academy of Orthotists and
   Prosthetists**
526 King Street
Suite 201
Alexandria, VA 22314
(703) 836-0788
(703) 836-0737 (fax)
http://www.oandp.org/

**American Academy of Physical Medicine and
   Rehabilitation**
One IBM Plaza
Suite 2500
Chicago, IL 60611-3604
(312) 464-9700
(312) 464-0227 (fax)
http://www.aapmr.org/

American Academy of Podiatric Sports Medicine
P.O. Box 723
Rockville, MD 20848-0723
(888) 854-3338
http://www.aapsm.org/about.html

American Orthopaedic Society for Sports Medicine
6300 North River Road
Suite 500
Rosemont, IL 60018
(847) 292-4900
(847) 292-4905 (fax)
http://www.sportsmed.org/

Arthroscopy Association of North America
6300 North River Road
Suite 104
Rosemont, IL 60018-4262
(847) 292-2262
(847) 292-2268 (fax)
http://www.aana.org/

Athletic Trainers Association of Florida
P.O. Box 12846
Tallahassee, FL 32317-2846
(850) 487-1879, ext. 5006
http://www.ataf.org/

Canadian Academy of Sport Medicine
Unit 14 - 1010 Polytek Street
Gloucester, Ontario, Canada K1J 9H9
(877) 585-2394
(613) 748-5792 (fax)
http://www.casm-acms.org/

Canadian Association for Health, Physical Education, Recreation and Dance
403-2197 Riverside Drive
Ottawa, Ontario, Canada K1H 7X3
(613) 523-1348
(800) 663-8708 (Canada only)
(613) 523-1206
http://www.cahperd.ca/

College Athletic Trainers' Society (CATS)
Thorp Reed & Armstrong, LLP
One Oxford Centre
301 Grant Street, 14th Floor
Pittsburgh, PA 15219
http://www.collegeatc.org/

Canadian Athletic Therapists' Association (CATA)
312-902 11th Avenue S.W.
Calgary, AB, Canada T2R 0E7
(403) 509-2282
(403) 509-2280 (fax)
http://www.athletictherapy.org/main.html

Diabetes Exercise and Sports Association
8001 Montcastle Drive
Nashville, TN 37221
(800) 898-4322
(615) 673-2077 (fax)
http://www.diabetes-exercise.org/

European Society of Sports Traumatology, Knee Surgery, and Arthroscopy
7, av. Krieg
case postale 139
1211 Geneva 17 Switzerland
41-22-703-4808
41-22-347-4769 (fax)
http://www.esska.org/

Great Lakes Athletic Trainers Association
1199 Hadley Road
Mooresville, IN 46158
(317) 834-5143
(317) 831-9347 (fax)
http://www.glata.org/

Institute for Preventative Sports Medicine
P.O. Box 7032
Ann Arbor, MI 48107
(734) 434-3390
http://www.ipsm.org/

International Academy for Sports Dentistry
118 Faye Street
Farmersville, IL 62533
(800) 273-1788 (U.S.A. only)
(217) 227-3431
http://www.acadsportsdent.org/

International Association of Arthroscopy, Knee Surgery and Orthopedic Sports Medicine
2678 Bishop Drive
Suite 250
San Ramon, CA 94583-2338
(925) 807-1197
(925) 807-1199 (fax)
http://www.isakos.com/

International Federation of Orthopaedic Manipulative Therapists
81 Queens Road
London SW19 8NR
England
44-208-879-1567
44-208-944-7734 (fax)
http://www.omt.org/homepage/ifomt/ifomt.htm

International Federation of Sports Medicine
P.O. Box 25137
1307 Nicosia, Cyprus
(357) 22-663-762
357-22-664-669 (fax)
http://www.fims.org/fims/frames.asp

International Society of Biomechanics in Sport
1199 Hadley Rd.
Mooresville, IN 46158
(317) 834-5143
(317) 831-9347 (fax)
http://www.uni-stuttgart.de/External/isbs/

**International Society of Exercise and
    Immunology (ISEI)**
Institute of Sportsmedicine
University of Paderborn
Warburger Str. 100
33098 Paderborn
Germany
http://www.isei.de/

Japanese Athletic Trainers' Organization
c/o Sony Enterprise
Shinagawa Intercity B-11F
2-15-2 Konan, Shinagawa-ku
Tokyo 108-6111 Japan
81-3-5769-6645
81-3-5769-6676 (fax)
http://www.jato-trainer.org/

National Athletic Trainers Association
2952 Stemmons Freeway
Dallas, TX 75247
(214) 637-6282
(214) 637-2206
http://www.nata.org/

National Collegiate Athletic Association
700 West Washington Street
P.O. Box 6222
Indianapolis, IN 46206-6222
(317) 917-6222
(317) 917-6888 (fax)
http://www.ncaa.org/

**National Operating Committee on Standards
    for Athletic Equipment**
P.O. Box 12290
Overland, KS 66282-2290
(913) 888-1340
(913) 888-1065 (fax)
http://www.nocsae.org/

National Safety Council
1121 Spring Lake Drive
Itasca, IL 60143-3201
(630) 285-1121
(630) 285-1315 (fax)
http://www.nsc.org/

**National Sports Medicine Institute of the
    United Kingdom**
32 Devonshire Street
London W1G 6PX
44-0-20-7908-3636

44-0-20-7908-3635 (fax)
http://www.nsmi.org.uk/

National Strength and Conditioning Association
3333 Landmark Circle
Lincoln, NE 68504
(402) 476-6669
(888) 746-2378
(402) 476-7141 (fax)
http://www.nsca-cc.org/

National Youth Sports Safety Foundation
One Beacon Street
Suite 3333
Boston, MA 02108
(617) 277-1171
(617) 722-9999
http://www.nyssf.org/

New Zealand Sports Medicine
40 Logan Park Drive
P.O. Box 6398
Dunedin, New Zealand
64-3-477 7887
64-3-477 7882
http://sportsmedicine.co.nz/

Orthopaedic Research Society
6300 North River Road
Suite 727
Rosemont, IL 60018
(847) 698-1625
(847) 823-4921 (fax)
http://www.ors.org/

**President's Council on Physical Fitness
    and Sports**
Department W
200 Independence Avenue SW, Room 738-H
Washington, D.C. 20201-0004
(202) 690-9000
(202) 690-5211 (fax)
http://www.fitness.gov/

Sport Physiotherapy Canada
1600 James Naismith Drive
Gloucester, Ontario K1B 5N4 Canada
http://www.sportphysio.ca/aboutus/involve.htm

**United Kingdom Association of Doctors
    in Sport**
22 Alder Avenue
Wakefield
West Yorkshire WF2 0TZ England
44-1924-239-642
44-1924-371-793
http://www.ukadis.org/

United States Olympic Committee
National Headquarters
One Olympic Plaza

Colorado Springs, CO 80909
(719) 866-4500
http://www.usoc.org/

World Council on Orthopaedic Sports Medicine

2678 Bishop Drive, Suite 250
San Ramon, CA 94583-2338
(925) 807-1197
(925) 807-1199 (fax)
http://www.isakos.com/wcosm.html

World Federation of Athletic Training and Therapy

Department of Exercise Science
Ramsey Center, 300 River Road
Athens, GA 30602-6554
(706) 542-3148
(706) 542-3148 (fax)
http://www.wfatt.org/

APPENDIX VI
SPORTS MEDICINE SCHOOLS

Sports medicine refers to many different areas of exercise and sports science that relate both to performance and care of injury. Within sports medicine are areas of specialization such as clinical medicine, orthopedic medicine, exercise physiology, biomechanics, physical therapy, athletic training, sports nutrition, sports psychology, and more. Many schools and universities have programs in sports medicine, and many professionals use the title sports medicine. The term, however, has multiple meanings. People as diverse as team physicians, orthopedic surgeons, exercise physiologists, biomechanists, physical therapists, athletic trainers, and sports nutritionists might call themselves sports medicine professionals.

Consequently, studying sports medicine means studying one of these particular fields that combine medical principles and science with sport and physical performance. The first question, then, if one is interested in studying sports medicine, is not how and where to study sports medicine, but which of these fields of study is of interest. Once the focus is narrowed to a particular field of study, the requirements for certification in the field must be determined.

Many professions in sports medicine require a certification, and each profession has different requirements for the certification process. The main reason for requiring a certification is to protect the profession and guarantee that the practitioner is qualified in the field of practice. The best way to find out about these requirements is to learn about the organizations and associations that regulate the certification process for each profession.

This appendix does not provide an exhaustive list of schools that offer sports medicine programs and degrees. To find such a list, consult the following two directories: *The American College of Sports Medicine's 2003 Directory of Graduate Programs in Sports Medicine and Exercise Science* and *The American College of Sports Medicine's 2003 Directory of Undergraduate Programs in Sports Medicine and Exercise Science*. To order, contact the ACSM Communications and Public Information Department at publicinfo@acsm.org or check your local library.

SPORTS MEDICINE PROGRAMS ENDORSED BY THE AMERICAN COLLEGE OF SPORTS MEDICINE

Appalachian State University
Exercise Science Major
Bachelor of Science
Admissions Office
Boone, NC 28608
(828) 262-2120
(828) 262-3296 (fax)
admissions@appstate.edu

Ball State University
Exercise Science Major
Bachelor of Science
Muncie, IN 47306
(765) 285-8300
http://www.bsu.edu
askus@bsu.edu

East Stroudsburg University
Exercise Science Professional Major
Bachelor of Science
200 Prospect Street
East Stroudsburg, PA 18301
(570) 422-3542
(570) 422-3933 (fax)
undergrads@po-box.esu.edu

Florida Atlantic University
Exercise Science and Health Promotion Major
Bachelor of Science

777 Glades Road
Boca Raton, FL 33431
(561) 297-2458
http://www.fau.edu

Montana Tech of the University of Montana
Applied Health Science Major
Bachelor of Science
1300 West Park Street
Butte, MT 59701-8997
(406) 496-4178
admissions@mtech.edu
http://www.mtech.edu

Morehead State University
Exercise Science Major
Bachelor of Science
Howell McDowell 301
Morehead, KY 40351
(606) 783-2000
admissions@morehead-st.edu

North Dakota State University
Human Performance and Fitness Major
Bachelor of Science
P.O. Box 5454
Fargo, ND 58105-5454
(701) 231-8643
nuadmiss@plains.nodak.edu

Northeastern University
Exercise Physiology Major
Bachelor of Science
150 Richards Hall
Boston, MA 02115-5096
(617) 373-2200
admissions@neu.edu

Ohio State University
Exercise Science Education Major
Bachelor of Science
Lincoln Tower, Third Floor
Columbus, OH 43210-1200
(614) 292-3980
telecounseling@fa.adm.ohio-state.edu

Santa Fe Community College
Exercise Science Major
Associate of Applied Science
Admissions Office
Santa Fe, NM 87501
http://www.santafe.cc.fl.us

Slippery Rock University of Pennsylvania
Exercise Science Major
Bachelor of Science
Maltby Center
Slippery Rock, PA 16057
(724) 738-2015
apply@sru.edu

South Dakota State University
Health Promotion Major
Bachelor of Science
P.O. Box 2201
Brookings, SD 57007
(605) 688-4121
sdsuadms@adm.sdstate.edu

University of Georgia
Exercise and Sport Science Major
Bachelor of Science
Admissions Office
Athens, GA 30602
(706) 542-3000
undergrad@admissions.uga.edu

University of Mary
Exercise Science Major
Bachelor of Science
7500 University Drive
Bismarck, ND 58504
(800) 288-629
marauder@umary.edu

University of Pittsburgh
Movement Science Major
Bachelor of Science
4337 Fifth Avenue
First Floor, Masonic Temple
Pittsburgh, PA 15213
(412) 624-7488
oafa@pitt.edu

University of Texas at Arlington
Exercise Science Major
Bachelor of Science
P.O. Box 19111
701 South Nedderman Drive, Room 110
Davis Hall
Arlington, TX 76019
(817) 272-3251
admissions@uta.edu

University of Wisconsin
Adult Fitness/Cardiac Rehabilitation Major
Master of Science
716 Langdon Street
La Crosse, WI 53706
(608) 262-3961
on.Wisconsin@mail.admin.wisc.edu

Youngstown State University
Exercise Science Major
Bachelor of Science
One University Plaza
Youngstown, OH 44555-0001
(330) 742-2000
(330) 742-3674 (fax)
enroll@ysu.edu

GENERAL SPORTS MEDICINE PROGRAMS

Arkansas State University
P.O. Box 1630
State University, AR 72467
(870) 972-3024
admissions@chickasaw.astate.edu

California State University, Chico
400 West First Street
Chico, CA 95929
(530) 898-4428
info@csuchico.edu

California State University, Long Beach
Brottman Hall
1250 Bellflower Boulevard
Long Beach, CA 90840
(562) 985-4641
http://www.csulb.edu

College of William and Mary
P.O. Box 8795
Williamsburg, VA 23187-8795
(757) 221-4223
admiss@facstaff.wm.edu

Columbia University
Mail Code 4101, Lewisohn Hall
2970 Broadway
New York, NY 10027-9829
(212) 854-2772
gsdegree@columbia.edu

Indiana State University
210 North Seventh Street
Terre Haute, IN 47809-1401
(812) 237-2121
admisu@amberindstate.edu

Miami University Sports Medicine
Oxford, OH 45056
(513) 529-2531
admission@muohio.edu

Middle Tennessee State University
Murfreesboro, TN 37132
(615) 898-2111
admissions@mtsu.edu

Minnesota State University
209 Wrigley Administration Center
Mankato, MN 56001
(507) 389-6670
admissions@mankato.msus.edu

Montclair State University
Valley Road and Normal Avenue
Upper Montclair, NJ 07043-1624

(800) 331-9205
msuadm@saturn.montclair.edu

Northern Illinois University
Admissions Office
DeKalb, IL 60115-2854
(815) 753-0446
admission-info@niu.edu

Southern Illinois University at Carbondale
Mail Code 4710
Carbondale, IL 62901-4710
(618) 536-4405
admrec@siu.edu

Ohio State University
Lincoln Tower, Third Floor
Columbus, OH 43210-1200
(614) 292-3980
telecounseling@fa.adm.ohio-state.edu

Temple University
Admissions Office
Philadelphia, PA 19122-1803
(215) 204-7200
tuadm@vm.temple.edu

University of Kentucky
100 W. D. Funkhouser Building
Lexington, KY 40506
(606) 257-2000
admission@pop.uky.edu

University of Nevada, Las Vegas
Box 451021
4505 Maryland Parkway
Las Vegas, NV 89154-1021
(702) 895-3443
http://www.unlv.edu

University of Oregon
1217 University of Oregon
Eugene, OR 97403-1217
(541) 346-3201
uoadmit@oregon.uoregon.edu

University of Tulsa
600 South College Avenue
Tulsa, OK 74104-3189
(918) 631-2307
admission@utulsa.edu

University of Wisconsin–Eau Claire
P.O. Box 4004
Eau Claire, WI 54702-4004
(715) 836-5415
ask-uwec@uwec.edu

West Virginia University
P.O. Box 6009
Morgantown, WV 26506-6009
(304) 293-2121
wvuadmissions@arc.wvu.edu

SPECIFIC SPORTS MEDICINE PROGRAMS

Biomechanics
Stanford University–Biomechanical Engineering Division
Stanford, CA 94305-9991
(650) 723-2091
undergrad.admissions@forsythe.stanford.edu

University of Florida
College of Health and Human Performance
P.O. Box 114000
Gainesville, FL 32611-4000
(352) 392-1365
http://www.ufl.edu

Exercise Physiology
University of California, Chico
400 West First Street
Chico, CA 95929
(530) 898-4428
info@csuchico.edu

West Virginia University
P.O. Box 6009
Morgantown, WV 26506-6009
(304) 293-2121
wvuadmissions@arc.wvu.edu

Orthopedics
Emory University
Atlanta, GA 30322-1100
(404) 727-6036
admiss@unix.cc.emory.edu

Louisiana State University
Health Sciences Center
433 Bolivar Street
New Orleans, LA 70112-2223
(504) 568-1829
http://www.lsu.edu

Ohio State University
Lincoln Tower, Third Floor
Columbus, OH 43210-1200
(614) 292-3980
telecounseling@fa.adm.ohio-state.edu

Temple University
Admissions Office
Philadelphia, PA 19122-1803
(215) 204-7200
tuadm@vm.temple.edu

University of Alabama at Birmingham
260 HUC
1530 3rd Avenue South
Birmingham, AL 35294-1150

(205) 934-8221
UndergradAdmit@uab.edu

University of Arkansas
200 Silas H. Hunt Hall
Fayetteville, AR 72701-1201
(501) 575-5346
uafadmis@comp.uark.edu

University of Florida
P.O. Box 114000
Gainesville, FL 32611-4000
(352) 392-1365
http://www.efl.edu

University of Missouri at Columbia
225 Jesse Hall
Columbia, MO 65211
(573) 882-7786
mu4u@missouri.edu

University of New Mexico
Albuquerque, NM 87131-2046
(505) 277-2446
apply@unm.edu

University of Rochester Medical Center
P.O. Box 270251
Rochester, NY 14627-0001
(716) 275-3221
admit@admissions.cc.rochester.edu

Yale University School of Medicine
P.O. Box 208234
New Haven, CT 06520-8324
(203) 432-9300
undergraduate.admissions@yale.edu

Physical Therapy
George Washington University
Admissions Office
Washington, DC 20052
(202) 994-6040
gwadm@gwis2.circ.gwu.edu

Medical College of Georgia
1120 Fifteenth Street
Augusta, GA 30912
(706) 721-2725
underadm@mail.mcg.edu

Northeastern University
150 Richards Hall
Boston, MA 02115-5096
(617) 373-2200
admissions@neu.edu

Nova Southeastern University
3301 College Avenue
Fort Lauderdale, FL 33314

(954) 262-8001
ncsinfo@polaris.nova.edu

Slippery Rock University
Maltby Center
Slippery Rock, PA 16057
(724) 738-2015
apply@sru.edu

South West Texas State University
Admissions Center
San Marcos, TX 78666
(512) 245-2364
admissions@swt.edu

University of Delaware
116 Hullihen Hall
Newark, DE 19716

(302) 831-8123
admissions@udel.edu

University of Tennessee
131 Hooper Hall
Chattanooga, TN 37403-2598
(423) 755-4662
patsy-reynolds@utc.edu

University of Washington
P.O. Box 355840
Seattle, WA 98195-5840
(206) 543-9686
http://www.washington.edu

APPENDIX VII
SPORTS MEDICINE JOURNALS

Web sites for the following journals can be found online, although most have a primary print edition. For more information or to locate other publications, check MedBioWorld's listings of orthopedic and sports medicine journals at http://www.medbioworld.com/.

American Journal of Sports Medicine
Bruce Reider, M.D., Managing Editor
675 Peter Jefferson Parkway
Suite 470
Charlottesville, VA 22911
(434) 975-0864
(434) 975-0865 (fax)
breider@ajsm.org
http://www.ajsm.org/

Arthroscopy Journal
Anne Stewart Skulskie, Managing Editor
CompRehab Plaza
131 Miller Street
Winston-Salem, NC 27103
(336) 716-8458
(336) 716-8448 (fax)
askulskie@ec.rr.com

Athletic Therapy Today
Gary Wilkerson, Editor
University of Tennessee at Chattanooga, Dept. 6606
615 McCallie Avenue
Chattanooga, TN 37403-2598
Gary-Wilkerson@utc.edu

British Journal of Sports Medicine
Centre for Sports Medicine Research & Education
School of Physiotherapy
Level 1, 200 Berkeley Street
Parkville, Victoria 3052 Australia
(613) 8344-4118
(613) 8344-3771
http://www.bjsm.bmjjournals.com/misc/contact.shtml
bjsm@bmjgroup.com

Clinical Biomechanics
Spinal Research Unit, University of Huddersfield
c/o 30 Queen Street
Huddersfield HD1 2SP, United Kingdom
44-1-484-535-200
44-1-484-435-744 (fax)
http://www.elsevier.nl/locate/clinbiomech
Kim@spineresearch.org.uk

Clinical Journal of Sports Medicine
University of Calgary
Sport Medicine Centre
2500 University Drive NW
Calgary, AB T2N IN4 Canada
(403) 220-8947
(403) 210-9393 (fax)
http://www.cjsportmed.com/
cjsm@ucalgary.ca

Current Sports Medicine Reports
Current Science, Inc.
400 Market Street, Suite 700
Philadelphia, PA 19106
(800) 427-1796
(215) 574-2266
http://www.current-reports.com/feedback.cfm?RE=
  Current%20Sports%20Medicine%20Reports
info@current-sports.com

International Journal of Sports Medicine
Georg Thieme Verlag
Rüdigerstraße 14
Postfach 301120
70451 Stuttgart Germany
http://www.thieme.de/sportsmed/

International Orthopaedics
Springer-Verlag Heidelberg
Tiergartenstr. 17
D-69121 Heidelberg Germany
http://www.springerlink.com/app/home/journal.asp?
  wasp=9cxu7yfa5x6ynk91255w&referrer=parent&
  backto=linkingpublicationresults,id:100518,1

Journal of Applied Biomechanics
Thomas S. Buchanan
Director, Center for Biomedical Engineering Research
University of Delaware
126 Spencer Lab
Newark, DE 19716
(302) 831-2410
(302) 831-3466 (fax)
http://www.humankinetics.com/products/journals/
    journal.cfm?id=JAB
buchanan@me.udel.edu

Journal of Athletic Training
Teresa Foster Welch
National Athletic Trainers' Association
2952 Stemmons Freeway
Dallas, TX 75247
(214) 637-6282
(214) 637-2206 (fax)
http://www.journalofathletictraining.org

*Journal of Orthopaedic & Sports Physical
    Therapy*
1111 North Fairfax Street
Suite 100
Alexandria, VA 22314-1436
(877) 766-3450
(703) 836-2210 (fax)
http://www.jospt.org
jospt@jospt.org

Journal of Prosthetics and Orthotics
526 King Street
Suite 201
Alexandria, VA 22314
(703) 836-0788
(703) 836-0737 (fax)
http://www.oandp.org/

Journal of Science and Medicine in Sport
ACHPER Inc.
214 Port Road
Hindmarsh, South Australia 5007
08-8340 3388
08-8340 3399 (fax)
http://www.achper.org.au/ajsm.htm
achper@achper.org.au

*Journal of Sports Medicine and Physical
    Fitness*
Swets Backsets Service
P.O. Box 810
2160 SZ Lisse, The Netherlands
31-0-252-435-111
31-0-252-415-888 (fax)
http://www.swets.nl/backsets/catalogue_result_
    0022-4707.htm
backsets@swets.nl

Journal of Sports Science and Medicine
Department of Sports Medicine
Medical Faculty of Uludag University
16059 Bursa, Turkey
90-224-442-81-96
90-224-442-87-27 (fax)
http://www.jssm.org
hakan@uludag.edu.tr

Knee Surgery, Sports Traumatology, Arthroscopy
Springer-Verlag Heidelberg
Tiergartenstr. 17
D-69121 Heidelberg, Germany
http://www.springerlink.com/app/home/journal.asp?
    wasp=9cxu7yfa5x6ynk91255w&referrer=parent&
    backto=linkingpublicationresults,id:100518,1

Medicine & Science in Sports & Exercise
Kent B. Pandolf, Senior Research Scientist
U.S. Army Research
Institute of Environmental Medicine
Natick, MA 07560-5007
(508) 233-4832
(508) 233-5298 (fax)
http://www.ms-se.com/
kent.pandolf@na.amedd.army.mil

Orthopedics Today
6900 Grove Road
Thorofare, NJ 08086
(856) 848-1000
(856) 853-5991 (fax)
http://www.slackinc.com/bone/ortoday/othome.asp
orthoday@slackinc.com

Physical Therapy in Sport
Kevin Foreman, Associate Dean
Professions Allied to Medicine
University of the West of England
Bristol, United Kingdom
http://www.harcourtinternational.com/journals/ptsp/
board.cfmptis@pettylane.freeserve.co.uk

The Physician and Sportsmedicine
4530 West 77th Street
Minneapolis, MN 55435
(952) 835-3222
(952) 835-3460 (fax)
http://www.physsportsmed.com/

*Research in Sports Medicine: An International
    Journal*
Department of Sports Science & Physical Education
G05 Kwok Sports Building, The Chinese University of
Hong Kong
Hong Kong
(852) 2609-6082
http://www.tandf.co.uk/journals/titles/15438627.html

Science and Sport
Elsevier
23 rue Linois
75724 Paris, Cedex 15 France
33-1-71-72-46-46
33-1-71-72-46-64 (fax)
http://www.elsevier.com/inca/publications/store/5/0/5/
    8/2/2/

Sports Medicine
Wolters Kluwer Health
Pharma Solutions Division

4 Gatehall Drive, 2nd Floor
Parsippany, NJ 07054
(973) 267-7210
(973) 267-7860
http://www.adis.com/page.asp?objectID=55

Sports Medicine and Arthroscopy Review
Lippincott Williams & Wilkins
530 Walnut Street
Philadelphia, PA 19016
(215) 521-8300
http://www.sportsmedarthro.com/

APPENDIX VIII
SPORTS MEDICINE WEB SITES

SEARCH ENGINES

Search for specific topics of interest at the following sports medicine search engines. The best way to search is to type in the most distinct keywords possible for your search topic. For example, if you are looking for information on common ankle injuries, you might want to search under "Achilles tendonitis" to draw the most information on that type of common ankle injury. Then you could do another search under "ankle sprain" for sites that specifically address this type of injury. If you want information specifically on taping ankle injuries, for example, search under "taping ankle injuries."

eSportmed.com
http://www.esportmed.com/

MedNets Orthopedic Journals
http://www.mednets.com/orthopedjournals.htm

Medscape
http://www.medscape.com/px/urlinfo

National Sports Medicine Institute of the United Kingdom
http://www.nsmi.org.uk/

Orthogate
http://www.owl.orthogate.com/

Sports Information Resource Center
http://www.sportsquest.com/

SportsMedicine.com
http://www.sportsmedicine.com/

DISCUSSION LISTSERVS

A discussion list is like an Internet P.O. box for specific subjects. Individuals who subscribe to the discussion list, which is also sometimes called a Listserv, can receive e-mail messages from other subscribers. This is a great way to interact with other professionals or interested persons from all around the world. Once subscribed to a discussion list, users can also send messages to the discussion list for others to reply to. Below are a few recommended lists. To subscribe, just follow the directions below for sending an e-mail to the list.

Web Sites to Find Discussion Lists or Newsgroups
YahooGroup
http://www.groups.yahoo.com/

Liszt (mailing directory)
http://www.liszt.com/

MSN Group
http://www.groups.msn.com/

Athletic Training Discussion List (ATHTRN-L)
E-mail address: LISTPROC@LISTS.INDSTATE.EDU
Subject: (leave this line blank)
Message: SUBSCRIBE ATHTRN-L Firstname Lastname

AthleticTraining_Education List (AT_Education)
E-mail address: athletic_training_education-subscribe@yahoogroups.com
Subject: (leave this line blank)
Message: (leave this line blank)

Christian Sports Medicine List (ChristianSportsMed)
Email address: christiansportsmed-subscribe@yahoogroups.com
Subject: (leave this line blank)
Message: (leave this line blank)

Ethnically Diverse Athletic Trainers (LEDAT)
E-mail address: LEDAT-subscribe@yahoogroups.com
Subject: (leave this line blank)
Message: (leave this blank)

High School Athletic Trainer List (HS-ATC)
E-mail address: HS-ATC@LAWRENCEVILLE.ORG
Subject: SUBSCRIBE
Message: Firstname Lastname

Physical Therapy Education (APTA Education Section)
E-mail address: aptaeducationsubscribe
@yahoogroups.com
Subject: (leave this line blank)
Message: (leave this blank)

Physical Therapy Manager List (PTManager)
E-mail address: ptmanager-subscribe@yahoogroups.com
Subject: (leave this line blank)
Message: (leave this line blank)

Student Athletic Trainers' Association (SATA)
E-mail address: student_athletic_trainers_association-
subscribe@yahoogroups.com
Subject: (leave this line blank)
Message: (leave this blank)

Super Training List (SuperTraining)
E-mail address: supertrainingsubscribe
@yahoogroups.com
Subject: (leave this line blank)
Message: (leave this line blank)

INDIVIDUAL SPORTS MEDICINE SITES

About: Sports Medicine
http://www.sportsmedicine.about.com/

About: Orthopedics - Sports Medicine
http://www.orthopedics.about.com/msub22.htm?once=
true&

American College of Sports Medicine
http://www.acsm.org/

Athletic Trainer.Com
http://www.athletictrainer.com

Body IQ
http://www.bodyiq.com/

Boomeritis - Sports Injuries
http://www.boomer-it is.org

Canadian Academy of Sport Medicine
http://www.casm-acms.org/

eSportMed.com
http://www.esportsmed.com/

ESPN Training Room
http://www.espn.go.com/trainingroom/index.html

Gatorade Sports Science Institute
http://www.gssiweb.com

Hardin Meta Directory (Internet Health Sources)
http://www.lib.uiowa.edu/hardin/md

Health South
http://www.healthsouth.com

Health Sports Medicine Center (University of Wisconsin)
http://www.uwsportsmedicine.org

The Hughston Clinic
http://www.hughston.com/

International Federation of Sports Medicine (FIMS)
http://www.fims.org/

Medical Matrix
http://www.medmatrix.org/index

Medicine on the Net
http://www.Corhealth.com/motn/motnhome4.asp

Methodist Sports Medicine Center
http://www.methodistsports.com/

Mississippi Sports Medicine & Orthopedic Center
http://www.msmoc.com

Nicholas Institute of Sports Medicine
http://www.nismat.org

PubMed
http://www.ncbi.nlm.nih.gov/pubmed/medline.html

Sports Doc
http://www.medfacts.com/sprtsdoc.htm

Sports Medicine - Australia
http://www.ausport.gov.au/sma

SportsMed - British Columbia
http://www.sportmedbc.com/sportmed.php

SportsMed CEU (School Health)
http://www.sportsmedceu.com/main.html

Sports-Med.com
http://www.sports-med.com/

Sports Medicine Concepts
http://www.sportsmedicineconcepts.com

Sports Medicine Digest
http://www.sportsmeddigest.com

Sports Medicine Shop
http://www.sportsmedshop.com

Sport Quest.com
http://www.sportquest.com

Sports Rehab.com
http://www.sportsrehab.com

SportsMed Web
http://www.rice.edu/~jenky/mednav.html

The Stone Clinic
http://www.stoneclinic.com

Student ATC
http://www.11.ewebsity.com/adamhopkins/main.asp

Tendinosis.org
http://www.tendinosis.org/

Tulane Institute of Sports Medicine
http://www.som.tulane.edu/departments.orthopaedics/
    sportsmed

Virtual Sports Injury Clinic
http://www.sportsinjuryclinic.net

SPORTS NUTRITION SITES

Harvard Eating Disorders Center
http://www.hedc.org

National Eating Disorders Association
http://www.nationaleatingdisorders.org

Nutrition, Exercise, & Wellness (University of Arizona)
http://www.ag.arizona.edu/NSC/new/index.htm

Nutrition, Health, & Medicine
http://www.osu.orst.edu/food-resource/nutri.html

Sports Nutrition Guidelines
http://www.hmse.memphis.edu/faculty/kreider/
    Nutrition.Nutindex.htm

Sports Nutrition (Health-Nexus)
http://www.doctors.health-nexus.com/sports_
    nutrition.com

Sports Nutrition Information Resources
http://www.wellcentered.com/sntg/resources.html

BIBLIOGRAPHY

GENERAL

Anderson, Marcia K. *Fundamentals of Sports Injury Management.* Hagerstown, Md.: Lippincott, Williams & Wilkins, 2002.

Beim, Gloria, and Ruth Winter. *The Female Athlete's Body Book: How to Prevent and Treat Sports Injuries in Women and Girls.* New York: McGraw-Hill/Contemporary Books, 2003.

Brukner, Peter, Karim Khan, and John Sutton. *Clinical Sports Medicine.* New York: McGraw-Hill, 2002.

Delee, Jesse, and David Drez, eds. *Delee & Drez's Orthopaedic Sports Medicine: Principles and Practice.* Philadelphia: W. B. Saunders, 2003.

Feinberg, Joseph H., and Neil I. Spielholz, eds. *Peripheral Nerve Injuries in the Athlete.* Champaign, Ill.: Human Kinetics, 2003.

Griffith, H. Winter. *Complete Guide to Sports Injuries: Hot to Treat Fractures, Bruises, Sprains, Strains, Dislocation, Head Injuries.* New York: Perigee, 1997.

Ireland, Mary, and Aurelia Nattiv, eds. *The Female Athlete.* Philadelphia: W. B. Saunders, 2003.

Irvin, Richard, Duane Iversen, and Steven Roy. *Sports Medicine: Prevention, Assessment, Management & Rehabilitation of Athletic Injuries* (2nd Ed.). Philadelphia: Benjamin/Cummings, 1998.

Kolt, Gregory S., and Lynn Snyder-Mackler, eds. *Physical Therapies in Sport and Exercise.* Philadelphia: Churchill Livingstone, 2003.

Landry, Gregory L., and David T. Bernhardt. *Essentials of Primary Care Sports Medicine.* Champaign, Ill.: Human Kinetics, 2003.

Levy, Allan M. *Sports Injury Handbook: Professional Advice for Amateur Athletes.* New York: John Wiley & Sons, 1993.

Micheli, Lyle J. *Sports Medicine Bible: Prevent, Detect, and Treat Your Sports Injuries Through the Latest Medical Techniques.* New York: HarperResource, 1995.

Miller, Mark D., et al. *Surgical Atlas of Sports Medicine.* Philadelphia: W. B. Saunders, 2003.

———. *Review of Sports Medicine & Arthroscopy.* Philadelphia: W. B. Saunders, 2002.

Ross, Michael J. *Maximum Performance: Sports Medicine for Endurance Athletes.* Charleston, S.C.: Velo Press, 2003.

Rouzier, Pierre A. *The Sports Medicine Patient Advisor.* Amherst, Mass.: SportsMed Press, 1999.

Starkey, Chad. *Evaluation of Orthopedic and Athletic Injuries.* Philadelphia: F. A. Davis, 2001.

BASEBALL

Andres, James R., ed. *Injuries in Baseball.* Hagerstown, Md.: Lippincott Williams & Wilkins, 1998.

Croce, Pat. *Baseball Player's Guide to Sports Medicine.* Champaign, Ill.: Human Kinetics, 1987.

Rogers, Marc A., et al. *Sports Medicine for Coaches and Athletes: Older Individuals and Athletes Over 50.* London: Dunnitz Martin, 2000.

Shamoo, Adil E., Charles E. Silberstein, and Robert M. Germeroth. *Sports Medicine for Coaches and Athletes: Baseball.* London: Dunnitz Martin, 2000.

BASKETBALL

Bassett, Frank H. *Basketball Injuries and Treatment.* Hagerstown, Md.: Lippincott, Williams & Wilkins, 1999.

McKeag, Douglas, ed. *Basketball* (*Handbook of Sports Management and Science*). Oxford, England: Blackwell, 2003.

Wright, John D. *Basketball* (*Sports Injuries: How to Prevent, Diagnose & Treat*). Brookshire, Tex.: Mason Crest, 2003.

BICYCLING

Burke, Ed. *Cycling Health and Physiology: Using Sports Science to Improve Your Riding and Racing.* Montpelier, Vt.: Vitesse Press, 1998.

Cabutan, Ross R. *Sport of Bicycling—Helmet Laws, Head, & Body Injuries & Accident Prevention: Index & Reference Book of New Information.* Washington, D.C.: ABBE, DC, 1996.

Friel, Joe. *The Cyclist's Training Bible: A Complete Training Guide for the Competitive Road Cyclist.* Charleston, S.C.: Velo Press, 1996.

Pavelka, Ed, ed. *Bicycling Magazine's Complete Book of Road Cycling Skills: Your Guide to Riding Faster, Stronger, Longer, and Safer.* Emmaus, Pa.: Rodale Press, 1998.

FOOTBALL

Ekstrand, Jan, ed. *Football Medicine.* New York: Routledge, 2002.

Fevre, Dave. *Collision Sports: Injury and Repair.* Philadelphia: Butterworth-Heinemann Medical, 1998.

Spinks, Warwick, et al., eds. *Science and Football IV.* New York: Routledge, 2001.

HOCKEY

Bompa, Tudor O., and Dave Champers. *Total Hockey Conditioning: From Pee-Wee to Pro.* Westport, Conn.: Firefly Books, 2003.

Horrigan, Joseph M., E. J. Kreis, and Luc Robitaille. *Strength, Conditioning, and Injury Prevention for Hockey.* New York: McGraw-Hill/Contemporary Books, 2002.

Twist, Peter, and Pavel Bure. *Complete Conditioning for Ice Hockey.* Champaign, Ill.: Human Kinetics, 1996.

RUNNING

Ellis, Joe. *Running Injury-Free: How to Prevent, Treat and Recover from Dozens of Painful Problems.* Emmaus, Pa.: Rodale Press, 1994.

Fox, James D., and Rick McGuire. *Save Your Knees.* San Diego, Calif.: DTP, 1988.

Glover, Bob, and Murray Weisenfeld. *The Injured Runner's Training Handbook: The Coach's and Doctor's Guide for Prevention, Running Through, and Coming Back from Injury.* New York: Penguin, 1985.

Hawley, John A., ed. *Running (Handbook of Sports Medicine and Science).* Oxford, England: Blackwell Science, 2000.

Higdon, Hal. *Hal Higdon's Smart Running: Expert Advice on Training, Motivation, Injury Prevention, Nutrition, and Good Health for Runners of Any Age and Ability.* Emmaus, Pa.: Rodale Press, 1998.

Mangi, Richard, Peter Jokl, and O. William Dayton. *The Runner's Complete Medical Guide.* New York: Simon & Schuster, 1979.

Micheli, Lyle J., and Mark D. Jenkins. *Healthy Runner's Handbook.* Champaign, Ill.: Human Kinetics, 1998.

Noakes, Tim, and Stephen Granger. *Running Injuries.* New York: Oxford University Press, 2003.

O'Connor, Francis, and Robert Wilder. *Textbook of Running Medicine.* New York: McGraw-Hill Professional, 2001.

Scott, Dagny. *Runner's World Complete Book of Women's Running: The Best Advice to Get Started, Stay Motivated, Lose Weight, Run Injury-Free, Be Safe, and Train for Any Distance.* Emmaus, Pa.: Rodale Press, 2002.

Weisenfeld, Murray, and Barbara Burr Weisenfeld. *The Runner's Repair Manual.* New York: St. Martin's, 1981.

SKIING

Ekeland, Arne, et al., eds. *Sports Medicine for Coaches and Athletes: Skiing.* London: Dunitz Martin, 2000.

Leach, Robert E. *Alpine Skiing (Handbook of Sports Medicine and Science).* Oxford, England: Blackwell Science, 1994.

Muller, Eric, et al., eds. *Science and Skiing.* New York: Routledge, 1997.

Rusko, Heikki. *Handbook of Cross-Country Skiing: Olympic Handbook of Sports Medicine.* Oxford, England: Blackwell Science, 2002.

SOCCER

Farrow, Pete. *Soccer (Sports Injuries: How to Prevent, Diagnose & Treat).* Brookshire, Tex.: Mason Crest, 2003.

Fevre, David. *Collision Sports: Injury and Repair.* Philadelphia: Butterworth-Heinemann Medical, 1998.

Garrett, William E., Jr., Donald T. Kirkendall, and S. Robert Contiguglia, eds. *U.S. Soccer Sports Medicine Book.* Hagerstown, Md.: Lippincott, Williams & Wilkins, 1996.

Reilly, Thomas, ed. *Science and Soccer.* New York: Routledge, 2002.

Shamoo, Adil E. *Sports Medicine for Coaches and Athletes: Soccer.* London: Dunitz Martin, 1995.

Smith, Alan G. *Soccer Injuries: Prevention and First Aid.* Ramsbury, England: Crowood Press, 1995.

SWIMMING

Costill, David L. *Swimming (Handbook of Sports Medicine and Science).* Oxford, England: Blackwell Science, 1992.

Miyashita, M., Y. Mutoh, and A. B. Richardson, eds. *Medicine and Science in Aquatic Sports (Medicine and Sport Science, vol. 39).* Basel: S. Karger Publishing, 1994.

Stager, Joel M., and David Tanner. *Swimming (Handbook of Sports Management and Science).* Oxford, England: Blackwell Science, 2003.

Troup, J. P., et al. *Biomechanics and Medicine in Swimming.* New York: Routledge, 1996.

TENNIS

Croce, Pat. *Tennis Player's Guide to Sports Medicine.* Champaign, Ill.: Human Kinetics, 2003.

Levisohn, Steven R., and Harvey Simon. *Tennis Medic: Conditioning, Sports Medicine and Total Fitness for Every Player.* Mosby, 1984.

Levy, Allan M., and Mark L. Fuerst. *Tennis Injury Handbook : Professional Advice for Amateur Athletes.* New York: John Wiley & Sons, 1999.

Renstrom, Per, ed. *Tennis: Olympic Handbook of Sports Medicine.* Oxford, England: Blackwell Science, 2002.

TRIATHLON

Fitzgerald, Matt. Triathlete Magazine's *Complete Triathlon Training Book: The Training, Diet, Health, Equipment, and Safety Tips You Need to Do Your Best.* New York: Warner Books, 2003.

Friel, Joe. *The Triathlete's Training Bible: A Complete Training Guide for the Competitive Multisport Athlete.* Charleston, S.C.: Velo Press, 1998.

VOLLEYBALL

Dearing, Joel. *Volleyball Fundamentals.* Champaign, Ill.: Human Kinetics, 2003

Reeser, Jonathan, and Roald Bahr, eds. *Volleyball (Handbook of Sports Medicine and Science).* Oxford, England: Blackwell Science, 2003.

INDEX

Boldface page numbers
indicate major treatment
of a subject.

A

AAASP (Association for the
Advancement of Applied
Sports Psychology) 199–200
abdominal muscles,
strengthening in pregnancy
60
abrasions **1**
    corneal **50–51**
    wrestling and 241
ACA Sports Council 271
acetazolamide (Diamox), for
    acute mountain sickness 7
Achilles tendon
    anatomy of 264
    in calf muscle injuries
        37
    rupture **2–3,** 263
    stretch for **3**
Achilles tendinitis **3–5**
    bicycling and 232
    running and 235
AC joint injury. *See* acromio-
    clavicular (AC) joint, injury
ACL injury
    See anterior cruciate liga-
        ment (ACL) injury
acromioclavicular (AC) joint
    266
    injury **5–6, 193–195**
        dislocation 44–45
activity level, increasing, and
    injury prevention 113

acupuncture, for cervical
    radiculopathy 43
acute mountain sickness **6–7**
adductor magnus strain **85**
adductors, of thigh, and
    piriformis syndrome 171
adenosine diphosphate (ADP),
    creatine and 52
adenosine triphosphate (ATP),
    creatine and 52
adhesive capsulitis **78–80**
adolescents
    dehydration in 56
    hamstring injury in 90
    iliopsoas tendinitis in
        107–109
    and meal planning in bas-
        ketball 243–244
    medial condylar fracture of
        elbow 138–139
    Osgood-Schlatter disease
        154–156
    osteochondritis dissecans
        161–162
    participation in sports
        224–226
    risk of injury in 225
    Sever's disease **190**
    slipped capital femoral epi-
        physis **197–198**
    sports psychology tips for
        201
    swimming and 256
    testicular torsion in
        212–213
aerobic training/exercise **7–9**
    after hip dislocation 100

vs. anaerobic 9
    benefits of, with congestive
        heart failure 50
    for femoral neck fractures
        72–73
    for osteoarthritis 160
    running and 233
African-Americans, slipped
    capital femoral epiphysis
    197–198
age. *See also* aging
    femur fractures and 73
    and skiing injuries 238
aging
    and AC joint injury 194
    flexibility and 77
    and herniated disk 96–98
    and injury prevention 113
    low back pain and 127,
        128, 185
    and lumbosacral disk
        injuries 128
    and posterior tibial tendini-
        tis 174–175
    and rotator cuff tear in
        shoulder dislocation
        192–193
    and skin cancer 195
    weight training and 203,
        220
    and wrist injuries **220–222**
    yips and **223–224**
AIDS, anabolic steroids for
    9–10
air quality, and running safety
    234

alcohol consumption
    and avascular femoral head
        necrosis 22, 24
    and back pain 129
alcohol consumption
    golf and 249, 250
    and post-exercise recovery
        254
    and swimming safety 240
alignment problems
    and femoral neck fractures
        72
    and jumper's knee 118
    and overuse injuries 165
    and patellofemoral pain
        syndrome 180–182
allergies
    contrast media and 47–48
    and exercise-induced
        asthma 18, 19
allograft, for ACL
    reconstruction 16
altered mental status,
    concussion 48–49
altitudes, high
    pregnancy and 61
    proper techniques for
        ascending to 7
    running safety at 234
    skiing safety and 238
altitude sickness **6–7**
amenorrhea **68–69**
    athletic **20–21**
    in female athlete triad
        67–69
    and femoral neck fractures
        70–71
    primary *vs.* secondary 20
American Academy of Ortho-
    pedic Surgeons 266, 271
American Academy of Orthotists
    and Prosthetists 271
American Academy of
    Pediatrics, children and
    boxing 31
American Academy of Physical
    Medicine and Rehabilitation
    271

American Academy of Podiatric
    Sports Medicine 272
American Alliance for Health,
    Physical Education,
    Recreation & Dance 271
American College of Sports
    Medicine
    contact information 271
    endorsed sports medicine
        programs 275–276
*American Journal of Sports
    Medicine* 281
American Massage Therapy
    Association 271
American Orthopaedic Society
    for Sports Medicine 272
American Osteopathic Academy
    of Sports Medicine 271
American Physical Therapy
    Association 271
American Physiological Society
    271
American Psychological
    Association 200
American Society of Exercise
    Physiologists 271
anabolic steroids **9–11**
    cortisone *vs.* 51
    and sudden death 205
anaerobic activities, *vs.* aerobic
    exercise 9
anaphylaxis, contrast media
    and 48
anatomic abnormalities
    and femoral neck fractures
        72
    and mountain biking
        injuries 145
    and overuse injuries **165**
    and patellofemoral pain
        syndrome 168
    and running injuries
        233–234
androgenic effects, of male
    hormones 10
anemia
    and exercise in pregnancy
        62

    and fatigue 66
    iron deficiency **114–115**
ankle
    anatomy of 264
    injuries
        ankle fracture 12–13
        ankle sprain 13–14
        common **264**
        osteochondritis disse-
            cans 161–162
        peroneal tendinitis
            169–170
        posterior tibial tendini-
            tis 174–175
        prevention of **114**
        running and 234
        tibialis posterior syn-
            drome 215–216
ankle brace **114**
ankle fracture **12–13**
ankle sprain **13–14**
    avulsion fractures and 75
anorexia **14–16,** 68
    athletic amenorrhea and
        21
anterior cruciate ligament
    (ACL) injury **16,** 263
    skiing after 236
    wrestling and 241
anterior dislocation, of shoulder
    192
anterior hip dislocations 98
anterior knee pain. *See*
    patellofemoral pain syndrome
anterior tibial tendon 264
anticatabolic effect, of anabolic
    steroids 10
antiseptics, for abrasions 1
anxiety, and yips 223–224
apophysitis
    calcaneal **190**
    medial **125–127**
Appalachian State University
    275
appetite suppression, ephedrine
    and 59
arches, of foot 264, 265
arch pain **16–17**

arch supports. *See also* orthotics
    for posterior tibial tendinitis
        175
Arkansas State University 277
arm
    injuries/disorders
        biceps tendinitis 28
        little league elbow
            125–127
        thoracic outlet syn-
            drome **214–215**
    weakness
        with burners/stingers
            35
        in cervical radiculopa-
            thy 42
arthritic spurs, cervical
    radiculopathy 42
arthritis
    after hip dislocation 100
    anabolic steroids for 9–10
    degenerative (*See*
        osteoarthritis)
    glucosamine for **82–83**
    and knee bursitis 121
arthrocentesis, for osteoarthritis
    160
arthrography
    for Baker's cyst 25
    for frozen shoulder 79
arthroscope **17**
    as diagnostic tool 18
arthroscopy **17–18**
    for AC joint injury 194
    for meniscus injuries 140
    for osteochondritis disse-
        cans 161
Arthroscopy Association of
    North America 272
Arthroscopy Journal 281
Association for the
    Advancement of Applied
    Sports Psychology (AAASP)
    199–200
associations, sports medicine,
    contact information **271–274**
asthma
    anabolic steroids for 10

chronic, and exercise-
    induced asthma 18, 19
    exercise-induced **18–20**
athletes, sports psychology tips
    for 201
athlete's foot **20**
athletic amenorrhea **20–21**
athletic "jet lag" **162–165**
athletic performance. *See*
    performance
Athletic Therapy Today 281
athletic trainer 21–22
Athletic Trainers Association of
    Florida 272
attitude, sports psychology and
    199–201
Australia
    golf competition in 248
    soccer training in 252–253
autograft, for ACL
    reconstruction 16
avascular necrosis
    of femoral head **22–24**
        with hip dislocation
            100
    scaphoid fractures and
        183–184
avulsion fractures **74–75**

B
back. *See also* back pain
    anatomy of 264
    injuries/conditions
        common **264**
        diving and 239
        facet syndrome 65–66
        herniated disk **96–98**
        lumbosacral disk
            injuries **128–130**
        lumbosacral facet syn-
            drome **130–133**
        rhomboid muscle
            injury **177**
        running and 234, 235
        stress fracture 203
        whiplash **220**
    strengthening in pregnancy
        60

back pain. *See also* low back
    pain
    causes of 128–129,
        130–132
    herniated disk and 97
    in lumbosacral disk injuries
        128–130
Baker's cyst **25**
balance, pregnancy and 61
ballet
    athletic amenorrhea 20–21
    female athlete triad 67–69
    FHL tenosynovitis 77–78
    gluteal strain 83
    hamstring injury 90–91
    hip flexor injury 101–102
    iliopsoas tendinitis
        107–109
    sciatica **184–186**
    sesamoiditis 189–190
    stress fracture 203–204
Ball State University 275
banned substances
    anabolic steroids 9–11
    caffeine 37
    ephedrine 59–60
barbells 202, 219
basal cell carcinoma 195
baseball
    ankle sprain 13–14
    biceps tendinitis 28
    blisters 29–30
    blowout fracture 30–31
    bursitis 35–36
    common injuries in 267
    eye injury and 31
    hamate fracture 87–89
    infraspinatus syndrome
        111–112
    injury risk and prevention
        in 226
    little league elbow 125–127
    lumbosacral facet syndrome
        130–133
    nasal fractures 149–150
    osteochondritis dissecans
        161–162
    rotator cuff tear 178–179

baseball *(continued)*
    and rotator cuff tendinitis
        179–180
    safety tips for **229**
    sesamoiditis 189–190
    testicular injury 212–213
    thoracic outlet syndrome
        214–215
    trigger finger 216
    wrist injuries **220–222**
    yips **223–224**
baseball finger **25–26**
basketball
    Achilles tendon rupture
        2–3
    ACL injury 16
    ankle fracture 12–13
    ankle sprain 13–14
    blowout fracture 30–31
    characteristics of **243**
    common injuries in 267
    corneal abrasion 50–51
    eye injury and 31
    groin strain 85
    hip dislocation 98–101
    injury risk and prevention
        in 226
    jammed finger **117–118**
    MCP joint dislocations
        140–141
    nutrition in **243–245**
    Osgood-Schlatter disease
        154–156
    plantar fascitis 172–173
    safety tips for **229–230**
    tibialis posterior syndrome
        215–216
biceps tendon, and swimmer's
    shoulder 209
biceps tendinitis **28**
bicycles
    and bicycling safety
        230–231
    choosing 230
    ill-fitting
        and injury **113**
        and mountain biking
            injuries 145–146

insuring proper fit of
    230–231
stationary 231–232
bicycle seat, and bicycling safety
    231
bicycle seat neuropathy **28–29**
bicycling
    abrasions 1
    AC joint injury 5–6,
        193–195
    bicycle seat neuropathy
        28–29
    characteristics of **245–246**
    common injuries in 267
    equipment and injury pre-
        vention **113**
    exercise-induced asthma
        18–20
    first century ride, training
        tips 269–270
    hip flexor injury 101–102
    iliotibial band syndrome
        109–111
    jumper's knee 118–119
    mountain biking **144–146**
    nasal fractures 149–150
    nutrition for **245–248**
    painful plica 167–168
    patellofemoral pain syn-
        drome **180–182**
    safety tips for **230–232**
    shoulder dislocation
        191–193
    shoulder separation
        193–195
    in triathlons 259–260
big toe 264
    turf toe and 216–217
bike gloves 232
biomechanical problems
    and iliotibial band syn-
        drome 109–110
    and osteitis pubis 157
    and overuse injuries 165
    and running injuries
        233–234
biomechanics, sports medicine
    programs 278

biopsy, of skin cancer 196–197
bleeding, cryotherapy for 53
blepharospasm 223
blisters **29–30**
blood loss, femur fractures and
    73
blood pressure
    ephedrine and 59
    and exercise in pregnancy
        62
blood tests, for osteoarthritis
    160
blood volume, in pregnancy
    61–62
blowout fracture **30–31**
body coils, for MRI 136
body fat levels
    in cyclists 246
    in long-distance runners
        250
    in middle-distance runners
        252
    in soccer players 253
    in sprinters 255
    in tennis players 258
    in triathletes 261
body image, and female athlete
    triad 68, 69
body temperature
    and exercise in pregnancy
        62
    in heat stroke 95
    in hypothermia 104–105
body weight
    optimal, for performance
        69
    recording, in log book 27
bone graft, for avascular
    femoral head necrosis 23
bone growth-plate injuries. *See*
    growth-plate injuries
bone loss
    anorexia and 15
    and stress fractures 70
bone scans, for AC joint injury
    194
boutonniere deformity, with
    jammed finger 117, 118

bowling, in pregnancy 61
boxer's fracture **31–32**
boxing
    children and 31
    eye injury and 31
    stress fracture 203
boys. *See* male(s)
braces/bracing
    for calf muscle injuries 38
    and injury prevention 113
    to prevent ankle sprains
        13–14
brachial plexus injury 35
brain injuries
    acute mountain sickness
        6–7
    concussion **48–49**
    hyponatremia and 103
    second-impact syndrome
        48, **186–189**
breaststroke, and MCL injury
    137
breaststroker's knee **121–122**
breathing
    pregnancy and 61
    proper technique while
        stretching 204
    relaxed, and performance
        27
breathing problems
    acute mountain sickness
        6–7
    asthma, exercise-induced
        18–20
    in congestive heart failure
        49
    and contrast dye allergy 48
brick sessions 259, 260
British Journal of Sports Medicine
    281
broken nose **149–150**
bronchodilator, for exercise-
    induced asthma 19
bruises
    of hamstring 90–91
    hip pointer 102
    thigh bruise **213–214**
    wrestling and 241

bucket handle tear 139
buddy taping, for MCP joint
    dislocations 141
bulimia **32–34,** 68
bunion **34–35**
bunionectomy 34
burners/stingers **35**
burnout **162–165**
bursa sacs 35
    in shoulder 266
bursitis **35–36**
    Baker's cyst 25
    iliopsoas bursitis 107, 108
    knee bursitis **121–122**
    pes anserine bursitis
        121–122
    pre-patella, wrestling and
        241
    running and 235
buttocks pain
    gluteal strain 83
    in piriformis syndrome
        170–171

C

caffeine
    ephedrine with 59
    and sports performance **37**
    and yips 224
calcaneal apophysitis **190**
calcaneus 264, 265
calcium, for overtraining
    syndrome 164
calf muscle injuries **37–39**
California State University
    277
calorie consumption
    for fatigue prevention 66
    in pregnancy 61
Canadian Academy of Sport
    Medicine 272
Canadian Association for
    Health, Physical Education,
    Recreation and Dance 272
Canadian Athletic Therapists'
    Association (CATA) 272
cancer
    and back pain 129, 185

MRI for detection of
    136–137
    skin cancer **195–197**
carbohydrates
    before basketball game 244
    in beverages 57
    for bicycling 246, 247
    complex **46**
    creatine loading and 52
    for fatigue prevention 66
    for golf 249
    for long-distance running
        recovery 250
    for middle-distance run-
        ning 252
    for pregnancy 61
    replacement, and sports
        performance 27
    for soccer training 253
    in sports drinks 57
    for sprinting 254–255
    types of 39
carbohydrate loading **39**
    for bicycling event
        247–248
    for triathlons 260
cardiac pacemakers, and MRI
    135
cardiac problems. *See* heart
    disease
cardiovascular activities. *See*
    aerobic training/exercise
cardiovascular system
    aerobic training/exercise
        and 233
    changes, in pregnancy
        61–62
    screening, for sudden death
        prevention 205
    weight training for 202,
        219
careers
    for orthopedists 153–154
    in physical therapy 170
    in sports nutrition 199
    in sports psychology 200
carpal tunnel syndrome **39–41**
carpus injuries **220–222**

cartilage
    in osteoarthritis 158–160
    in osteochondritis dissecans
        161–162
    restoration, glucosamine
        for **82–83**
    superior labrum lesion
        206–207
cast
    for Achilles tendon rup-
        tures 3
    for ankle fractures 12
    for boxer's fracture 32
    for fifth metatarsal fracture
        75
    for scaphoid fracture 183
    for stress fracture 203
    for wrist injury 222
catecholamines, and exercise
    intolerance in congestive
    heart failure 50
CAT scan. *See* computerized
    axial tomography (CAT) scan
century ride, first, training tips
    269–270
cerebral edema
    in acute mountain sickness
        6–7
    hyponatremia and 103
certification
    sports medicine 275
    for sports psychologists
        199–200
cervical discogenic pain
    syndrome **41–42**
cervical fusion, for facet
    syndrome 65
cervical radiculopathy **42–44**
charley horse **146–147,**
    213–214
children
    boxing and 31
    dehydration and 55, 56, 57
    heat and 57
    and heat-related illnesses
        92, 93, 95
    little league elbow in
        125–127

medial condylar fracture of
    elbow 138–139
nasal fractures in 149
Osgood-Schlatter disease
    154–156
osteochondritis dissecans
    161–162
participation in sports
    224–226
prevention of bicycle seat
    neuropathy in 29
risk of injury in 225
Sever's disease **190**
slipped capital femoral epi-
    physis **197–198**
sports psychology tips for
    201
wrist injuries in 221
cholesterol, high, and sudden
    death 205
chondromalacia patellae. *See*
    patellofemoral pain
    syndrome
chronic otitis externa 207
cigarettes, and back pain
    129
circuit program, of weight
    training 202
clavicle 266
    injuries **44–45**
        shoulder separation
            193–195
cleaning, of wrestling
    equipment 241
climbing, in pregnancy 61
Clinical Biomechanics 281
Clinical Journal of Sports Medicine
    281
clothing/dress
    for frostbite prevention
        78
    for hypothermia prevention
        105
    to prevent heat-related ill-
        nesses 92, 94
    for skiing safety 238
    for skin cancer prevention
        197

coaches
    sports psychology tips for
        201
    and youth participation in
        sports 224
cocaine, and sudden death 205
cognitive functioning, repetitive
    head injury and 187
cold air, and exercise-induced
    asthma 19
cold exposure, and frostbite 78
colds
    and fatigue 67
    overtraining syndrome and
        165
    in swimmers 257
cold therapy. *See* ice therapy
collateral ligament injuries
    with jammed finger 117,
        118
    of knee
        lateral **123–124**
        medial **137–138**
    wrestling and 241
College Athletic Trainers'
    Society (CATS) 272
College of William and Mary
    277
collision sports, and AC joint
    injury 5–6, 193–195
Columbia University 277
comminuted fracture, of wrist
    222
communication skills, in
    athletic trainers 22
compartment syndrome **45–46**
    hamstring injury and 91
    Lisfranc fracture-dislocation
        and 124
    with medial condylar frac-
        ture of elbow 138–139
    running and 235
    vs. shin splints 190–191
competition
    basketball 243
    bicycling 245
    golf 248
    mental rehearsal for 27

soccer 253
sports psychology and 199–201
sprinting 254
swimming 256
tennis 257
wrestling 240
youth participation in 224
complex carbohydrates 39, **46**
complex dislocation, MCP joint dislocations 141
compression **178**
compulsive exercise **46–47**
computerized axial tomography (CAT) scan **47–48**
for head injury 187
MRI *vs.* 137
concussion **48–49,** 263
grading of 187
condylar fracture of elbow, medial **138–139**
congestive heart failure, and exercise **49–50**
consciousness, loss of, with concussion 48, 187
conscious sedation, for medial condylar fracture of elbow 139
contact information
associations and organizations **271–274**
sports medicine journals **281–283**
sports medicine schools **275–279**
contact sports
burners/stingers 35
and hip dislocation 101
in youth sports 225
contractions, uterine, exercise and 62
contrast media
allergic reactions to 47–48
in CAT scan 47–48
for MRI 136
contusions. *See* bruises
cool down, for injury prevention **112–113**

core decompression, for avascular femoral head necrosis 23
core skills, of sport 26
Cormack, Allan 48
corneal abrasion **50–51**
coronary artery disease, and sudden death 205
coronary spasm, and sudden death 205–206
corticosteroids
and avascular femoral head necrosis 22, 24
cortisone **51**
and hamstring injury 90–91
injection **51**
for cervical radiculopathy 43
for FHL tenosynovitis 77–78
for lumbosacral disk injuries 130
for painful plica 167–168
for sciatica 186
for tennis elbow 212
for trigger finger 216
for swimmer's ear 208
cortisol **10**
cortisone **51**. *See also* corticosteroids
cramps
gassy, carbohydrate loading and 39
heat 91–93
muscle **146–147**
creatine and 52
creatine monohydrate **51–53**
cross-training
after minor injuries 26
after stress fracture 203
for iliopsoas tendinitis 109
for peroneal tendinitis 169
cryotherapy **53**. *See also* ice therapy
Current Sports Medicine Reports 281

cutting and jumping motions
Achilles tendon rupture and 2–3
Osgood-Schlatter disease 154–156
cycling. *See* bicycling

D

Damadian, Raymond 136–137
dancing. *See* ballet
Danis-Weber classification, for ankle fractures 12
death
caffeine and 37
ephedrine and 60
sudden death **205–206**
decongestants, for nasal fractures 150
deformity, in blowout fracture 31
degenerative arthritis. *See* osteoarthritis
degenerative disk disease
cervical discogenic pain syndrome 41–42
facet syndrome and 65
phases of 128
dehydration **55–57**
basketball and 244
bicycling and 246–247
caffeine and 37
creatine and 52
and fatigue 66–67
golf and 249
and heat-related illnesses 92, 93, 95
and hypothermia 105
and muscle cramps 146
and sports performance 27
triathlons and 261
wrestling and 241
depression, in overtraining syndrome 164
deviated septum **151**
dexamethasone (Decadron), for acute mountain sickness 7
DEXA scan, for athletic amenorrhea 21

diabetes
>contrast dye and 48
>creatine and 52
>glucosamine supplements
>>and 83
>
>*vs.* lumbosacral disk injuries
>>129
>
>*vs.* metatarsalgia 142
>sports nutrition for 199
>and swimmer's ear 207

Diabetes Exercise and Sports
>Association 272

diarrhea, and dehydration 55,
>56, 57

diet, treatment plan for bulimia
>33

Dietary Supplement Health and
>Education Act (1994) 52

discography
>cervical, for degenerative
>>discogenic disease 42
>
>for herniated disk 97
>for lumbosacral disk
>>injuries 130

discussion lists, sports medicine
>285–286

disks, intervertebral. *See*
>intervertebral disks

dislocations
>with clavicle fracture
>>44–45
>
>with hamate fracture 88
>hip dislocation 98–101
>with jammed finger 117,
>>118
>
>Lisfranc fracture-dislocation
>>**124–125**
>
>metacarpophalangeal
>>(MCP) joint dislocations
>>**140–141**
>
>shoulder dislocation
>>**191–193**

disordered eating. *See* eating
>disorders

diving
>athletic amenorrhea 20–21
>cervical spine injuries 41
>safety tips for 239–240

dorsal dislocation, with jammed
>finger 117, 118

double vision, in blowout
>fracture 31

drafting, in triathlons 259

drinking. *See also* fluid
>intake/replacement
>>during soccer, tips for 254
>>during tennis, tips for 258
>>recommended frequency
>>>for 56

drugs, and hyponatremia 103

dumbbells 202, 219

dystonia, focal **223–224**

E

ear injuries/infections
>frostbite 78
>swimmer's ear **207–208**

East Stroudsburg University
>275

eating disorders
>anorexia 14–16
>athletic amenorrhea and
>>21
>
>bulimia nervosa 32–34
>compulsive exercise and
>>46–47
>
>in female athlete triad
>>67–69
>
>sports nutrition for 199

ecchymosis 90

eczema, and swimmer's ear 207

efforts, high-intensity, in
>interval training 27

elbow
>anatomy of 84, 125, 265
>injuries/conditions
>>bursitis 35–36
>>common **264–265**
>>golfer's elbow **83–85**
>>little league elbow
>>>**125–127**
>>
>>medial condylar frac-
>>>ture **138–139**
>>
>>minor, general treat-
>>>ment principles for
>>>26

osteochondritis disse-
>>>cans 161–162
>>
>>tennis elbow **211–212**

electrical stimulation, for
>cervical radiculopathy 43

electrolyte(s)
>hyponatremia and
>>102–104
>
>loss, and muscle cramps
>>146
>
>replacement 55–57

electromyography
>for herniated disk 97
>for lumbosacral facet syn-
>>drome 132

elevation **178**

Emory University 278

emotions, and sports
>psychology 200, 201

encephalopathy, second-impact
>syndrome and 186

endurance
>aerobic training/exercise
>>and 9
>
>caffeine and 37
>carbohydrate loading and
>>39
>
>maintaining, after minor
>>injuries 26
>
>water loss and 27

endurance training/events
>hyponatremia and
>>102–104
>
>for iliopsoas tendinitis
>>108
>
>and iron deficiency anemia
>>114–115
>
>and muscle cramps
>>146–147
>
>running and 233

energy
>from complex carbohy-
>>drates 46
>
>creatine and 52
>ephedrine and 59
>nutritional deficiencies and
>>66
>
>sports drinks for 57

environment, and running
    safety 234
Ephedra equisetina 59
ephedrine **59–60**
    and heatstroke 53
epicondyles, of elbow 84,
    265
epicondylitis
    lateral **211–212**
    medial **83–85**
epidural steroid injections
    for lumbosacral disk
        injuries 130
    for sciatica 186
epiphysial injuries. *See* growth-
    plate injuries
equipment
    for baseball safety 229
    for basketball safety
        229–230
    and bicycle seat neuropathy
        29
    for bicycling 230–231
    for bursitis prevention
        36
    cleaning of, in wrestling
        241
    for concussion prevention
        49
    for eye protection 31, 51
    for head injury prevention
        188–189
    and injury prevention
        113
    and LCL injury 124
    and MCL injury 138
    for mountain biking 145
    for nose injury prevention
        151
    and overuse injuries 165
    and PCL injury 174
    to prevent blowout fracture
        31
    for skiing safety 236–238
    for soccer safety 239
    for strength training 202
    and tennis elbow preven-
        tion 212

for testicular injury preven-
    tion 213
and training for first
    marathon or century ride
    269
for volleyball safety 240
for weight training 219
for wrestling safety 241
erectile dysfunction, bicycle seat
    neuropathy 28–29
estrogen deficiency
    amenorrhea and 21
    and bone mineral content
        70
    in female athlete triad 69
European Society of Sports
    Traumatology, Knee Surgery,
    and Arthroscopy 272
eversion ankle sprains 13–14
exercise(s)
    after hip dislocation
        100–101
    for calf muscle injuries 38
    compulsive **46–47**
    congestive heart failure and
        49–50
    for hamstring injury pre-
        vention 91
    and iron depletion 114
    for lumbosacral facet syn-
        drome 132–133
    for osteitis pubis 158
    during pregnancy **60–63**
    stabilizing, for herniated
        disk 97
    and sudden death 204–205
exercise-induced asthma
    18–20
exercise intolerance, congestive
    heart failure and 49–50
exercise physiology, sports
    medicine programs 278
exercise program(s)
    aerobic, beginning 9
    cardiovascular screening for
        205
    for painful plica 167
    of weight training 202

extrinsic muscles, of foot 264,
    265
eye injuries/conditions
    blepharospasm 223
    blowout fracture 30–31
    corneal abrasion 50–51
eyewear, protective 31, 51

F
face shields 31
facet syndrome **65–66**
    lumbosacral **130–133**
facial injuries
    blowout fracture 30–31
    frostbite 78
    nasal fractures 149–150
    wrestling and 240–241
fascia, of iliotibial (IT) band
    109
fascial hernias, in compartment
    syndrome 45
fat
    body levels (*See* body fat
        levels)
    dietary, golf and 249
fatigue
    congestive heart failure and
        49, 50
    and middle-distance run-
        ning 252
    monitoring of, for over-
        training syndrome 164
    in overtraining syndrome
        163
    post-viral 67
    prevention **66–67**
        in golf 249
    and skiing injuries 238
feet injuries/conditions. *See*
    foot, injuries/conditions
female(s)
    adolescent, swimming and
        256
    anorexia in 14
    athletic amenorrhea in
        20–21
    bulimia in 32–34
    female athlete triad 67–69

female(s) (continued)
femoral neck fracture 263
frozen shoulder 78–80
iliopsoas tendinitis
107–109
iron deficiency anemia
114–115
iron deficiency in 66
distance running and
250–251
Osgood-Schlatter disease
154–156
osteoarthritis 158–160
osteochondritis dissecans
161–162
posterior tibial tendinitis
174–175
RDA for iron for 66
and skiing injuries 238
sprinters, body fat level in
255
stress fractures in 70
swimmers, iron deficiency
in 257
triathletes, carbohydrates
for 260
wrist injuries in 221
female athlete triad **67–69.** *See
also* anorexia
athletic amenorrhea in 21
and femoral neck fractures
70–71
and stress fractures 70
femoral neck fracture **69–73,**
263
femur injuries/fractures
73–74
avascular femoral head
necrosis **22–24**
femoral neck fractures
69–73
slipped capital femoral epiphysis **197–198**
stress fracture 203, 263
ferritin tests, for iron deficiency
anemia 114–115
fever, and dehydration 55, 56,
57

FHL tenosynovitis. *See* flexus
hallucis longus (FHL)
tenosynovitis
fiber, complex carbohydrates 46
fibula fracture
ankle fracture 12–13
stress fracture 203
fifth metacarpal fracture **31–32**
fifth metatarsal fractures **74–75**
figure skating
athletic amenorrhea 20–21
female athlete triad 67–69
Osgood-Schlatter disease
154–156
finger injuries
baseball finger 25–26
boxer's fracture 31–32
common 266
frostbite 78
gamekeeper's thumb
81–82, 238
with hamate fracture 88
jammed finger **117–118**
metacarpophalangeal
(MCP) joint dislocations
140–141
trigger finger 216
finger pain, in thoracic outlet
syndrome 214–215
fitness program development
and injury prevention 113
weight training in 202
fixation, for femoral neck
fractures 72
flat feet. *See* overpronation
flexibility **75–77**
aging and 77
and injury risk 76–77
and overuse injuries 165
training (*See*
stretches/stretching)
flexus hallucis longus (FHL)
tenosynovitis 77–78
Florida Atlantic University
275–276
fluid intake/replacement
55–57. *See also* drinking
basketball and 244

for fatigue prevention
66–67
for golf 249
inadequate, dehydration
and 55
in long-distance running
events 251
for middle-distance run-
ning 252
for running safety 234
in soccer 254
and sports performance
27
in tennis 258
fluid loss 55–57
basketball and 244
bicycling and 246–247
golf and 249
in heat exhaustion 93
in soccer 253, 254
and sports performance 27
in swimming 256–257
in tennis 258
in triathlons 261
focal dystonia **223–224**
food deprivation, wrestling and
241
foot
anatomy of 264, 265–266
injuries/conditions
arch pain **16–17**
athlete's foot **20**
blisters **29–30**
bunion **34–35**
common **265–266**
FHL tenosynovitis
77–78
fifth metatarsal frac-
tures **74–75**
foot-strike hemolysis
114
frostbite **78**
hammer toe **89**
and iliotibial band syn-
drome 109–110
Lisfranc fracture-dislo-
cation **124–125**
metatarsalgia **141–143**

peroneal tendinitis **169–170**

plantar fascitis **172–173**

posterior tibial tendinitis **174–175**

running and 234–235

sesamoiditis **189–190**

Sever's disease **190**

stress fracture 203

tibialis posterior syndrome **215–216**

turf toe **216–217**

football

Achilles tendon rupture 2–3

AC joint injury 5–6, 193–195

ACL injury 16

ankle sprain 13–14

and avascular femoral head necrosis 22

biceps tendinitis 28

burners/stingers 35

cervical radiculopathy 44

cervical spine injuries 41

common injuries in 267

concussion 48–49

corneal abrasion 50–51

creatine and 53

femur fractures 73–74

groin strain 85

hamstring injury 90–91

head injuries in 188–189

and heat-related illnesses 92, 94

hip dislocation 98–101

hip pointer 102

injury risk and prevention in 225–226

little league elbow 125–127

lumbosacral facet syndrome 130–133

MCP joint dislocations 140–141

neck strain in 150–151

osteitis pubis 156–158

PCL injury 173–174

rotator cuff tear 178–179

shoulder dislocation 191–193

shoulder separation **193–195**

whiplash **220**

foot-strike hemolysis 114

footwear. *See* shoes

fractures. *See also* stress fractures

ankle fracture **12–13**

with baseball finger 25–26

blowout fracture **30–31**

boxer's fracture **31–32**

clavicle fracture **44–45**

comminuted 222

femoral neck fracture **69–73**

femur fractures **73–74**

fifth metacarpal fracture **31–32**

fifth metatarsal fractures **74–75**

gamekeeper's fracture 81

hamate fracture **87–89**

with hip dislocation 99, 100

medial condylar fracture of elbow **138–139**

in mountain biking 144

nasal fractures **149–150**

scaphoid fracture **183–184,** 263–264

of sesamoids 189

wrist fractures **220–222**

free weights 202, 219

frostbite **78**

ice therapy and 178

frozen shoulder **78–80**

fungus infection

athlete's foot **20**

swimmer's ear **207–208**

G

gadolinium 136

gait abnormalities

and femoral neck fractures **72**

with iliopsoas tendinitis 108

gamekeeper's fracture 81

gamekeeper's thumb **81–82,** 238

gangrene, in frostbite 78

gastrocnemius muscle, in calf muscle injuries 37

gastroenteritis, dehydration and 55

gastrointestinal disturbances

creatine and 52

in long-distance runners 251

genitals, pain and numbness in 28–29

George Washington University 278

girls. *See* female(s)

glenohumeral joint 79, 266. *See also* shoulder

gloves

bike gloves 232

and injury prevention 113

weight gloves 202, 219

glucosamine **82–83**

glucose, complex carbohydrates and 46

gluteal strain **83**

glycogen

carbohydrate loading and 39

complex carbohydrates and 46

sports drinks and 57

goggles

blowout fracture 31

corneal abrasion 51

and injury prevention 113

golf

characteristics of **248**

common injuries in 267

hamate fracture 87–89

lumbosacral facet syndrome 130–133

neck strain in 150–151

nutrition in **248–250**

in pregnancy 61

wrist injuries **220–222**

golfer's elbow **83–85**

gout
  vs. metatarsalgia 142
  vs. turf toe 216
grafting
  for ACL reconstruction 16
  for osteochondritis disse-
    cans 162
  for skin cancer 197
Great Lakes Athletic Trainers
  Association 272
grip, after wrist injury 222
groin pain 108
  in hip flexor injury
    101–102
groin strain **85**
growth
  and hamstring injury 90
  and iliopsoas tendinitis
    107–109
  and little league elbow
    125–126
  and nutrition in basketball
    243–244
  and nutrition in swimming
    256
growth hormone disorders, and
  slipped capital femoral
  epiphysis 198
growth-plate injuries
  and little league elbow 125
  Osgood-Schlatter disease
    155
  Sever's disease **190**
  slipped capital femoral epi-
    physis **197–198**
  and youth participation in
    sports 225
guards, and injury prevention
  113
gymnastics
  athletic amenorrhea 20–21
  blisters 29–30
  female athlete triad 67–69
  gluteal strain 83
  hamstring injury 90–91
  hip dislocation 98–101
  iliopsoas tendinitis
    107–109

injury risk and prevention
  in 226
medial condylar fracture of
  elbow 138–139
Osgood-Schlatter disease
  154–156
osteochondritis dissecans
  161–162
safety tips for **232–233**
wrist injuries **220–222**

H
hallux 264
hallux valgus **34–35**
hamate fracture **87–89**
hammer toe **89**
hamstrings
  flexibility, measurement of
    76
  injury **90–91**
  and knee bursitis 121, 122
  and patellofemoral pain
    syndrome 168
  sciatica **184–186**
  stretching 27
    for painful plica 167
    for patellofemoral pain
      syndrome 169
hamstring tendinitis **91**
  running and 235
hand injuries/conditions
  baseball finger **25–26**
  bicycling and 232
  blisters **29–30**
  boxer's fracture **31–32**
  carpal tunnel syndrome **40**
  common **266**
  frostbite 78
  gamekeeper's thumb
    81–82
  metacarpophalangeal
    (MCP) joint dislocations
    140–141
  rock climbing and 221
  stress fracture 203
  thoracic outlet syndrome
    214–215
  trigger finger 216

writer's cramp 223
yips **223–224**
handlebars, and bicycling safety
  231
hand pain, in thoracic outlet
  syndrome 214–215
head injuries
  concussion **48–49**
  grading of 187
  long-term effects of 188
  second-impact syndrome
    48, **186–189**
  wrestling and 240–241
healthy lifestyles, sports
  nutrition and 199
heart attack
  and congestive heart failure
    49
  heart remodeling after
    49
heart disease
  exercise with 205
  pregnancy with 63
  and sudden death
    205–206
heart rate
  aerobic training/exercise
    and 8, 233
  ephedrine and 59
  maximum, determination
    of 232
  in pregnancy 61–62
  resting 27
  stationary bikes and 232
  and yips 223
heart rate monitor test, for
  overtraining syndrome
  164
heat cramps **91–93**
heat exhaustion **93–94**
heat illness/injury
  dehydration and 55
  long-distance running
    events and 251
  prevention of 92–93, 94,
    96
heat-induced muscle cramps
  146

heat stroke **94–96**
 creatine and 53
 ephedrine and 53, 60
heat therapy 178
heavy-resistance training,
 anabolic steroids and 10
heel 265
heel pads, for Sever's disease
 190
heel pain
 plantar fascitis 172
 in Sever's disease **190**
helmets
 and bicycling safety 231
 for concussion prevention
  49
 and injury prevention
  113
 for mountain biking 144,
  145
hematoma 213
herniated disk **96–98**
 vs. burners/stingers 35
 cervical radiculopathy
  42
 low back pain and 128
herpes simplex, wrestlers and
 241
high altitudes. *See* altitudes,
 high
high blood pressure, and
 exercise in pregnancy 62
high-speed sports, and hip
 dislocation 101
hiking
 acute mountain sickness
  6–7
 arch pain 16–17
 blisters 29–30
 corneal abrasion 50–51
 in pregnancy 61
hills
 and body fat levels of
  cyclists 246
 and running safety 234
 and training for first
  marathon or century ride
  269

hip
 anatomy of 98
 injuries/conditions
  avascular femoral head
   necrosis **22–24,** 100
  femoral neck fractures
   69–73
  hip dislocation 98–101
  hip flexor injury
   101–102
  hip pointer 102
  osteitis pubis
   156–158
  and osteitis pubis 157
  pain of 71
  running and 234, 235
  slipped capital femoral
   epiphysis **197–198**
hip dislocation 98–101
hip flexor injury 101–102
hip pointer 102
hockey
 AC joint injury 5–6,
  193–195
 burners/stingers 35
 cervical spine injuries 41
 common injuries in 267
 concussion 48–49
 femur fractures 73–74
 groin strain 85
 neck strain in 150–151
 osteitis pubis 156–158
 rotator cuff tear 178–179
 shoulder separation
  193–195
hop test, for femoral neck
 fractures 71
hormone replacement therapy
 (HRT), for female athlete
 triad 69
horse riding, testicular injury
 212–213
hot treatment, for neck strain
 150
hot tub, for overtraining
 syndrome 164
Hounsfield, Godfrey 48
humerus 266

humidity
 and heat-related illnesses
  92, 93, 95
 and running safety 234
hunger flatting 247
hurdling
 flexibility and 76
 gluteal strain 83
hydration. *See* drinking; fluid
 intake/replacement
hypertrophic cardiomyopathy,
 and sudden death 205
hyponatremia **102–104**
hypothermia **104–105**
 skiing and 236
hypothyroidism, and slipped
 capital femoral epiphysis 198

I
ice hockey. *See* hockey
ice therapy **53, 178**
 for ankle fracture 12
 for fifth metatarsal fracture
  75
 and frostbite 178
 for MCL injury 137
 for minor injuries 26
 for plantar fascitis 172
 for rhomboid muscle injury
  177
 for tennis elbow 211
iliac crest injury 102
iliopsoas bursitis 107, 108
iliopsoas strain 101–102
iliopsoas tendinitis 101, **107–109**
iliotibial band restriction, and
 peroneal tendinitis 169
iliotibial band syndrome
 109–111
illness
 and fatigue 67
 overtraining syndrome and
  165
 in swimmers 257
imaging techniques
 CAT scan **47–48**
 MRA 135
 MRI **135–137**

immobilization
    for Achilles tendon rup-
        tures 3
    for ankle fractures 12
    for gamekeeper's thumb
        81, 82
    for jammed finger 117
    for Osgood-Schlatter dis-
        ease 156
    for scaphoid fractures
        183–184
    for turf toe 217
immune system
    aerobic training/exercise
        and 9
    and fatigue 67
    in swimmers 257
impetigo, wrestlers and 241
implants, metal, and MRI
    135
impotence, bicycle seat
    neuropathy 28–29
Indiana State University 277
infants
    dehydration and 55, 56
    heat and 57
infections
    athlete's foot 20
    of blisters 30
    with knee bursitis 122,
        123
    skin, wrestling and 241
    swimmer's ear 207–208
    urinary tract, vs. testicular
        injury 213
inflammation, cortisone
    injections for 51
infraspinatus muscle, in rotator
    cuff tear 178
infraspinatus syndrome
    111–112
injuries. See also specific injuries
    commonly misdiagnosed
        263–264
    evaluation of, in game set-
        ting 153
    guidelines for managing
        235–236

minor, general treatment
    principles for 26
old, and injury prevention
    113
risk for, flexibility and
    76–77
and secondary osteoarthri-
    tis 159
injury prevention 112–114,
    229–241
    in baseball 229
    in basketball 229–230
    in bicycling 230–232
    in gymnastics 232–233
    in running 233–236
    in skiing 236–239
    in soccer 239
    in swimming 239–240
    in volleyball 240
    in weight training
        202–203
    in wrestling 240–241
Institute for Preventative Sports
    Medicine 272
International Academy for
    Sports Dentistry 272
International Association of
    Arthroscopy, Knee Surgery
    and Orthopedic Sports
    Medicine 272
International Federation of
    Orthopaedic Manipulative
    Therapists 272
International Federation of
    Sports Medicine 272
International Journal of Sports
    Medicine 281
International Olympic
    Committee
    and caffeine 37
    and ephedrine 59
International Orthopaedics 281
International Society of
    Biomechanics in Sport 273
International Society of
    Exercise and Immunology
    (ISEI) 273
interval training 27

intervertebral disks
    anatomy of 96
    cervical discogenic pain
        syndrome 41–42
    facet syndrome and 65–66
    herniated disk 96–98
        vs. burners/stingers 35
        cervical radiculopathy
            42
        low back pain and 128
    lumbosacral disk injuries
        128–130
intradiskal electrothermy
    (IDET), for lumbosacral disk
    injuries 130
intrauterine growth retardation
    (IUGR), and exercise in
    pregnancy 62–63
intrinsic muscles, of foot 264,
    265
inversion injuries
    ankle sprains 13–14
    and peroneal tendinitis
        169–170
    and posterior tibial tendini-
        tis 175
iodine allergy, and contrast
    media 47–48
iron
    deficiency
        and fatigue 66
        in long-distance run-
            ners 250–251
    food sources of 115
    for overtraining syndrome
        164
    RDAs for 66
    status
        in basketball players
            244
        in cyclists 246
        in long-distance run-
            ners 250–251
        in middle-distance run-
            ners 252
        in sprinters 255–256
        in swimmers 257
    supplements 246

iron deficiency anemia
114–115
Ironman triathlons
hyponatremia and
102–104
nutrition and 259–261
training for 259
ischemia, and sudden death
205–206
isometric exercises, for
hamstring injury prevention
91

J

jammed finger **117–118**
Japanese Athletic Trainers'
Organization 273
javelin throwing, bursitis
35–36
jerks **223–224**
jogging. *See also* running
common injuries in
234–235
in pregnancy 61
joint mice 161
joints
degeneration of, Lisfranc
fracture-dislocation and
124
injuries (*See also* specific
injuries)
arthroscopy for 17–18
in pregnancy 60
relaxin and 61
Jones fractures **74–75**
Journal of Applied Biomechanics
282
Journal of Athletic Training 282
*Journal of Orthopaedic & Sports
Physical Therapy* 282
Journal of Prosthetics and Orthotics
282
*Journal of Science and Medicine in
Sport* 282
*Journal of Sports Medicine and
Physical Fitness* 282
*Journal of Sports Science and
Medicine* 282

journals, of sports medicine
281–283
jumper's knee **118–119**
jumping
Achilles tendon rupture
and 2–3
arch pain 16–17
gluteal strain 83
groin strain 85
Morton's neuroma
143–144
Osgood-Schlatter disease
154–156
patellofemoral pain syn-
drome 180–182
Sever's disease 190
shin splints 190–191
stress fracture 203–204
turf toe 216–217

K

kicking
hip flexor injury 101–102
osteitis pubis 156–158
kidney disease
contrast dye and 48
creatine and 52
kidney function, and
hyponatremia 103
knee
injuries/conditions,
wrestling and 240–241
locking, in meniscus
injuries 140
stressful activities for 119
knee brace 113
for jumper's knee 118
knee bursitis **121–122**
knee injuries/conditions
anterior cruciate ligament
(ACL) injury **16**
arthroscopic surgery for 18
Baker's cyst **25**
bicycling and 232
and hip dislocation 99
jumper's knee **118–119**
knee bursitis 35–36,
121–122

lateral collateral ligament
(LCL) injury **123–124**
medial collateral ligament
(MCL) injury **137–138**
meniscus injuries
139–140
minor, general treatment
principles for 26
Osgood-Schlatter disease
154–156
osteochondritis dissecans
161–162
painful plica **167–168**
patellofemoral pain syn-
drome **168–169,
180–182**
posterior cruciate ligament
(PCL) injury **173–174**
prevention of **113**
runner's knee **180–182**
running and 234, 235
ski bindings and 237
knee pads
for Osgood-Schlatter dis-
ease 156
for painful plica 168
for volleyball 240
for wrestling 241
knee pain
in adolescents 154–156
lateral, and iliotibial band
syndrome 110
*Knee Surgery, Sports Traumatology,
Arthroscopy* 282

L

lab tests, for osteoarthritis
160
lacerations, skiing and 238
lacrosse
blowout fracture 30–31
groin strain 85
testicular injury 212–213
laminectomy, for herniated disk
97
lateral collateral ligament (LCL)
injury **123–124**
wrestling and 241

lateral epicondyle, of elbow 84, 265
lateral epicondylitis **211–212**
lateral longitudinal arch 265
LCL injury. *See* lateral collateral ligament (LCL) injury
leg injuries
    calf injuries **37–39**
    running and 235
leg-length discrepancy
    and femoral neck fractures 70, 71
    and osteitis pubis 158
lesions, and skin cancer 197
lidocaine challenge test, for iliopsoas tendinitis 108
life span, aerobic training/exercise and 9
ligaments
    general looseness in 192
Lisfranc fracture-dislocation **124–125**
Listservs, sports medicine 285–286
little league elbow **125–127**
long-distance events, carbohydrate loading for 39
longitudinal arch, of foot 16–17
loss of consciousness 187
    concussion and 48
loss of flexibility, with aging 77
loss of memory, concussion and 48
loss of sleep, and fatigue 66–67
Louisiana State University 278
low back pain **127–128**
    evaluation of 184–185
    and exercise in pregnancy 62
    herniated disk and 96, 97
    lumbosacral disk injuries **128–130**
    lumbosacral facet syndrome 130–133
    in mountain biking 146
    sciatica **184–186**

lower back
    anatomy of 264
    pregnancy and 61
lumbar disk disease 41
lumbosacral disk injuries **128–130**
lumbosacral facet syndrome **130–133**
lumbosacral radiculopathy. *See* sciatica
lumbosacral strain, running and 235
lungs
    injuries/conditions
        acute mountain sickness 6–7
        asthma, exercise-induced 18–20
        pregnancy and 61

M

magnesium
    and muscle cramps 146
    for overtraining syndrome 164
magnetic resonance angiogram (MRA) 135
magnetic resonance imaging (MRI) **135–137**
    for AC joint injury 194
    for degenerative discogenic disease 42
    for head injury 187
    for iliopsoas tendinitis 108
    for infraspinatus syndrome 111
    for meniscus injuries 140
    for rotator cuff tendinitis 180
    for sciatica 185
ma huang 59–60
    and heatstroke 53
male(s)
    AC joint injury 193–195
    adolescent, swimming and 256
    anorexia in 14

bicycle seat neuropathy in 28–29
femur fractures and 73
iron deficiency anemia in 115
medial condylar fracture of elbow 138–139
Osgood-Schlatter disease 154–156
osteitis pubis 156–158
osteochondritis dissecans 161–162
RDA for iron for 66
slipped capital femoral epiphysis **197–198**
sprinters, body fat level in 255
testicular injury **212–213**
triathletes, carbohydrates for 260
male hormones, effects of 10
malignant otitis externa 207
mallet finger **25–26**
manipulation under anesthesia, for frozen shoulder 80
marathon, first, training tips 269–270
March fractures. *See* stress fractures
martial arts, hip flexor injury 101–102
massage, for overtraining syndrome 164
maximum heart rate, determination of 232
MCL. *See* medial collateral ligament (MCL) injury
MCP joint dislocations. *See* metacarpophalangeal (MCP) joint dislocations
medial apophysitis **125–127**
medial collateral ligament (MCL) injury **137–138**
    wrestling and 241
medial condylar fracture of elbow **138–139**
medial epicondylitis **83–85**
medial longitudinal arch 265

medial malleolus, tibialis posterior syndrome 215–216

medial stress syndrome
running and 235
vs. shin splints 190–191

Medical College of Georgia 278

medical history, of back pain 128–129

medication, for minor injuries 26

Medicine & Science in Sports & Exercise 282

melanoma 195

memory, loss of, concussion and 48

men. *See* male(s)

meniscus injuries **139–140**

menopause, early, and low back pain 129, 185

menstruation
cessation of (*See* amenorrhea)
nutrition and 21

mental health, aerobic training/exercise and 8

mental skills, sports psychology and 199

mental status, altered, concussion 48–49

metabolic endocrine disorders, and slipped capital femoral epiphysis 198

metabolism
ephedrine and 59
pregnancy and 61

metacarpal fracture, fifth **31–32**

metacarpophalangeal (MCP) joint dislocations **140–141**

metal, and MRI 135

metastatic cancer, and back pain 129, 185

metatarsals 264, 265

metatarsal fractures, fifth **74–75**

metatarsalgia **141–143**
running and 234

metatarsal stress fractures 203–204

Miami University Sports Medicine 277

microfracture, femur fracture 73

Middle Tennessee State University 277

mid-shaft fractures **74–75**

minerals, complex carbohydrates 46

Minnesota State University 277

minor injuries, general treatment principles for 26

mitts, and injury prevention 113

moles, and skin cancer 197

moleskin, for blisters 30

Montana Tech of University of Montana 276

Montclair State University 277

Morehead State University 276

Morton's neuroma 143–144

motor sports, femur fractures 73–74

motor vehicle accidents, PCL injury 173–174

mountain bike, choosing 230

mountain biking **144–146**. *See also* bicycling

mountain climbing, acute mountain sickness 6–7

MRA (magnetic resonance angiogram) 135

MRI. *See* magnetic resonance imaging (MRI)

multidetector scanners 47

multidirectional release ski bindings 237

muscle atrophy
in congestive heart failure 50
in infraspinatus syndrome 111–112

muscle cramps **146–147**
creatine and 52
heat cramps 91–93

muscle fatigue, and femoral neck fractures 70

muscle health, aerobic training/exercise and 9

muscle mass
anabolic steroids and 10
cortisol and 10
creatine and 51–53

muscle tone, weight training to improve 202, 219

musculoskeletal changes, in pregnancy 61

myelography, for herniated disk 97

N

nasal fractures **149–150**

National Athletic Trainers Association 21–22, 273

National Collegiate Athletic Association 273
and ephedrine 59

National Operating Committee on Standards for Athletic Equipment 273

National Safety Council 273

National Sports Medicine Institute of the United Kingdom 273

National Strength and Conditioning Association 273

National Youth Sports Safety Foundation 273

navicular fracture **183–184**, 263–264

neck injuries/conditions
burners/stingers 35
cervical discogenic pain syndrome **41–42**
cervical radiculopathy **42–44**
diving and 239
facet syndrome 65–66
herniated disk 97
neck sprain **220**
neck strain **150–151**
spasmodic torticollis 223

neck pain
cervical discogenic pain syndrome 41–42

neck pain *(continued)*
    cervical radiculopathy 42
    facet syndrome 65–66
neck sprain **220**
neck strain **150–151**
needle sterilization 30
nerve block, for infraspinatus
    syndrome 112
nerve conduction studies
    (NCS), for lumbosacral facet
    syndrome 132
nerve injuries/damage
    bicycle seat neuropathy
        28–29
    bicycling and 232
    in blowout fracture 31
    burners/stingers 35
    carpal tunnel syndrome
        39–41
    cervical radiculopathy
        42–44
    in compartment syndrome
        45–46
    and femoral neck fractures
        71
    hammer toe 89
    herniated disk and 97
    with hip dislocation 99
    infraspinatus syndrome
        111–112
    Morton's neuroma
        143–144
    sciatica **184–186**
    in surgery for hamate frac-
        ture 88
    thoracic outlet syndrome
        214–215
neuroendocrine disorder,
    overtraining syndrome
    162–165
neuropathy, and lumbosacral
    disk injuries 129
neurotransmitter release, and
    exercise in pregnancy 62
neurovascular injuries/damage
    with clavicle injuries
        44–45

with medial condylar frac-
    ture of elbow 138–139
thoracic outlet syndrome
    214–215
neutral spine position 133
newsgroups, sports medicine
    285–286
New Zealand Sports Medicine
    273
nifedipine, for acute mountain
    sickness 7
noncontact sports, in youth
    sports 225
nonmelanoma skin cancer 195
nonsteroidal anti-inflammatory
    medications, for minor
    injuries 26
norepinephrine, and exercise in
    pregnancy 62
North Dakota State University
    276
Northeastern University 276,
    278
Northern Illinois University 277
nosebleeds 151
nose injuries **151**
    frostbite 78
    nasal fractures 149–150
Nova Southeastern University
    278–279
nuclear magnetic resonance
    imaging. *See* magnetic
    resonance imaging (MRI)
numbness
    in arm with
        burners/stingers 35
    in blowout fracture 31
    in carpal tunnel syndrome
        40
    of cervical radiculopathy
        43
    and lumbosacral disk
        injuries 129
    in perineal region 28–29
nutrition
    and athletic amenorrhea
        21

for basketball players
    243–245
for cyclists **245–248**
and fatigue 66–67
fluid replacement **55–57**
for golfers **248–250**
for long-distance runners
    250–251
for middle-distance runners
    251–252
monitoring, for bulimia 33
and overtraining syndrome
    164
for soccer players **252–254**
sports nutrition **198–199,**
    243–261
    Web sites 287
and sports performance 27
for sprinters **254–256**
for swimmers **256–257**
for tennis players **257–259**
and training for first
    marathon or century ride
    270
for triathletes **259–261**
Web sites 287

O

obesity
    and back pain 129
    and slipped capital femoral
        epiphysis 197–198
Ohio State University 276, 277,
    278
oral contraceptives, for female
    athlete triad 69
oral rehydrating solutions, *vs.*
    sports drinks 56
organizations, sports medicine,
    contact information **271–274**
Orthopaedic Research Society
    273
orthopedic medicine 153–154.
    See also sports medicine
    sports medicine programs
        278
Orthopedics Today 282

orthopedic surgeons 154
orthotics
    for arch pain 17
    for femoral neck fractures
        72
    for jumper's knee 118
    for metatarsalgia 142
    for patellofemoral pain syn-
        drome 181–182
    for posterior tibial tendinitis
        175
    for Sever's disease **190**
Osgood-Schlatter disease (OSD)
    154–156
    and knee bursitis 121
osteitis pubis **156–158**
osteoarthritis **158–160**
    after hip dislocation 100
    avascular femoral head
        necrosis and 22–24
    glucosamine for **82–83**
    meniscus injuries and
        139–140
osteochondritis dissecans
    161–162
    and knee bursitis 121
    vs. Osgood-Schlatter disease
        155–156
osteoporosis 69
    anorexia and 15
    athletic amenorrhea and 21
    and back pain 129, 185
    in female athlete triad
        67–69
    and wrist injuries 221
osteotomy, for avascular
    femoral head necrosis 24
otitis externa **207–208**
overhead activities
    and rhomboid muscle
        injury 177
    and rotator cuff tendinitis
        179–180
    superior labrum lesion and
        206–207
overheating, long-distance
    running events and 251

overpronation
    arch pain 16–17
    and femoral neck fractures
        72
    and iliotibial band syn-
        drome 109–110
    and jumper's knee 118
    and patellofemoral pain
        syndrome 168
    for patellofemoral pain syn-
        drome 182
    and posterior tibial tendini-
        tis 174–175
    shin splints 190
    and tibialis posterior syn-
        drome 215
overstretching 204
overstriding, and hamstring
    injury 90
overtraining
    and fatigue 66
    shin splints 190–191
    and sports performance 27
    swimmer's shoulder
        208–209
overtraining syndrome
    162–165
    compulsive exercise and
        46–47
overuse injury **165–166**
    arch pain **16–17**
    biceps tendinitis **28**
    bursitis **35–36**
    carpal tunnel syndrome
        39–41
    grading of 166
    hamstring tendinitis **91**
    hip flexor injury **101–102**
    iliopsoas tendinitis
        107–109
    infraspinatus syndrome
        111–112
    jumper's knee **118–119**
    little league elbow
        125–127
    MCL injury **137–138**
    medial epicondylitis **83–85**

    in mountain biking 145
    Osgood-Schlatter disease
        154–156
    and osteoarthritis 159
    plantar fascitis **172–173**
    rhomboid muscle injury
        177
    rotator cuff tear **178–179**
    rotator cuff tendinitis
        179–180
    runner's knee **180–182**
    and sesamoiditis 189
    shin splints 190–191
    stress fracture **203–204**
    swimmer's shoulder
        208–209
    tennis elbow **211–212**
veruse injury (continud)
    tibialis posterior syndrome
        215–216
    trigger finger 216
    wrist injuries **220–222**
overuse syndrome, in youth
    sports 225

            P
pacemakers, and MRI 135
pads
    and injury prevention 113
    for metatarsalgia 142
    for mountain biking 145
    for Sever's disease **190**
pain
    aerobic training/exercise
        and 9
    in avascular femoral head
        necrosis 22, 23
    back pain (See back pain)
    carpal tunnel syndrome 40
    cervical discogenic pain
        syndrome 41–42
    of cervical radiculopathy
        42, 43
    cortisone injections for 51
    cryotherapy for 53, 1787
    evaluation of, in sciatica
        184–185

pain *(continued)*
    and femoral neck fractures
        70, 71
    and frozen shoulder 79
    of hip dislocation 98, 99
    infraspinatus syndrome
        111–112
    low back pain (*See* low back
        pain)
    of lumbosacral disk injuries
        128–129
    in lumbosacral facet syn-
        drome 130–132
    metatarsalgia 141–143
    patellofemoral pain syn-
        drome **168–169**
    sciatica **184–186**
    in slipped capital femoral
        epiphysis 198
    in stress fracture 203
    surgical incisions and
        17–18
    in swimmer's shoulder
        209
    in testicular injury
        212–213
    in thoracic outlet syndrome
        214–215
    and training for first
        marathon or century ride
        269
painful arc syndrome **179–180**.
    See also rotator cuff tendinitis
painful plica 167–168
parents
    sports psychology tips for
        201
    and youth participation in
        sports 224
passive straight leg raise test,
    for flexibility 76
patellar malalignment. *See*
    patellofemoral pain syndrome
patellar tendinitis **118–119**
patellofemoral pain syndrome
    168–169, 180–182
    bicycling and 232

    vs. Osgood-Schlatter disease
        155–156
    running and 235
PCL injury. *See* posterior
    cruciate ligament (PCL)
    injury
pedal rate, and bicycling safety
    231
pedals, and bicycling safety 231
pelvis. *See also* hip
    biomechanics, abnormal,
        and osteitis pubis 157
    strengthening muscles in
        pregnancy 60
performance
    basic tips for 26–27
    caffeine and 37
    carbohydrate loading for
        39
    creatine and 51–53
    dehydration and 55
    golf, nutrition and 249
    sports nutrition and 198,
        199
    weight and 69
    yips and 223–224
performance anxiety, and yips
    223–224
perineal region, pain and
    numbness in 28–29
periodization of workouts 164
peritenonitis **4**
peroneal tendinitis **169–170**
pes anserine bursitis **121–122**
pH, and swimmer's ear 207,
    208
phalanges 264, 265
physical therapy **170**. *See also*
    sports medicine
    for AC joint injury
        194–195
    for femoral neck fractures
        72
    for herniated disk 97
    for hip dislocation
        100–101
    for little league elbow 126

    for lumbosacral disk
        injuries 130
    for sciatica 185, 186
    for shoulder dislocation
        192
    sports medicine programs
        278–279
Physical Therapy in Sport 282
Physician and Sportsmedicine 282
pins
    for slipped capital femoral
        epiphysis 198
    for wrist injury 222
PIP joint injuries **117–118**
piriformis syndrome **170–172**
pitching
    bursitis 35–36
    safety tips for 229
placenta previa, and exercise in
    pregnancy 62
plantar fascitis **172–173**
    running and 234
pole vaulting, gluteal strain 83
posterior cruciate ligament
    (PCL) injury **173–174**
posterior dislocations
    of hip 98
    of shoulder 192
posterior tibial tendon 264
posterior tibial tendinitis
    174–175
    running and 234
posture
    and herniated disk 97
    and lumbosacral disk
        injuries 130
    and thoracic outlet syn-
        drome 215
post-viral fatigue 67
potassium, and muscle cramps
    146
pre-game/event meals
    for basketball 244
    for bicycling 247
    for long-distance running
        251
    for soccer 253

for sprinting 255
for triathlons 260
pre-game pep talk 201
pregnancy
  amenorrhea and 21
  CAT scan and 47
  exercise during **60–63**
  MRI in 136
  physical changes during
    61–62
  RDA for iron in 66
  twin, and exercise 63
pre-patella bursitis, wrestling
  and 241
President's Council on
  Physical Fitness and Sports
  273
preterm labor, and exercise in
  pregnancy 62
prevention of injury. *See* injury
  prevention
primary amenorrhea 68
programs, sports medicine
  275–279
protective equipment
  for mountain biking 145
  for nose injury prevention
    151
protective eyewear 31
protein, dietary
  and fatigue prevention
    66
  menstruation and 21
  for sprinting 255
proximal bony avulsions, of
  hamstring 90–91
proximal interphalangeal (PIP)
  joint injuries **117–118**
pseudoepinephrine 59
pseudo-Jones fracture **74–75**
pseudomonas osteomyelitis of
  temporal bone, *vs.* swimmer's
  ear 207
psychology, sports **199–201**
  for yips 224
pubic symphysis, inflammation
  of **156–158**

pudendal nerve injury, bicycle
  seat neuropathy 28–29
pulmonary congestion,
  congestive heart failure and
  49
pulmonary edema, in acute
  mountain sickness 6–7
pulmonary function testing, for
  exercise-induced asthma 19
pulse rate. *See* heart rate

Q

Q-tip abusers, and otitis externa
  207–208
quadriceps contusion **213–214**
quadriceps strengthening
  for knee bursitis 122
  for painful plica 168
  for patellofemoral pain syn-
    drome 169, 181, 182

R

race car driving, hip dislocation
  98–101
racing bike, choosing 230
racket sports
  medial epicondylitis
    83–85
racquetball
  blowout fracture 30–31
  corneal abrasion 50–51
  hamate fracture 87–89
radiculopathy
  cervical 42–44
  lumbosacral (*See* sciatica)
  and lumbosacral disk
    injuries 128–130
radiography
  for nasal fractures 149
  for Osgood-Schlatter dis-
    ease 155
radio waves, in MRI 135, 136
range of motion
  exercises, for shoulder dis-
    location 192
  in frozen shoulder 78–79
  stretching and 204

rearview mirrors, and bicycling
  safety 231
recommended dietary
  allowances, for iron 66
recovery
  after basketball game 245
  from bicycling event 248
  from long-distance running
    250
  during soccer training 253
  and triathlons 260
reduction
  for hip dislocation 99–100
  for MCP joint dislocations
    141
reflexes, and femoral neck
  fractures 71
rehabilitation
  after head injuries 188
  after LCL injury 123
  after minor injuries 26
  for lumbosacral facet syn-
    drome 133
rehabilitation The (continued
  programs **170**
  for running injuries 236
  for stress fracture 203
  weight training in 202,
    219
relaxation, and sports
  performance 27
relaxin, effects of 61
remodeling process, and
  overuse injuries 165
repetitive motion injury
  39–41
*Research in Sports Medicine: An
  International Journal* 282
resistance training, iliopsoas
  tendinitis 107–109
respiratory rate, in pregnancy
  61
rest **178**
  insufficient, in overtraining
    syndrome 162
  for MCL injury 137
  for minor injuries 26

rest (continued)
    for overtraining syndrome
        164
    and physiologic improve-
        ment 162
    for plantar fascitis 172
    and sports performance 27
    for stress fracture 203
resting heart rate 27
retropatellar pain. See
    patellofemoral pain syndrome
return to play
    after calf muscle injury 38
    after clavicle injury 45
    after frozen shoulder 80
    after hip flexor injury 102
    after jumper's knee 119
    after LCL injury 123–124
    after MCL injury 137–138
    after piriformis syndrome
        171
    after second-impact syn-
        drome 187
    after shin splints 191
    after tennis elbow 212
    after thigh bruise 214
    decisions to, team physi-
        cians and 153
    with jammed finger 118
    with osteochondritis disse-
        cans 162
rhomboid muscle injury 177
RICE (rest, ice, compression,
    elevation) 177–178
    for MCL injury 137
ringworm, wrestlers and 241
road bike, choosing 230
road rash 1
rock climbing, hand injuries
    221
rodeo, shoulder dislocation
    191–193
rollerblading, wrist injuries
    220–222
rotator cuff 266
    and swimmer's shoulder
        208–209

rotator cuff tear 178–179
    vs. AC joint injury 5–6,
        194
    in shoulder dislocation
        192–193
    and superior labrum lesion
        206–207
rotator cuff tendinitis 179–180
    vs. infraspinatus syndrome
        111
    and superior labrum lesion
        206–207
rowing
    common injuries in 267
    iliopsoas tendinitis
        107–109
    rhomboid muscle injury
        177
rugby
    AC joint injury 5–6,
        193–195
    cervical spine injuries 41
    concussion 48–49
    hamstring injury 90–91
    hip dislocation 98–101
    shoulder dislocation
        191–193
    shoulder separation
        193–195
rule changes, for head injury
    prevention 188–189
runner's knee 180–182. See also
    patellofemoral pain syndrome
running. See also sprinting
    Achilles tendinitis 4, 235
    arch pain 16–17
    athletic amenorrhea 20–21
    calf muscle injuries 37–39
    carbohydrate loading for 39
    characteristics of
        long-distance 250
        middle-distance 251
    common injuries in
        234–235, 267
        causes of 233–234
        guidelines for manag-
            ing 235–236

compartment syndrome
    45–46, 235
corneal abrasion 50–51
female athlete triad 67–69
femoral neck fractures
    69–73
FHL tenosynovitis 77–78
first marathon, training tips
    269–270
flexibility and 76
and gastrointestinal prob-
    lems 251
gluteal strain 83
groin strain 85
hamstring injury 90–91,
    235
hip dislocation 98–101
iliopsoas tendinitis
    107–109
iliotibial band syndrome
    109–111
jumper's knee 118–119
long-distance
    characteristics of 250
    nutrition for 250–251
middle-distance
    characteristics of 251
    nutrition for 251–252
Morton's neuroma
    143–144
nutrition in
    for long-distance run-
        ners 250–251
    for middle-distance
        runners 251–252
painful plica 167–168
PCL injury 173–174
and piriformis syndrome
    171
plantar fascitis 172–173,
    234
safety tips for 233–236
sciatica 184–186, 235
sesamoiditis 189–190
Sever's disease 190
shin splints 190–191,
    235

stress fracture 203–204,
234–235
ultra-distance 250
running surface
ideal 234
shin splints and 191
ruptured disk. *See* herniated disk

S
saddle numbness 28–29
safety devices, and injury
prevention 113
safety tips **229–241**
for baseball **229**
for basketball **229–230**
for bicycling **230–232**
for gymnastics **232–233**
for running **233–236**
for skiing **236–239**
for soccer **239**
for swimming **239–240**
for volleyball **240**
for wrestling **240–241**
salt tablets, for heat stroke 95
Santa Fe Community College
276
sartorius strain **85**
scaphoid fractures **183–184,**
263–264
scapula 266
SCFE. *See* slipped capital
femoral epiphysis (SCFE)
schools, sports medicine
275–279
sciatica **184–186**
and exercise in pregnancy
62
herniated disk and 97
in piriformis syndrome
170–172
running and 235
sciatic nerve injury, with hip
dislocation 100
Science and Sport 283
SC joint injuries. *See*
sternoclavicular (SC) joint
injuries

seafood allergy, and contrast
media 47–48
search engines, sports medicine
285
seat belts
for concussion prevention
49
for injury prevention 31
secondary amenorrhea 68–69
secondary osteoarthritis 159
second-impact syndrome (SIS)
48, **186–189**
sedation
for medial condylar frac-
ture of elbow 139
for MRI 136
seizures, and low back pain
129, 185
septal hematoma, nasal
fractures *vs.* 149
septum, deviated **151**
sesamoid bones 265
sesamoiditis 189–190
Sever's disease **190**
sexual dysfunction, bicycle seat
neuropathy 28–29
shin guards, for soccer safety
239
shin splints 190–191
compartment syndrome *vs.*
45
running and 235
shoes
and ankle injury preven-
tion 114
arch pain and 17
for basketball 229
and bunion prevention
34–35
and femur fractures 73, 74
for fifth metatarsal fracture
75
and hammer toe 89
and iliotibial band syn-
drome 109–110
and injury prevention
113

and metatarsalgia 141–143
and Morton's neuroma
143–144
for patellofemoral pain syndrome 181–182
for peroneal tendinitis prevention 169–170
and plantar fascitis 172
for posterior tibial tendinitis
175
and running injuries 233
and sesamoiditis 189
for Sever's disease **190**
shock absorption of 233
for soccer safety 239
and turf toe 216
shoulder
anatomy of 79, 191–192,
266
injuries/conditions
acromioclavicular joint
injury **5–6, 193–195**
arthroscopic surgery for
18
biceps tendinitis **28**
burners/stingers **35**
bursitis **35–36**
clavicle injuries **44–45**
common **266**
frozen shoulder
78–80
infraspinatus syndrome
111–112
minor, general treat-
ment principles for
26
in mountain biking
144
prevention of **114**
rotator cuff tear
178–179
shoulder dislocation
191–193
shoulder instability
192
superior labrum lesion
206–207

shoulder (continued)
  swimmer's shoulder
    208–209
  thoracic outlet syn-
    drome **214–215**
  instability 192
  stability of 111
shoulder dislocation **191–193**
  anterior vs. posterior 192
  superior labrum lesion and
    206
shoulder impingement
  syndrome **208–209**
shoulder pain
  infraspinatus syndrome
    111–112
  in shoulder dislocation
    192, 193
shoulder separation **193–195**.
  See also acromioclavicular
  (AC) joint, injury
simple carbohydrates 39, 46
simple dislocation, MCP joint
  dislocations 141
Sinding-Larsen-Johansson (SLJ)
  disease, vs. Osgood-Schlatter
  disease 155–156
SIS. See second-impact
  syndrome (SIS)
sit and reach test, for flexibility
  76
skating, scaphoid fractures
  183–184
skis 238
ski bindings
  choosing 237
  and LCL injury 124
  multidirectional release
    237
  and PCL injury 174
  and skiing safety 236–237
ski boots 237–238
skier's thumb 81–82, 238
skiing
  ACL injury 16
  acute mountain sickness
    6–7

attitudes in, and injury
  238–239
common injuries in 267
exercise-induced asthma
  18–20
femur fractures 73–74
hip dislocation 98–101
LCL injury 123–124
MCL injury 138
PCL injury 173–174
in pregnancy 61
rotator cuff tear 178–179
safety tips for **236–239**
shoulder dislocation
  191–193
skills 26
skin
  anatomy of 195
  blood flow to, and heat-
    related illnesses 92, 93
  ice therapy and 178
  problems/injuries
    abrasions 1
    athlete's foot 20
    blisters 29–30
    frostbite 78
    skin cancer **195–197**
    skin infections 241
    wrestling and 241
skin cancer **195–197**
skin grafting, for skin cancer
  197
ski poles 238
sleep
  lack of, and fatigue 66–67
  for overtraining syndrome
    164
  and training for first
    marathon or century ride
    269
slipped capital femoral
  epiphysis (SCFE) **197–198**
    vs. Osgood-Schlatter disease
    156
slipped disk. See herniated disk
Slippery Rock University of
  Pennsylvania 276, 279

snapping hip syndrome
  107–109
snow conditions, and ski
  injuries 238
soccer
  ankle sprain 13–14
  blowout fracture 30–31
  carbohydrate loading for
    39
  cervical spine injuries 41
  characteristics of **252–253**
  common injuries in
    267–268
  FHL tenosynovitis 77–78
  groin strain 85
  hamstring injury 90–91
  head injuries in 188–189
  hip flexor injury 101–102
  iliopsoas tendinitis
    107–109
  injury risk and prevention
    in 226
  nutrition in **252–254**
  Osgood-Schlatter disease
    154–156
  osteitis pubis 156–158
  safety tips for **239**
sodium
  and heat exhaustion 93
  and heat stroke 95
  hyponatremia and
    102–104
  in sports drinks 57
softball, injury risk and
  prevention in 226
South Dakota State University
  276
Southern Illinois University at
  Carbondale 277
South West Texas State
  University 279
spasmodic torticollis 223
speed, water loss and 27
speed skating, tibialis posterior
  syndrome 215–216
spinal cord injury, vs.
  burners/stingers 35

spinal stenosis, running and 235
spine
    low back pain and
        127–128
    lower, anatomy of 127
    neutral spine position 133
spiral scanners 47
splinting
    for baseball finger 25–26
    for boxer's fracture 32
    for carpal tunnel syndrome
        40
Sport Physiotherapy Canada
    273
sports drinks **57**
    absorption of 57
    basketball and 244
    for bicycling 247
    for hyponatremia preven-
        tion 104
    oral rehydrating solutions
        vs. 56
sports medicine
    ACSM endorsed programs
        275–276
    associations and organiza-
        tions **271–274**
    basic practices at home **26**
    careers for orthopedists 153
    certification 275
    discussion Listservs
        285–286
    general programs **277**
    journals **281–283**
    schools **275–279**
    search engines 285
    specific programs **278–279**
    Web sites **285–287**
Sports Medicine 283
*Sports Medicine and Arthroscopy
    Review* 283
sports nutrition **198–199,
    243–261**. *See also* nutrition
    Web sites 287
sports performance. *See*
    performance

sports psychology 199–201
    for yips 224
sprains
    treatment for 141
sprinting
    characteristics of **254**
    FHL tenosynovitis 77–78
    flexibility and 76
    gluteal strain 83
    groin strain 85
    hamstring injury 90–91
    Morton's neuroma
        143–144
    nutrition for **254–256**
    osteitis pubis 156–158
Spurling test, for cervical
    radiculopathy 43
squamous cell carcinoma 195
squash
    hamate fracture 87–89
    hamstring injury 90–91
stabilization phase, of
    degenerative disk disease
    128
stabilizing exercises, for
    herniated disk 97
stamina, aerobic
    training/exercise and 9
Stanford University—
    Biomechanical Engineering
    Division 278
state of mind, sports psychology
    and 199–201
stationary bikes 231–232
stenosing tenosynovitis **216**
sterilization, of needle 30
sternoclavicular (SC) joint
    injuries, dislocations 44–45
steroids. *See also* corticosteroids
    anabolic 9–11
        vs. cortisone 51
    and avascular femoral head
        necrosis 22
stimulants
    caffeine 37
    ephedrine 59–60
stingers/burners **35**

stirrup splint, for peroneal
    tendinitis 169
stitches, for abrasions 1
strength
    creatine and 51–53
    and overuse injuries 165
strength training **201–203,
    219–220**
    for AC joint injury 194
    after hip dislocation
        100–101
    anabolic steroids and 10
    for cervical radiculopathy
        43
    goals for 202, 219
    for iliopsoas tendinitis 108
    infraspinatus syndrome
        111–112
    for knee bursitis 122
    for lumbosacral facet syn-
        drome 133
    for patellofemoral pain syn-
        drome 169
    in pregnancy 60–61
    for shoulder dislocation
        192.
    shoulder separation in 194
    and sports performance 27
    for sprinting 254
    for wrist injury prevention
        222
stress fractures **203–204**
    vs. acute fracture 70
    anorexia and 15
    athletic amenorrhea and
        21
    compartment syndrome *vs.*
        45
    definition of 73
    disordered eating and
        67–68
    femoral neck fractures
        69–73
    femur fractures **73–74**
    fifth metatarsal fracture 75
    in metatarsalgia 142
    muscle fatigue and 70

stress fractures *(continued)*
        running and 234–235, 235
        of shin bone *vs.* knee bursi-
            tis 121
        vs. shin splints 190
        women and 70
stretches/stretching **204**
        for Achilles tendon **3**
        after hip dislocation 100
        for ankle injury prevention
            114
        for calf muscle injury pre-
            vention 38
        for cervical radiculopathy
            43
        for iliotibial band syndrome
            110
        for injury prevention **113**
        and injury risk 77
        knee 113
        for knee bursitis 122
        for lumbosacral facet syn-
            drome 132–133
        for muscle cramps 146,
            147
        for patellofemoral pain syn-
            drome 169
        for piriformis syndrome
            prevention 172
        for plantar fasciitis 172
        for shoulder injury preven-
            tion 114
        and sports performance 27
        static *vs.* ballistic 76
        for wrist injury prevention
            222
student athletic trainers 22
subluxation, definition of 192
subscapularis muscle, in rotator
    cuff tear 178
Sudafed 59
sudden death **205–206**
sugars 46
        in sports drinks 57
sunglasses 51, 197
sunlight, and skin cancer 195,
    197

sunscreen
        and injury prevention 113
        and skin cancer prevention
            197
superior labrum lesion
        206–207
supplements
        creatine **51–53**
        glucosamine **82–83**
        iron 246
        for middle-distance run-
            ning 252
        for overtraining syndrome
            164
        for sprinters 256
suprascapular nerve
        compression 111–112
supraspinatus muscle, in rotator
    cuff tear 178
supraspinatus tendon, in rotator
    cuff tear 178
supraspinatus tendinitis
        179–180. *See also* rotator cuff
        tendinitis
surfaces, playing
        ideal for running 234
        shin splints and 191
        for soccer safety 239
        and turf toe 216, 217
surfing, in pregnancy 61
surgeons, orthopedic 154
surgery
        for Achilles tendon rupture
            3
        for AC joint injury 6,
            194–195
        for ACL injury 16
        arthroscopic **17–18**
            for meniscus injuries
                140
        for avascular femoral head
            necrosis 23–24
        for bunion 34
        for carpal tunnel syndrome
            40–41
        for cervical discogenic pain
            syndrome 41–42

for cervical radiculopathy
    43
for clavicle fracture 44–45
for facet syndrome 65
for femoral neck fractures
    72
for gamekeeper's thumb
    81–82
for hamate fracture 88
for hammer toe 89
for herniated disk 97
for hip dislocation 99–100
for infraspinatus syndrome
    112
for knee bursitis 122
for LCL injury 123
for lumbosacral disk
    injuries 130
for MCL injury 137
for meniscus injuries
    140
for nasal fractures 150
for osteochondritis disse-
    cans 161
for PCL injury 173–174
for rotator cuff tendinitis
    180
for sciatica 185–186
for skin cancer 197
for slipped capital femoral
    epiphysis 198
for trigger finger 216
sweat, insufficient, and heat-
    related illnesses 92, 93, 95
sweat losses
    golf and 249
    swimming and 256–257
    tennis and 258
    in triathlons 261
swelling
    in compartment syndrome
        45–46
    cortisone injections for
        51
    cryotherapy for 53
swimmer's ear **207–208**
swimmer's shoulder **208–209**

swimming
    carbohydrate loading for
        39
    cervical radiculopathy 42,
        44
    characteristics of **256**
    common injuries in 268
    knee bursitis **121–122**
    MCL injury 137–138
    nutrition for **256–257**
    in pregnancy 61
    and rotator cuff tendinitis
        179–180
    safety tips for **239–240**
    for shoulder dislocation 192
    stroke mechanics 209
    superior labrum lesion and
        206–207
    swimmer's ear **207–208**
    swimmer's shoulder
        208–209
    thoracic outlet syndrome
        214–215
synovial plica syndrome
    167–168
systemic lupus, and avascular
    femoral head necrosis 22

T
talus 264, 265
talus fracture 12–13
taping
    for ankle injury prevention
        114
    for MCP joint dislocations
        141
    to prevent ankle sprains
        13–14
    for turf toe 217
tarsal bones 264, 265
tarso-metatarsal fracture-
    dislocation **124–125**
team physician 153
teams, sports psychology tips
    201
team sports 26
    youth participation in 224

technique, and overuse injuries
    165
temperature, and running
    safety 234
Temple University 277, 278
tendinitis
    Achilles tendinitis **3–5**
    biceps tendinitis **28**
    hamstring tendinitis **91**
    iliopsoas tendinitis 101,
        107–109
    patellar tendinitis
        118–119
    peroneal tendinitis
        169–170
    posterior tibial tendinitis
        174–175
    rotator cuff tendinitis
        179–180
        vs. infraspinatus syn-
            drome 111
    running and 235
    sesamoiditis 189–190
    wrist extensor tendinitis
        211–212
    wrist flexor tendinitis
        83–85
    wrist tendinitis 220–222
tennis
    Achilles tendon rupture 2–3
    blowout fracture 30–31
    bursitis 35–36
    cervical radiculopathy 42
    characteristics of **257**
    common injuries in 268
    corneal abrasion 50–51
    hamate fracture 87–89
    hamstring injury 90–91
    infraspinatus syndrome
        111–112
    nutrition in **257–259**
    plantar fascitis 172–173
    in pregnancy 61
    rhomboid muscle injury
        177
    and rotator cuff tendinitis
        179–180

thoracic outlet syndrome
    214–215
    trigger finger 216
    wrist injuries **220–222**
tennis elbow **211–212**
    vs. golfer's elbow 84
tennis elbow strap
    for medial epicondylitis
        84–85
    for tennis elbow 211
tennis leg 37–38
tennis racquet, and tennis
    elbow prevention 212
teres minor muscle, in rotator
    cuff tear 178
testicular injury **212–213**
    rupture 212–213
    torsion 212–213
testosterone, effects of 10
tetanus, and abrasions 1
thigh bruise **213–214**
thigh injuries, running and 235
thigh wrap, for groin strain 85
thirst, dehydration and 56
thoracic outlet syndrome (TOS)
    214–215
throwing
    biceps tendinitis 28
    and frozen shoulder 80
    little league elbow
        125–127
    medial epicondylitis **83–85**
    off season, for shoulder
        injury prevention **114**
    superior labrum lesion and
        206–207
thumb injuries
    gamekeeper's thumb
        81–82, 238
    metacarpophalangeal
        (MCP) joint dislocations
        140–141
tibia fracture
    ankle fracture 12–13
    stress fracture 203
tibialis posterior syndrome
    215–216

tinea pedis **20**
toe(s)
    anatomy of 264, 265
    injuries/conditions
        bunion 34–35
        flexus hallucis longus
            (FHL) tenosynovitis
            77–78
        frostbite 78
        hammer toe 89
        metatarsalgia 141–143
        sesamoiditis 189–190
        turf toe **216–217**
torticollis, spasmodic 223
TOS. *See* thoracic outlet
    syndrome (TOS)
total hip replacement, for
    avascular femoral head
    necrosis 24
touring bike, choosing 230
toxemia, and exercise in
    pregnancy 62
track and field
    hamstring injury 90–91
    iliopsoas tendinitis 107–109
    injury risk and prevention
        in 226
    nutrition for 251–252
training
    basketball 243
    bicycling 245
    golf 248
    interval 27
    for long-distance running
        250
    for middle-distance run-
        ning 251
    for physical therapists 170
    soccer 252–253
    for sports nutritionist
        198–199
    strength 27
    swimming 256
    tennis 257
    tips for first marathon or
        century ride 269–270
    for triathlons 259

training errors
    and femoral neck fractures
        70
    in mountain biking 145
    and overuse injuries 165
    and running injuries 233
training log
    for overtraining syndrome
        164–165
    and sports performance 27
trampoline jumping, cervical
    spine injuries 41
transcutaneous nerve
    stimulation (TENS), for
    frozen shoulder 80
transverse arch, of foot 16–17,
    265
traumatic avascular femoral
    head necrosis 22
traumatic injuries, femur
    fractures 73–74
traveling, nutrition and
    in basketball 245
    in golf 249–250
    in sprinting 255
    in tennis 259
    in triathlons 261
treatment principles, general 26
triathlons
    carbohydrate loading for 39
    characteristics of **259–260**
    hyponatremia and
        102–104
    nutrition for **259–261**
trigger finger **216**
tumors
    formation of 195
    Morton's neuroma
        143–144
turf toe **216–217**
twin pregnancy, exercise and 63
twisted testicle 212–213
twisting motions
    ACL injury 16
    lumbosacral facet syndrome
        130–133
twitches **223–224**

U
ulnar nerve injury, in surgery
    for hamate fracture 88
ultra-endurance events
    hyponatremia and
        102–104
    running 250
ultrasound, for iliopsoas
    tendinitis 108
ultraviolet (UV) radiation, and
    skin cancer 195, 197
United Kingdom Association of
    Doctors in Sport 273
United States Olympic
    Committee 273–274
University of Alabama at
    Birmingham 278
University of Arkansas 278
University of California, Chico
    278
University of Delaware 279
University of Florida 278
University of Georgia 276
University of Kentucky 277
University of Mary 276
University of Missouri at
    Columbia 278
University of Nevada, Las Vegas
    277
University of New Mexico
    278
University of Oregon 277
University of Pittsburgh 276
University of Rochester Medical
    Center 278
University of Tennessee 279
University of Texas at Arlington
    276
University of Tulsa 277
University of Washington 279
University of Wisconsin 276
University of Wisconsin—Eau
    Claire 277
unstable phase, of degenerative
    disk disease 128
urinary tract infection, *vs.*
    testicular injury 213

urine color, dehydration and
  56
uterine contractions, exercise
  and 62

V

vaginal bleeding, and exercise
  in pregnancy 62
vascularized fibula graft, for
  avascular femoral head
  necrosis 23
vegetarianism
    athletic amenorrhea and
      21
    and iron deficiency anemia
      115
vertebrae injuries/conditions
    cervical discogenic pain
      syndrome **41–42**
    facet syndrome **65–66**
    herniated disk **96–98**
    lumbosacral disk injuries
      128–130
    whiplash **220**
viral illness
    and fatigue 67
    overtraining syndrome and
      165
visualization, and sports
  performance 27
vitamins, complex
  carbohydrates 46
volar plate disruption, with
  jammed finger 117, 118
volleyball
    infraspinatus syndrome
      111–112
    Osgood-Schlatter disease
      154–156
    rhomboid muscle injury
      177
    and rotator cuff tendinitis
      179–180
    safety tips for **240**
volleyball shoulder **111–112**
vomiting, and dehydration 55,
  56, 57

W

walking
    arch pain 16–17
    calf muscle injuries
      37–39
    jumper's knee 118–119
    Morton's neuroma
      143–144
    patellofemoral pain syn-
      drome 180–182
    in pregnancy 61
warm-up
    for ankle injury prevention
      114
    hip dislocation and 101
    for injury prevention
      112–113
    and injury risk 77
    for knees 113
    for plantar fascitis
      172
    for shoulder injury preven-
      tion 114
    before stretching 204
water absorption 56
water intoxication **102–104**
water loss. *See* fluid loss
water polo, thoracic outlet
  syndrome 214–215
water retention, creatine and
  52
water-skiing
    and avascular femoral head
      necrosis 22
    hamstring injury 90–91
    hip dislocation 98–101
    in pregnancy 61
weakness
    of arm
        with burners/stingers
          35
        in cervical radiculopa-
          thy 42
    and lumbosacral disk
      injuries 129
weather
    and fluid loss in soccer 253

and running safety 234
and skiing safety 236
Web sites, sports medicine
  285–287
    associations and organiza-
      tions **271–274**
    journals **281–283**
    schools **275–279**
weekend warrior, calf muscle
  injuries in 37–38
weight
    optimal, for performance
      69
    recording, in log book
      27
weight belt 202, 219
weight control
    anorexia and 14–16
    bulimia and 32–34
    compulsive exercise and
      46–47
    soccer and 253
    wrestling and 241
weight gain
    carbohydrate loading and
      39
    and creatine 52
    sports nutrition for 199
weight gloves 202, 219
weight lifting. *See* strength
  training
weight loss 27
    aerobic training/exercise
      and 8, 9
    ephedrine and 59
    fluid replacement and 56
    in golf 249
    metastatic cancer and
      129
    for osteoarthritis 160
    sports nutrition for 199
weight machines 202, 219
weight training **201–203,
  219–220**. *See also* strength
  training
wellness practices, sports
  nutrition and 198–199

West Virginia University 277, 278
whip-kick technique, and MCL injury 137
whiplash **220**
        facet syndrome after 65
winter sports, and exercise-induced asthma 19
women. *See* female(s)
World Council on Orthopaedic Sports Medicine 274
World Federation of Athletic Training and Therapy 274
wound care 1
wrestling
        burners/stingers 35
        cervical spine injuries 41

common injuries in 240–241
        safety tips for **240–241**
wrist extensor tendinitis **211–212**
wrist flexor tendinitis **83–85**
wrist fractures 220–222
wrist injuries/conditions **220–222**
        carpal tunnel syndrome 39–41
        common 266
        hamate fracture **87–89**
        scaphoid fracture **183–184,** 263–264
        yips **223–224**
wrist tendinitis 220–222

writer's cramp 223
wryneck 223

X
X-rays. *See* radiography

Y
Yale University School of Medicine 278
yips **223–224**
young players. *See* adolescents; children
Youngstown State University 276

Z
zinc, for overtraining syndrome 164